The International Libra

INTEGRATIVE PSYCHOLOGY

Founded by C. K. Ogden

The International Library of Psychology

PHYSIOLOGICAL PSYCHOLOGY
In 10 Volumes

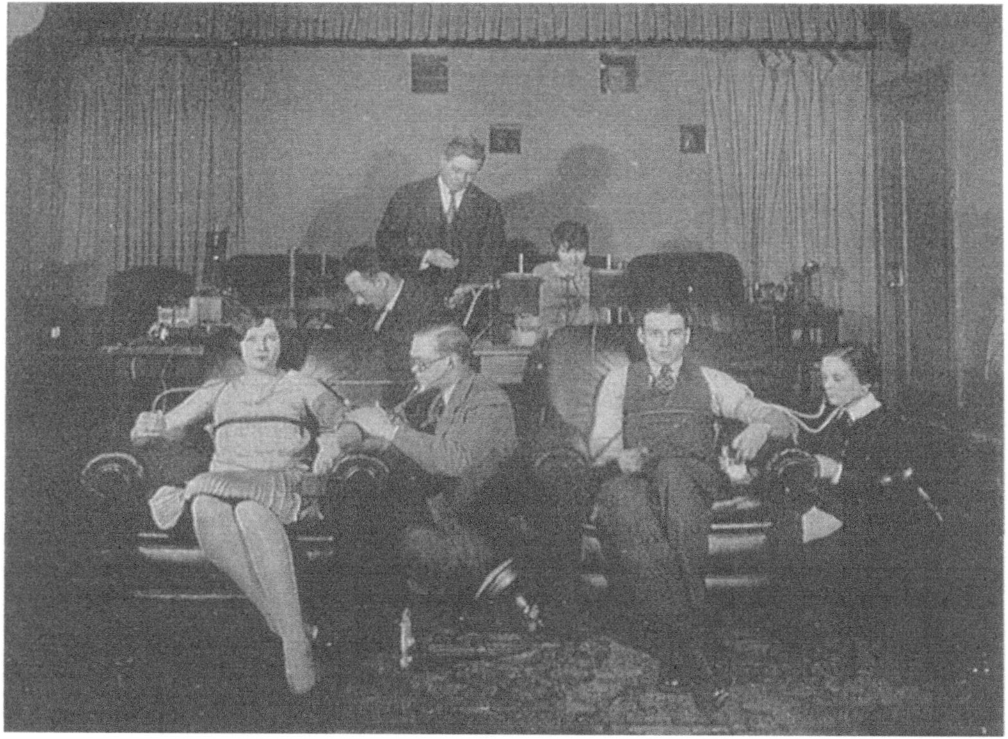

Fig. 45

EXPERIMENTAL SET-UP FOR MEASURING BODILY SYMPTOMS OF EMOTION *(See p. 485)*

INTEGRATIVE PSYCHOLOGY

A Study of Unit Response

WILLIAM M MARSTON, C DALY KING
AND ELIZABETH H MARSTON

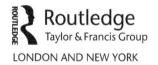

Routledge
Taylor & Francis Group

LONDON AND NEW YORK

First published in 1931 by
Routledge
2 Park Square, Milton Park, Abingdon, Oxfordshire OX14 4RN
711 Third Avenue, New York, NY 10017

First issued in paperback 2014

Routledge is an imprint of the Taylor and Francis Group, an informa business

The publishers have made every effort to contact authors/copyright holders
of the works reprinted in the *International Library of Psychology*.
This has not been possible in every case, however, and we would
welcome correspondence from those individuals/companies
we have been unable to trace.

These reprints are taken from original copies of each book. In many cases
the condition of these originals is not perfect. The publisher has gone to
great lengths to ensure the quality of these reprints, but wishes to point
out that certain characteristics of the original copies will, of necessity, be
apparent in reprints thereof.

British Library Cataloguing in Publication Data
A CIP catalogue record for this book
is available from the British Library

Integrative Psychology
ISBN 0415-21077-1
Physiological Psychology: 10 Volumes
ISBN 0415-21131-X
The International Library of Psychology: 204 Volumes
ISBN 0415-19132-7

ISBN 13: 978-1-138-87549-4 (pbk)
ISBN 13: 978-0-415-21077-5 (hbk)

CONTENTS

v

LIST OF FIGURES

FOREWORD

WHILE teaching General Psychology at such obviously dissimilar institutions as Radcliffe College, American University, Tufts College, Bentley School of Accounting, New York University, Central School for Physical Education, and Columbia University, I have encountered a student attitude which seems clearly attributable to the present state of this science. Students make two demands which psychology does not fulfil : a unified, organized subject matter, distinctively its own, and some practical knowledge about themselves, applicable to the personal problems of their everyday lives. Really, both are the same ; if sufficiently definite laws of human behaviour were presented to the student, he could apply some of them, at any rate, to himself.

Beginners in psychology, after completing the first year course, frequently express amazement and distrust because they must go to their final examinations with no unified idea of what psychology actually is. This, they say, is not true of first year courses in biology, chemistry, physiology, and the other sciences. In fact, much of the material taught in modern " objective " psychology courses, has been met previously in other college departments. Students inquire, with some apparent justification, why they should be given a small dose of physiology, another of biology, a third instalment of genetics, a fourth section of endocrinology, a fifth of statistics, and a sixth of psychiatry, with the whole, disconnected hodge-podge set down in the catalogue as a course in psychology.

This throwing together of assorted fragments is undesirable, not only to the college student but to any worker in the field who takes his vocation seriously. Psychology is a branch of science and its field can be defined. It does not need to be a gathering together of left-overs from the other sciences. The psychologist has a right to take his job seriously, and to tell the world without apology what he conceives that job to be. As a result of my own efforts to solve this problem, and to organize the field of psychology for my students, the plan of this book was conceived.

In the first place, it has seemed to me that psychology, to be practical, must have its own, elementary units of human behaviour. Psychology's units, or primary elements, should be discoverable in fact, according to available methods of experimentation, and objective, clinical observation. They should not be hidden in the genes of the germplasm like instincts, nor should they be artefacts of another science, like the conditioned reflex. The present volume takes its point of departure from a critical examination of various psychological, and semi-psychological attempts to classify fundamental, human activities ; and thereafter attempts to postulate elementary behaviour units which may serve psychology precisely as the atom, the electron, and the proton have served chemistry. Regardless of whether these concepts are metaphysically ultimate, there are essential chemical facts which correspond to protons and electrons, and there are, I believe, essential psychological facts which correspond to the four, elementary types of unit response postulated in this book.

In the second place, I cannot avoid the conclusion that consciousness is real ; and if it is, then consciousness is the one, important problem which psychology, and no other science, is called upon to solve. I believe that attaining consciousness of the right sort is, broadly speaking, the chief purpose of all normal, human strivings. If psychology could teach its students, objectively, the nature of consciousness, and how various sorts of consciousness are produced, it seems certain that this field of knowledge would become immediately the most humanly useful of the sciences. The present volume attempts to deal with consciousness in this way.

A majority of students to whom I have taught psychology as outlined in this book have manifested an active interest in the new unification of the subject as a distinctive science, and also have discovered practical value in attempting to analyze and reconstruct their own experiences and behaviour according to the system proposed. A few teachers of psychology, who have not fully informed themselves, at first hand, concerning the innovations which I have ventured to make, have advanced the criticism that my treatment of the science is highly theoretical. It is. So was the reorganization of chemistry upon the basis of the atomic theory, and the comparatively recent secession of neurology as a separate field of study, made possible by the neuronic theory. But the further implication of these critics that my treatment is based upon "theoretical" subject matter is wholly erroneous, and seems attributable to an inability or unwillingness to consider new implications from previously established facts. For example, it is heresy, at the moment, to question Pavlov's concept of the conditioned reflex. I do question it, and discard it as far as psychology is concerned. But I do not discard the facts and experimental procedures which gave rise, in Pavlov's mind, to the concept mentioned. In my own mind, considering these facts for psychology and *not* for physiology, new interpretations occur, and are presented in the present volume. A careful check-up of the actual material here used, will show, I believe, a more detailed and comprehensive adherence to experimental findings in neurology and physiology than frequently is found in the current type of General Psychology. Many theoretical implications, however, will be found quite dissimilar to those of other sciences because, after all, psychology is entitled to its own internal unity, and its own, distinctive point of view. Both are essential if psychology is to advance as other sciences have done.

My collaborators, C. D. King and E. H. Marston, whose general points of view in the matters above discussed are very similar to my own, have been working with me during the last two years in a joint effort to assemble and simplify the facts and theories which we regard as most essential to psychology, and to reorganize this material along the lines suggested. The resulting treatment, as here presented, is not to be regarded as exhaustive, or even as satisfactorily complete, but only as a skeleton outline of objective psychology, which carries the true unity and meaning of the science as we see it.

We are indebted especially to Elizabeth H. Marston, who supervised the illustrations in this book ; to the several authors and publishers who kindly permitted us to reprint drawings, as indicated in legends beneath the figures in question ; and to Mrs. Elizabeth Brayton, who prepared the the illustrations for press. We also acknowledge with sincere appreciation the assistance of Mrs. Olive Byrne Richard, who prepared for us the research material on " Bodily Symptoms of Emotion," contained in Chapter XVIII, and assisted generally in revising the book ; the aid of Mrs. Marjorie W. Huntley, who assisted in various phases of preparing the manuscript ; and the work of Miss Olga Ausperger in research and preparation of the manuscript. For many helpful suggestions and criticisms, I wish to thank colleagues and students at Tufts College, Columbia, and New York University ; and for editorial revision and valuable alterations in the text a grateful acknowledgment is due Dr. H. S. Hatfield, who has been kind enough to take a personal interest in my work.

WILLIAM MOULTON MARSTON.

New York City,
December 21, 1930.

INTEGRATIVE PSYCHOLOGY

CHAPTER I

The Integrative Psychology of You

Introductory

Human, adult psychology is the science of " You." Please distinguish " You " from . " I." The older psychology, and the psychology of the self-styled and self-trained " psychologists " of every day life and of the popular lecture platform, is the psychology of " I." Any normal adult, without scientific training or interest, may become a disciple of the " I " school of psychology. " *I* am not afraid to tell my employer what I think of him," says this type of " psychologist." " *I* voted the Republican ticket because their candidate is the ablest man " " *I* kicked my dog last night because he jumped up on me." " *I* gave my secretary a raise because her work deserved it." And so on.

Now comes the psychologist who has been trained in the scientific study of " You." " *You*," he asserts, " have never told your employer what you really think of him. You have been restrained by a number of influences, chief among which is your necessity for keeping your job." " *You*," continues the objective psychologist, " voted the Republican ticket as a result of several different causes. Chiefly, perhaps, because your father, and your father's father were Republicans before you, and because you have formed a fixed habit of thought requiring such action." " As for your dog, *you* kicked him last night because you knew your wife was away and you would have to get your own dinner. Many's the time you have caressed your dog warmly when he jumped upon your chest and licked your face with his tongue." " *You* raised your secretary's pay because she is a very beautiful and charming young woman and because she used her beauty skilfully to captivate you. This despite the fact that she

I B

made a stupid mistake in her work last week, which cost you a great deal of trouble and embarrassment."

The " I," while trying to make honest and accurate reports concerning his own behaviour and motives, really does something quite different. " I " involuntarily describes his own conduct as being of a sort he believes his auditor will approve of. Or " I " is so made that he is capable of truthful self-observation only when the truth coincides with self-interest for one reason or another (perhaps a truth about a fault is needed to cure it) ; or, more rarely, when carried " out of himself " by passionate submission to a person or being whom he has exalted above himself. Moreover, " I " changes his behaviour, more or less, when he deliberately tries to watch himself. Thus he may alter his reactions to such an extent that the very bit of behaviour that he especially desires to observe is placed outside the range of his attention, or is totally suppressed. When you are feeling unusually happy on occasion, try to observe your happiness and analyze it. The moment you begin to succeed, you will find your happiness beginning to disappear. " I " simply cannot observe himself, or any part of himself, without becoming a different " I " from that which he set out to observe.

On the other hand, a psychologist trained to observe " You " encounters none of these difficulties. He is not prejudiced by hope or fear concerning the results of his observations. He may find you to be a much greater, more admirable person than he expected. But he does not even pause to make judgment concerning your greatness, nor to admire your unexpected virtues. He simply notes down the facts he has found out about the behaviour of one " You," and proceeds to compare these facts with similar observations of the behaviour of subjects Smith, Jones, and Barry. This professional student of " You " is out to discover the laws and principles which make " You " what you are, and which explain all your reactions naturally, in terms of cause and effect. " You " are not a single, isolated individual to him, but only one member of a more or less homogeneous species or genus. To the scientific psychologist, " You " is a generic term for everybody outside the organism of the psychological observer. The one thing he insists upon is that " You " shall be observed and described objectively, and that " I " cannot possibly observe himself in that way. His interest is concerned about the way " You " behave, and about the circumstances which evidently cause you to behave in that way. Then he tries to reproduce those same circumstances again, on another occasion, and to observe whether " You " act in precisely the same way " You " did the first time. If he finds, after a sufficient number of trials, that the same circumstances always cause " You " to act in just the same way, then this scientific student of " You " formulates a *psychological law* which states that " You " are so constituted that " You " react thus and so when confronted with such and such influences. The fact that this psychologist has been observing " You " in a quiet way designed not to obtrude itself upon your attention, has not changed your behaviour in the least, although it must have changed to such an extent that no law could have been discovered, had your " I " tried to observe its own actions.

Psychological Law

Let us suppose now that our psychologist has been observing a baby. The psychologist observes that each time he opens the infant's hand forcibly and presses the fingers back against its resistance, the child responds with all its might by trying to squeeze its fingers down again against its hand, in the action known as " gripping." After trying this experiment again and again, and noting that the infant always reacts in precisely the same way, the psychologist formulates a law, something like this : Antagonistic pressure tending to open Baby Jones' hand causes Baby Jones to grip with increased strength.

Thus we seem to have formulated one psychological law, which may be expected to hold on all occasions for Baby Jones. But is this a law of " You," the chosen object which psychology has undertaken to describe scientifically ? Evidently not. Surely psychology cannot limit itself to Baby Jones. Perhaps Baby Jones is not like Baby Smith, or Baby Brown, or even the other babies in the Jones family. It is the task of psychology to find, if possible, laws of behaviour which will hold for all babies. And adults, also. And lower animals, perhaps ? How much is included in psychology's " You ? "

One way to answer the question would be as follows. Let us observe the simplest, most elementary activities of adult humans, children, babies, and animals possessing still simpler

organisms than those of the human race, and let us try to
discover just how large a group behave according to similar
laws and manifest identical types of elementary activities.
In other words, we are to find out how many different types
of animal organism, despite their differences, behave essentially
alike. All such basically similar organisms must be part and
parcel of the " You " which psychology undertakes to
describe.

Now suppose that the psychologist selects the " grasping "
law which he discovered in the reactions of Baby Jones, and
proceeds to investigate its applicability to other babies, adult
humans, and animals. He will find, undoubtedly, that the
law holds for all, or almost all, infants. It may thus be
accepted as a valid law of " infant psychology." Perhaps
he can demonstrate further that this law of the grip holds for
all, or almost all, children. He has therefore discovered a
valid law for " child psychology " also. With adults, a
psychological investigator may have a little more trouble,
especially in procuring experimental conditions that will make
the adult try, spontaneously, to keep his hand closed against
resistance. If there is no antagonism between the experimenter's manipulation of the hand and the adults' " set " or
tendency to grip the fingers together, then the law will not
hold. But if the adult can be brought to regard the contest
as a game, which he can win only by maintaining his grip upon
some object, then the same psychological law can be proved
for adults, as for infants and children. Our psychologist
has demonstrated, then, that one law of elementary activity,
at least, is common to human babies, children, and adults.

Now what about animals " lower," or less complicated
than humans ? Here we encounter differences of bodily
structure almost at once. The law of the grip, as initially
tested and formulated, had to do with the human hand. Most
animals below man have no hands. A dog, for example, grips
his food chiefly between his jaws. Suppose, then, that our
psychologist assumes the canine jaw-grip upon food to be
identical in function with the human hand-grip upon similar
materials, and proceeds to test the effect upon the dog's
behaviour of trying to pull a bone away from him. The dog
responds with his jaw muscles, just as the infant responded
with his hand muscles. He grips the bone tighter and tighter,
clamping his jaws together more and more energetically,

just as the child gripped his hand together tighter and tighter. If the experimenter pulls upward strongly enough on a rod which the infant has grasped, the baby's entire weight becomes suspended by the grip of that one hand upon the rod. In just the same way a dog may cling to a bone or to a rope or stick so firmly, that the experimenter may lift its entire body from the ground and swing it about, suspended by the jaw-grip alone. Evidently the dog is behaving in the same fundamental way as the child. Perhaps our psychologist, after a sufficient number of experiments with dogs, and with other animals of still simpler structure than canines, may conclude that the law of grip-resistance holds for many animal species below man.

The Limits of Psychological Law

How far down in the animal kingdom may this same elementary activity of grip-resistance be traced ? We cannot be quite certain. No research has been able to solve this particular point. But we do know something about the elementary activities of very simple animals, such as annelids or segmented worms, part of whose nervous system is made up of individual nerves, connected by junctions, or " synapses " as they are called, just like the nervous system of human beings. In considering the activities of such simple animals we again find ourselves confronted with radical changes in bodily structure. The segmented worms, for example, although their nervous system fundamentally resembles that of the higher animals, possess no hands, tentacles, or teeth with which to grip food or other objects. Therefore, when we try to apply to their behaviour the law of resistance to opposition which we have hitherto termed the " law of grip-resistance," we needs must seek some activity other than gripping which, when opposed, may result in increase of the activity tested. The chief elementary activity of annelids is crawling. This is accomplished in the customary worm fashion. A ripple of muscular activity runs from tip to tail, and stiff bristles projecting backward along the body ensure a forward movement of the annelid as a result of this muscular activity. The speed and vigour of crawling movements depend primarily upon the condition of the nervous system. When the worm is stimulated by resistance to any segment concerned in its crawling behaviour, with increased muscular activity required to surmount the obstacle, the nervous system becomes excited. As a result of such nervous excitement, the rate of conduction of the activity waves throughout the worm's body may increase from 25 mm. per second to 100 mm. per second. In other words, opposition to its crawling movements causes the worm to crawl four times as energetically as it did before. This result seems fairly comparable to the child's increase of hand-grip activity and to the dog's increase of jaw-clinching activity, as a result of opposition to these activities. It would seem, therefore, that a law of " increasing activity to overcome opposition " is common to the behaviour of segmented worms, vertebrate animals, human infants, human children, and human adults.

Have we reached the limits of the " You " in which psychology is interested ? Many psychologists and biologists would say no. There has been a tendency in recent years to include jelly-fishes and similar animals which possess a very elementary type of nervous system, and even amoeba, paramoecia, and other single-celled organisms which possess no nervous system at all, within the field of psychology. Biologists study these simple creatures, so why should we not expect to find a " psychology of the jelly-fish " and a " psychology of the amoeba," as well ? There seem to be two good reasons for drawing the line between annelids and jelly-fishes, between animals with synaptic nervous systems and animals with nerve-net nervous systems, or with no nervous systems at all. The first reason is, that different laws of behaviour necessarily result from the difference in nervous equipment. The second reason is, that there is no real " You " in the organism of a jelly-fish or of an amoeba, as we shall have occasion to remark presently.

If we try to follow the law of increase-of-activity-to-overcome-opposition down into the behaviour of jelly-fish, radiata (star-fish), or sea anemones, all of which possess nerve-nets but no synaptic nervous equipment like that of the higher animals and human beings, we immediately find ourselves at a loss as to how to proceed with our investigation. The reactions brought about by nerve-net mechanisms are so much slower than those we have been considering that we should have great difficulty in making sure that any observed increase of activity was really due to the conditions of opposition we had imposed. The rate of nervous transmission in sea anemones is, at most, about .2 meter per second ; that in jelly fishes about .5 meter per second ; while in human beings we find a rate of 125 meters per second. Furthermore, there is no mechanism in the nerve-net for bringing up energy reinforcements from other parts of the animal's body in order to increase its activity and overcome opposition. Altogether, we find that we are dealing with creatures basically different and with elementary activities which are not correlated and unified sufficiently to offer any hope of working out funda-mental laws in the least comparable with those resulting from the synaptic type of nervous organization.

Psychology's You Consists of Integrative Activities

We have just suggested that psychology's proper field includes only those living organisms which possess a synaptic type of nervous system. Of course selection of subject matter for any science and limitation of its field is largely a matter of convenience and expediency. But if the present use of the word psychology convinces us that this science is intended prinarily to examine and describe the characteristics of human beings which are peculiar to themselves and to similar organic forms, then we may easily limit the field by discovering first the peculiar characteristics of human beings not described by other sciences ; and second, the other species of animal organisms which possess these same peculiar characteristics.

We have made a preliminary survey of the behaviour and structural characteristics of human beings and lower animals down to the level of coelenterates and we have found at least one characteristic in common. All organisms within the range thus defined react toward outside stimuli *as a unit*. This unitary behaviour is made possible structurally by a special type of nervous system which is not continuous but composed of separate nerve cells joined by synapses. This synaptic type of nervous sytem makes possible a flexibility of connection between the nerves so that new connections can be made at any time to enable the organism to act as a unit with respect to any environmental stimulus. When, as in animals below the coelenterates, the nervous system is all-continuous in the form of a nerve net, then all reactions to outside stimuli are predetermined by the connections already existing. *No activities of special unification occur in response to environmental stimuli : and no structures devoted to special unification activities exist.*

Structures and activities designed to unify a given organism are generally termed *integrative structures* and *integrative activities*. Integration as a biological term refers to that special part of the organism's behaviour which tends to unite the entire organism functionally. In animal organisms possessing a nerve net system without synapses, these functional interconnections are rigidly established by the structure of the nerve net itself. There exist no spontaneously variable activities which are adaptively integrative in nature.

Synapses lying between the individual nerve cells in the nervous systems of human beings and higher animals may be regarded from our point of view as animated junction boxes. The junctional tissues in these synapses are themselves living protoplasm especially differentiated for the purpose of propagating *integrative energy*. It is this integrative energy generated by its own special structures which constitutes, according to our view, the peculiar characteristic of human and higher animal behaviour.

Let us recapitulate our position as follows. Psychology as a science is primarily devoted to those characteristics of behaviour which are peculiar to human beings. The human organism shares its physico-chemical reactions and behaviour with inanimate objects and plants. It shares its physiological and nervous reactions and behaviour with all other animal organisms, including unicellular animals of various types. But the human organism does *not* share its special integrative activities with animals below the order of coelenterates. Therefore, from our point of view, the " You " which it is expedient for psychology to investigate and describe is a " You " which is composed most importantly of integrative activity.

To illustrate what we mean by the integrative " You " of psychology, let us compare the reactions of a gyroscope and a human opponent in the game of football. Obviously psychology is interested in the behaviour of the football player ; and just as obviously psychology is not interested in the behaviour of the gyroscope. Yet both these reagents push back at us in much the same way when we attempt to disturb their existing state of balance.

Let us suppose that the gyroscope is spinning with its

vertical axis perpendicular to the ground. An observer
approaches and tries to push it over. The gyroscope immediately exerts an equal and opposite pressure against its human
opponent. In the same way the football player, crouched in
position on his own line, resists the attack of an opposing
linesman who tries to push him over. As a result of such
resistance the player retains his former position virtually
unchanged. From the point of view of a Watsonian behaviourist there could be no essential difference between the
reaction of the gyroscope and the reaction of the football
player. Both are mechanical responses designed to maintain
an existing equilibrium.

But from our point of view a tremendous difference exists
between the two responses. The gyroscope pushes back
against its opponent in a mechanically simple manner which
does not require any internal readjustment or integration
between its parts. The gyroscopic push-back results from
outside interference with a state of motion already going on.
But in the case of the football player resistance to his opponent
involves a great deal of special integrative activity within
his organism. Reserves of nervous energy not previously
functioning are connected with the parts of his brain and body
already active. These energy reinforcements are directed by
special integrative activities toward the particular portions
of the body where the greatest pressure from his opponent is
felt. The human push-back is not the result of interference
with a mechanical action already going on. It results instead
from a new integration of the entire organism which makes
fresh energy available and directs that energy toward the
points of greatest danger. It seems to us that it is this type
of integrative activity which sets human beings and higher
animals apart as the special objects of study for psychology.

Briefly, then, we are compelled to conclude that psychology
is not interested in jelly fishes, pollyps, and sea anenomes ;
much less in sponges, amoebas, and single-celled organisms
lacking all nervous systems whatsoever. Present evidence indicates that psychology's " You " is coextensive with organisms possessing in whole or in part synaptic nervous systems.
Thus we may say, somewhat loosely, that the proper sort of
creature for psychology to study is either a human being,
or an animal with a nervous system which operates on the
same selectively integrative principles as those on which the

human nervous system operates. Psychology is interested in discovering and formulating laws of behaviour which hold for all the different types of organisms included in this field of study from human down to segmented worms.

We propose to take the position in this book that *selectively integrative activities constitute the special or peculiar characteristics of the behaviour allotted to psychology*, as above outlined. Psychology, therefore, must interest itself primarily in integrative behaviour and its laws. Secondarily, psychology must seek to unravel other forms of behaviour which serve to initiate integrative activities or which result from, and therefore reveal, integrative activities which have previously occurred. In short, the proper subject matter for psychology is " You "; and " You " is essentially a group of selectively integrative structures and activities.

Consciousness : A Product of Integrative Activity

Psychology, physiology, and neurology are very closely intermingled and to a great extent overlap. At present it seems possible that some day psychology and neurology may be united, since the field of neurology properly includes a study of the structures which serve to integrate the synaptic nervous system and the functioning of these structures.

Nevertheless, it is our belief that psychology must go beyond neurology to find its own particular subject matter. An historical survey of psychology clearly shows that consciousness had always been assumed to constitute psychology's special field of study prior to the very recent advent of Behaviourism. Consciousness was formerly described in metaphysical or religious terms either as " mind " or "soul." J. B. Watson and other modern behaviouristic psychologists rightly maintain that it is unscientific to describe any physical phenomenon in mystic or subjective terms. Consciousness, they say, has always been described in this non-scientific manner. Therefore, they conclude, consciousness does not exist. Their premises are quite correct. Their conclusion is a childishly absurd *non sequitur*. We agree that consciousness must be studied and described objectively and scientifically. But we do not believe that any scientific psychology can escape its most important problem, that is, the study of consciousness, by naïvely asserting that this problem does not exist.

Some behaviourists may accuse us of misrepresenting them at this point. " We do not say there is no such thing as conciousness," they might argue : " We only say that we do not know anything about this thing you call consciousness, and therefore cannot talk about it." Accepting the sophistic argument at its face value, we may reply as follows : It is just as much of a *non sequitur* to say that we cannot talk about a thing because we do not know its real nature as it is to assert that a thing does not exist because it has been wrongly defined. The chemists and physicists do not really know what they are talking about when they mention electrons and protons, yet they do a great deal of talking about them just the same. No one yet knows the exact nature of an electric current or a ray of light but science has talked a great deal about these phenomena to very good effect. In the same way, while we do not pretend to know the ultimate nature of consciousness, it is quite possible to discuss its behaviour and its characteristics intelligently and scientifically, and to formulate a useful hypothesis about its physical nature.

We have said that neurology's task is the study of the nervous system which includes naturally the junctional tissues in the synapses and the individual functioning of these tissues. But neurology is not concerned with consciousness. It would seem to us, however, that consciousness appears whenever junctional tissues in the nervous system are activated. In other words, consciousness appears to correspond closely with the sum total of integrative activities which psychology is primarily interested in studying. The evidence for this connection between consciousness and integrative activity will be given in a later chapter. For the present we merely wish to point out that an objective or scientific study of the integrative activities of human beings and higher animals includes, *pari passu*, according to our view, an objective and scientific study of consciousness. We believe that psychology should lay chief emphasis upon the conscious aspect of integrative activities ; while neurology should emphasize chiefly the structural and functional aspects of selective integration in its relation to the nervous system.

To illustrate the practical dividing line between various sciences, let us consider the different types of phenomena which the same stimulus may evoke from a human body. Let us suppose first that a drop of concentrated nitric acid falls on the subject's hand at a place where no receptor organs for pain are affected by the action of the acid. Chemical reactions of the body cells composing skin and flesh immediately take place. In popular parlance, the skin is eaten away by the acid. Chemistry is interested. It is the province of the chemist to describe the atomic and molecular phenomena which have taken place. But neither neurology nor psychology as yet are called upon to study what has occurred.

Let us now suppose that the acid eats its way through the epidermis to a portion of the hand where sensory receptors are located. Let us further suppose that the afferent nerve trunk normally leading from the receptor organs thus stimulated to the sensory centres of the central nervous system has been severed at the elbow in a manner similar to that effected by Head and Boring. The afferent nerve trunk receives excitations from its receptor organs and reacts by propagating nervous impulses up to the point where the nerve has been cut at the subject's elbow. Neurology is certainly interested in the nervous phenomena that occur as a result of acid stimulation of the receptor organ. It is up to the neurologists to tell us what has happened in the receptor organs and afferent nerve fibres. But psychology need not be called in as yet to study what has occurred.

Suppose, however, that the nitric acid eventually reaches some deep lying sense organs which are connected directly to the central nervous system by afferent nerve trunks which have not been operated upon. The afferent nerve fibres are excited. They carry nervous impulses to junctional tissues, or " psychons " in the spinal cord and brain. These psychons themselves respond and excite in turn large groups of outward bound or efferent nerves. These nerve fibres carry impulses to the muscle fibres in the larynx, arms, and other parts of the body. The subject suddenly exclaims " Ow, my hand hurts ! " He shakes his hand violently, perhaps, in an attempt to get rid of the acid. When this attempt proves unsuccessful he rushes to the medicine closet, seizes an ammonia bottle, and applies the ammonia to his hand in order to neutralize the effect of the acid. All these actions of the subject are symptomatic of and result from a large amount of integrative activity which took place in the junctional psychons of the central nervous system. Psychology is interested immediately. It is the duty of the psychologist to study and explain the complicated reactions which appeared as a result of these integrative activities, and it is even more imperative for the psychologist to explain the integrative activities themselves which dictated the subject's final actions.

We may note that intense consciousness preceded these final actions *pari passu* with the integrative activities which we know also preceded them. Just before the subject shouted " Ow " he experienced a sharp, burning sensation. Just before he rushed for the ammonia bottle he experienced various hasty ideas about antidotes for acid burns and while he rushed for the bottle he doubtless became conscious of emotions of pressing desire and possibly of fear. It is certainly significant that these conscious experiences apparently occurred at precisely the same time that we know the integrative activities must have been taking place in his central nervous system. We believe that it is psychology's special task to study and explain these integrative-conscious phenomena.

Integrative Psychology Does Not Imply Control of the Organism by Environment

Does the idea of treating psychology as a physical science make it seem mechanical, materialistic, and inhuman ? All physical sciences—and psychology is one of them—must be completely impersonal in their methods of investigation. And the laws which they formulate must necessarily be impersonal too. But that is not the thing that really troubles people when they are told that human beings react mechanically to stimuli with which they come in contact. The annoying idea, to many people, is the thought that a human being, "made in the image of God," is *under the control of* chance stimuli, inanimate objects, and environmental influences which have the power to make or break human happiness and to build or destroy personality. Many people feel that there is something mistaken and decidedly destructive about the notion that man does not build his own destiny, nor even his own character. They resent the " materialistic " assertion that man is a machine that cannot do anything but react mechanically to whatever stimuli set it in motion.

Integrative psychology, inasmuch as it accepts the viewpoint of physical science, must regard the laws of the human organsmi as, in a sense, mechanical.   This use of the word mechanical, however, merely means that the integrative activities may be formulated into definite and invariable laws of cause and effect. If this were not so then we could never have any real psychology but only a combination of art, religion, and metaphysics. Certainly integrative psychology regards the laws of integrative activity and consciousness as invariable and exact. It maintains that these laws can be discovered and formulated by studying " You " from a completely objective point of view.

But all this is very far from maintaining that You are under the absolute control of your environment.   In fact, integrative psychology shows or attempts to show for the first time in a scientific way that human beings possess the ability to free themselves from environmental control and to use their environment to develop themselves in any way desired. · This ability is based upon the integrative activities themselves.   When the integrative activities of thought, which we shall consider in a later chapter, have been developed to a sufficient extent the human organism attains the power to direct its own destiny.   Of course in gaining this development the human brain is limited by its inherited physical characteristics.   It may also be greatly helped or hindered by environmental stimuli which are wholly outside its own control especially during the early years of childhood and youth.   But the potential capacity for self direction is present just the same in the integrative mechanisms and activities. If these are strongly enough developed, and normal enough, at any time of life, they are capable of utilizing environmental stimuli to enhance certain reactions and inhibit others ; to increase certain types of stimulation and remove other stimuli altogether ;   and to develop the integrative mechanisms themselves to the point where environmental stimuli may be more completely controlled.

In short, *we regard the integrative mechanisms of human beings as a spontaneously operating device whereby the human organism may be completely freed from environmental or materialistic control.*   The fact that this device is subject to invariable or mechanical laws enhances rather than diminishes its potentiality for self-freedom, because it can operate itself more effectively once it possesses an objective description of its own mechanisms.

All this would not be so if the integrative activities themselves were set in motion only by chance stimuli from the surrounding environment. In other words, if we conceive the integrative activities as a completely passive, inactive set of cog-wheels which depend for their impetus to activity upon outside influences, then such integrative mechanisms could give human beings no greater freedom from environmental control than that which the simple reflex or behaviouristic theory contemplates. But again, such is not the case. The integrative activities are kept in motion from before birth until after death by nervous energies activated from within the body itself. In a later chapter we shall devote considerable attention to an enumeration of the various stimulus mechanisms such as endocrines, organic pressures, nervous automatisms and other spontaneously acting stimuli which serve to activate the nervous system and compel continuous integration according to a self pattern dictated by the individual characteristics of the particular organism involved. Suffice it to say, at the moment, that human beings have evolved to the point where their own integrative activities are exercised and patterned very largely by spontaneously acting stimuli generated within their own organisms, throughout life. Therefore chance stimuli from the environment must meet and contend with this spontaneously set pattern of integrative activities which is already going on. The resultant integrations should be and can be controlled, in large part at least, by the organism's own spontaneous integrative activity.

In summary, our view is this. The integrative-conscious activities constitute a self-regulating and self-readjusting mechanism kept constantly in motion by the organism's own stimuli. This integrative-conscious mechanism is so designed that, once started, it is capable of utilizing all environmentally initiated influences to perpetuate and develop its own pattern. By means of this mechanism human beings, and to a much more limited extent higher animals, may regulate and control their own destinies and development, and free themselves from environmental or materialistic control.

CHAPTER II

Early Soul Theories

FROM the beginning of thought man has been deeply concerned over the explanation of those fundamental activities which are the main springs of human conduct. Loving, killing, running away, fearing, lying, playing, caring for children, vocalizing, self-locomotion, are activities shared by all. So, too, are sneezing, coughing, crying, swallowing, and breathing. What is their source?

To the primitive mind the answer was simple. The primitive man recognized within himself a something which he could not see but could feel ; something elusive, impulsive, and turbulent. He felt the air all around him. This, too, was an invisible force, to be reckoned with as sometimes benign and sometimes destructive. So he sensibly enough blamed " air " for all these invisible activities. When he took air in himself through his nostrils, did it not give him greater life and activity? Without doubt then the great Invisible without and the great Invisible within were one, namely air or spirit. When unleashed and free without him, it brought the cool breeze of summer, the stillness of the lake at twilight, the sandstorms of the desert, the gales of the sea. Within, the effect was equally varied. When his spirit was quiet, he " scratched with a stick in the mould " ; when warm within him, he sought his mate ; when driven to fury he gloated in gasping triumph over the final upward thrust that devA hated foe. This, however, was *his* air, *his* spirit, set apart from the air of the outer world. There was in his mind no doubt that the air which he had succeeded in capturing within his own bosom, had an individuality and a personality all its own. If he sneezed violently it might leave him and another take its place. Thus the movements of the spirit within him were sufficient explanation of all the fundamental activities which began with the first in-drawing of air at his birth and ended only when the air left his body at death.

Modern Soul Theories.

Somehow, although we have evolved widely different interpretations of this doctrine, we have never completely got away from it. Some leaders still say the soul, the sum total of our loves, our fears, our dreams, our hates, is the source of all activities. The activities of the soul are not a part of our brain, and not a part of our material environment. They are of a higher and finer vibration, different from the brain itself but still parallel to it. Regarding ourselves objectively the soul motivates us from within, a reservoir of energy which plays on the fibres of our being to our joy or our sorrow, according to the sort of a soul with which we happen to be endowed ; but looked at subjectively, the soul is outside the brain. When the brain is energized by a stimulus from the environment, the soul is similarly active. If the soul is disturbed, its energized condition somehow innervates the corresponding areas of the brain. What sort of gears, if any, connect the two ? The philosophical psychologists do not say. They merely take the primitive spirit and say, " This ' air ' of ours is not breath ; it is Hertzian waves, or still more subtle vibrations. What it does, we do also, and conversely what we do is reflected in our soul."

To those who find more mundane explanations sufficiently clear, the maintenance of this doctrine seems difficult and unnecessary. Yet many leaders have accepted it because they felt that no facts or evidence have yet been discovered which would substantiate a more tangible opinion. It was the doctrine of James, who taught always in terms of physiology ; so much so that his theories, apart from this doctrine of psychophysical parallelism, are just as objective and matter-of-fact as those of the most ardent of to-day's behaviourists, and yet he always preferred to recognize the soul as the source of our fundamental activities. This doctrine also builds the background from which spring two of our most modern psychological concepts, the Libido of Freud, Jung, and Adler, and the " hormic " urge of MacDougall. It must therefore be given careful study if we are to build a sound foundation for understanding the current theories concerning fundamental human activities.

C

Mechanistic Theories.

The psychological school most opposed to the philosophical group we have just been talking about are the Behaviourists. They take the primitive observation of the causal importance of air, and say, "Air? Quite so. The air rushing into the lungs of the new-born babe causes pain and a reflex cry. And this is an epitome of the organism's entire life activity. Some object in the environment presses a button which sets up a reflex or chain of reflexes or a conditioned reflex and we act accordingly. The whole matter is purely mechanical and is entirely determined by what buttons are pressed from the outside."

Between these extreme points of view there are many gradations. From the impulsive dispositions of MacDougall there is a transition to the inherited action tendencies of Woodworth; the progress continues thence to the biological concept of action tendencies, while Allport's prepotent reflexes are on the verge of the purely mechanistic concept of reflex response. All these theories, whether extreme or intermediary, emphasize concepts and lines of thought which are not necessarily the concern of psychology, rather than stress the integrative aspect of fundamental behaviour. Integration, or our ability to act as a unit instead of a mere collection of parts, results as a function of the psychon and is therefore, according to our ensuing analysis, the *sine qua non* of psychology. Human activities, or rather, the activities of all organisms with our type of nervous system, are determined by three factors: first, the continuous stream of reflex activity set up by chemical changes within our own bodies, second, the responses set up by the environment which interfere with those already going on, third, the integrative mechanism which unites the self-activated reflexes one with the other and combines these in turn with those set up by the environment. It is the purpose of this chapter to examine some of the most talked of theories which have been put forward to explain the well-springs of human conduct and show their relationships to the idea of a human being as a self-activated integrative unit.

The Dynamic School.

In the dynamic group we include those psychologists who base their principles of action upon the thesis that all human activity is energized from within by some vital force which is continuously striving toward some goal. Most psychologists of this school are also called "Instinctivists" because they say that the inherent impulse to action finds its outlet through specific action tendencies called instincts It should be born in mind, however, that the important factor is the impulsive striving. This is the source. The instincts are merely the avenues of outlet.

The Psychoanalysts.

The psychoanalysts more than any other present-day group utilize this principle of dynamic urge. They recognize the possibilities of many instincts but find in the conflict between the native strivings of the individual and the always opposed environment a sufficient basis for everything we think and feel and do.

Sigmund Freud first expounded his doctrine of psycho-analysis in 1895. Since then, arguments both for and against it have been so wide-spread and so heated, that many of the psychoanalytical terms have become household words. Freud is a physician. With a physician's privilege he spoke frankly his views on sex and so emphasized the importance of this basic urge that his teachings have been called by Janet the doctrine of Pansexuality. It was this very element, of course, that aroused popular interest both for and against Freud. Some people welcomed the discussion as an opportunity to bring to light their own sexual thoughts and feelings. Others, disgusted that the bars could be so easily and readily let down, fought against Freud. In either case, repressions were removed and psychoanalysis has obtained wide publicity without the aid of a press agent.

Freud's psychology is therefore primarily a therapeutic psychology. He is chiefly concerned with the diagnosis and cure of certain mental states and all his theories and principles are evolved on this basis. He postulates an inner source of energy that springs into action by way of the instincts. There are other instincts—he mentions "brutality," "cruelty", "the baser instincts", but the most important is sex. Since sex is our strongest instinct our energy is mostly sexual energy. Freud names the sum total of sexual energy, the Libido. The Libido is uninterruptedly striving for expression, constantly driving the individual toward some goal. It controls our physical action as well as our motives, our learning, and our thinking. In short, all our activities, and all the social extensions of our activities into art, sports, music, science, religion, and what not are energized through the Libido.

Freud's emphasis on sex resulted from his clinical experiences in treating neurotic patients. Early in his practice he discovered that if the patient began with some dream or with his symptoms and gave everything that came into his mind, sooner or later he would reveal some hitherto forgotten childhood wish or desire of a sexually unconventional sort. As the child became more conventionally minded, its ego, or the endo-psychic censor, repressed the original perverted sex wish, whereupon the sex energy, although not present in conscious form, was nevertheless active and in constant conflict with the ego, to the great distress and ill-health of the latter. As soon as the forgotten episode was revealed, the conflict ceased and the patient was relieved of his symptoms.

As an outcome of these observations, Freud defines three types of Consciousness ; first, the Conscious, which is made up of those sensations, thoughts and feelings of which we are immediately aware ; second, the Fore-conscious or Pre-conscious, which is made up of mental stuff not in the focus of consciousness at the moment but easily recallable ; the third, the Unconscious, a reservoir of all the undesirable sex ideas of which we were once conscious but which have since been repressed. The Unconscious can only be recalled by hypnosis, psychoanalysis or other extraordinary means.

Of these three, the Unconscious is the most important because the most dangerous. It is a realm of conflict from whence the dammed-up sex energy is constantly trying to escape and frequently succeeds by way of slips of the tongue, misspelling, dreams, absentmindedness and other unconscious but revealing activities. Apparently all the sex striving of childhood is unconventional. Freud says there are six types of perverted sex behaviour to be found during childhood and early adolescence. The earliest to appear is auto-sexual love or the self-arousal of erotic excitement. The next is homo-sexual love, or an erotic feeling for a person of the same sex, and the third is incestuous love, or an erotic drive toward a person of the opposite sex but in the same family, such as a boy's love for his mother or a girl's love for her father. In addition to these three perverse types of love activity which are normally to be expected in the life history of every individual, there may also be present masochism or an erotic desire to be cruelly subjugated by a lover, and sadism which is erotic excitement aroused by hurting or cruelly subjecting a lover ; and there is also exhibitionism which ranges from a desire to show off before the opposite sex to an erotic desire to expose the body to a lover. These unconventional sex desires may be either repressed or sublimated. If they are sublimated, the thwarted sex energy can be harnessed to some of the so-called higher activities ; the individual is happy and socially adjusted.

Many noted scholars who at one time or another have worked with Freud have disagreed with his emphasis on sex. The most noted of these is Dr. Carl Jung of Zurich. Jung accepts the basic energy principle which psychoanalysts share with many psychologists. Life is a constant flow of psycho-physical activity springing spontaneously from within. This self-energy is the power behind our activity and drives us continuously towards certain types of goals. It is Bergson's *élan vital*, called by Jung the Libido. The Libido according to Jung is not limited in its expression to sex activities. It also drives us toward egoistic goals and although there may be many other instinctive dispositions, only these two, the ego and sex are important. Through these two instruments the Libido is constantly seeking greater differentiations and greater individuality. In so doing it is constantly opposed by the environment, which places one obstacle after another in the pathway of success. The successful overcoming of environmental obstacles Jung calls " progression ". Some times, however, the Libido is not successful in its task. It is unable to win success and to reach the new goal. In such cases regression takes place. The Libido abandons the newer, more individual and progressive activity for responses on a lower level where it has previously found success. If the opposition is too great, the individual forsakes altogether the responsibilities of adult life and reverts to the attitudes and activities of childhood. In the extreme forms of regression only the racial residue remains, and the individual presently loses all his own peculiar activities, thoughts and feelings which have accrued in the course of personal development, and which differentiated him from the mass of his fellows. This interpretation of an all-inclusive life force has for its corollary a concept of the Unconscious which is also very different from Freud's. For Jung the Unconscious has two aspects ; there is the individual Unconscious and the collective Unconscious. The individual Unconscious includes in addition to repressed sex energies all the thousands of peripheral impressions to which we have been receptive during the course of our lives, but which we have never held in the focus of consciousness. Such impressions Jung maintains are not lost. They not only make their mark upon the physical nerve structure, but they also leave a psychic imprint in the individual Unconscious. The collective Unconscious is made up of racial symbols or archetypes and their effect is more far reaching than any of us realized. These archetypes may be thought of as inherited mental patterns characteristic of people with a common racial history. The people of every race have shared a common racial experience in a common racial environment. This has led to a gradual piling up of mental imagery and symbolism peculiar to these particular people, and has set actual physical and psychical limits to the range, extent and mode of their thinking. These archetypes are not verbalized, but spring up as a sort of thought-feeling of such strength that their influence upon our conduct is unescapable. The events and people of our dreams are racial symbols representing in primitive terms our stresses and worries. The content of the vast number of myths peculiar to each race is made up of those racial symbols, some common to one race only, others shared as thought forms with all mankind. These primordial images as potential thought-stuff make up the collective Unconscious. Together with the repressions and forgotten images acquired during the life history of the individual, they constitute the source of our whole life activities and their influence is continuous and inescapable.

Alfred Adler, originally a student of Freud but now widely diverging from his master in principle if not in practice, is the third of the psychoanalysts to venture an original opinion as to the nature of our fundamental activities. He does not offer an explanation of why we act as we do. He merely assumes certain innate tendencies or instincts, and sets about describing the interaction of these tendencies with the world. All of us have a desire to conquer our environment and be superior in intellectual attainment, depth and range of our emotional life, richness of imagination, speed and skill of reaction, power of physique, beauty of body; in short, we want to be perfect in everything we think, feel and do. If by any chance we discover that we aren't perfect, this discovery sets up a strong feeling of inferiority. With an accumulation of unpleasant experience, this feeling of inferiority becomes a complex, that is, a whole constellation of ideas as to how poor we are in this or that respect. The cause does not necessarily have to be real. A shy little girl frequently imagines that she is frightfully plain and quite unattractive to boys, when the truth of the matter is quite the reverse. However, if she is really convinced that she is neither beautiful nor charming she will seek consolation by trying to be very superior in other ways. She may, for instance, develop her intellect and win renown for her wit. Usually these compensations are moderately successful. Where they are not, the patient may become degenerate, take to drink or drugs or sex or crime, or become neurotic. He or she compensates by means of fantasy and day dreams and escapes the disappointments and disillusions of reality. Thus everything we do is purposive and *all life is striving for power.* Adler calls this doctrine Individual Psychology.

This short review of the psychologies of Freud, Jung, and Adler shows three essential elements for which the psychoanalysts stand. The first is the Libido, an inner source of energy, undifferentiated, psychic, inherent, unchangeable, the matrix of all instinctive activities. Second, conflict between the Libido and the environment. Third, reaction mechanisms built up as a result of this conflict. For Freud, the Libido is mostly sex and the mechanisms are repressions, sublimation and probably the Censor or the Ego, that weapon of the environment which labels sex undesirable. Jung emphasizes the Libido as the life force, the reservoir of all instincts, thoughts and feelings which must always find an outlet somewhere, somehow. The reaction mechanisms are unimportant compared with the fact that the life force is supreme and must always find an outlet. This outlet is provided by the instinctive dispositions and the archetypes which might be called thought-feeling dispositions. The influence of these two factors cannot be escaped. Adler on the other hand finds only the reaction mechanism important. The life energy is taken for granted, its purposive focus, defence mechanisms, and compensatory reactions provide an outlet for the will to power.

The emphasis on an inner reservoir, the energy always striving toward some end, is the most important concept psychoanalysis as a whole can give us. Freud's emphasis on the harmful results of suppressed sexual desires and his insistence on erotic experience as the ultimate purpose of human behaviour have done much to reveal the futility of the taboos placed on sex by civilized society. So, too, the Jungian archetypes have thrown a strong light on the extreme difficulty confronting us in the process of individualization and personal differentiation, but the Libido still remains the keynote of the contribution of psychoanalysis to modern psychology.

The Instinctivists.

In this discussion of fundamental activities, instincts are not to be thought of as completed and stereotyped performances springing like Athena full grown from the head of Zeus. Nor are they sharply marked from habit on the one hand and learning on the other. Instincts are merely native dispositions to certain types of activity. They set the goal and determine the mode of action but the specific act resulting therefrom depends on circumstances. Thus when accosted by a robber who is not greatly our superior in strength, we may draw a gun, swing a club, drive a stiletto, or dive in with our fists. In each case the goal is self-preservation, by active force, using whatever means are nearest at hand. From this instance it would seem as if the instinctive act were dependent upon environmental stimuli for its initial appearance. Such is not the case. We do not tend actively to defend ourselves and our property until the body has reached a certain maturity When it has, this instinct springs impulsively into action. and the little boy behaves aggressively whether the occasion warrants such response or not. The little boy has not learned to fight. He fights because he feels like it. His technique will undoubtedly improve with repetition, and if he is not deterred by some outside force stronger than he is, he may form the habit of bullying all environmental forces which appear to be weaker than he, but the original disposition to fight is innate and springs into action from within.

This point of view presumes a basic purposive drive

derived from an original reservoir of free energy constantly seeking outlets.

James

James was the first psychologist to insist that instincts are just as important in human behaviour as they are in animal behaviour. Biologists and psychologists previous to James had contrasted human and animal behaviour by saying that animals followed their instincts whereas humans are activated by reason. Man was supposedly void of instincts. James maintained that man has just as many instincts as the animals, and probably a great many more. Physically, James said, instinctive actions all conform to the general reflex type. Psychically an instinct is the faculty of acting in such a way as to produce certain ends without foresight of the ends and without previous education in the performance. Instincts are not to be confused with habit on the one hand or a learned response on the other. They are "implanted for the sake of giving rise to habits."[1] James based his latter conclusion upon the observed transiency of instincts. Ducklings if put into the water when very young will swim immediately. If kept from the water until mature they will flounder and flap much as hens do if they are put into water. There is apparently a time when their organisms are all set to swim. If they are given a chance to do so at this time, swimming will become an habitual means of locomotion. If they are not given a chance when the organism is ready they will never learn. James' idea of an instinct then, is not that of an exact end-response which always occurs on the presentation of a given stimulus. Originally an instinct is merely an impulse to action. It occurs spontaneously because we feel that the proposed action is the only natural and appropriate thing to do. Human beings according to James, have a great many of these natural impulses. Chief among these are :—sucking, biting, clasping, carrying objects to the mouth, crying, turning the head aside, holding the head erect, sitting up, standing, locomotion, vocalization, imitation, emulation or rivalry, pugnacity, anger, resentment, sympathy, hunting instinct, fear, appropriation or acquisitiveness, constructiveness, play, curiosity, sociability, and shyness, secretiveness, cleanliness, modesty, shame, love, jealousy, parental love. The natural

[1] *Principles of Psychology*, vol. II, p. 402.

impulses to action are never uniform and invariable. Many of them die out after a short period. They may be inhibited by other stronger instincts. After their first appearance they are modified by experience, by memory, associations, and habits. They remain, nevertheless, inherent, impulsive, spontaneous, self-activated springs of human actions.

The Purposivists

The essential purposive striving which differentiates living organisms from mechanical objects and which finds its outlet by way of instinct channels is accepted by William MacDougall as the basis of life. The *élan vital* or the will to live is the essential phenomenon whose manifestations we as psychologists have set out to discover. He differs from James in that he stresses the psychic aspects of conduct far more than he does the physical, and is more clear-cut and careful than the psychoanalysts in describing the expressions of the fundamental hormic urge.

MacDougall says[1] the human mind has certain inherited and innate tendencies which are the source of thought and action. These primary tendencies are the basis of all individual and racial development. They may vary from individual to individual and race to race in native strength ; that is, one tendency may be stronger than the others in any one individual or environment ; history and social contacts may favour the development of some tendencies at the expense of others, but the foundation, the main primary tendencies, are the same in all men and are also found in the more complex animals. These tendencies are of two sorts. The first class consists of general tendencies which might be termed the mechanics of the mind. In this class fall such mental processes as the tendency to imitate, suggestion and sympathy, the tendency to play, the tendency of every process to be repeated more readily after it has once occurred. The second class of tendencies are specific tendencies or instincts. Every instinctive action is the outcome of a purely mental process which has three aspects, the cognitive, affective and conative. That is to say, each instinctive response is initiated by some object in the environment. We recognize this object and it makes us afraid, or angry, or amorous, whereupon we act in a certain way toward the object or at least have an impulse

[1] *Social Psychology*, William McDougall, Boston, 1921, p. 44.

to do so. Though this process cannot be described in purely mechanical terms and is not to be looked upon as reflex, it nevertheless has some enduring nervous basis whose organization is inherited. It probably has the form of compound sensori-motor arcs and may centre in the lower thalamus.

Only the psychical side of instinct is of maximal importance, particularly the emotions accompanying the instinct. This alone remains unchanged. Thus we are always afraid of a loud noise, but after we learn that the source is harmless, a blow-out for instance, we do not run away. Nor do we punch our enemies when they rouse our wrath in the course of ordinary contacts, although the impulse to " knock his head off " still remains.

Each principal instinctive action has its characteristic constituent emotion. An emotion connected in this way with a principal instinct is called a primary emotion and plays such an important part in the total instinct that when MacDougall names an instinct he also gives its accompanying emotion. His list of principal instincts with their corresponding emotions includes flight-fear, curiosity—wonder, pugnacity—anger, self-abasement—subjection, self-assertion—elation, parental instinct—tender emotion. Some other instincts of less well defined emotional tendency are : sexual instinct, gregariousness, instinct of acquisition, instinct of construction. In explaining each class he discusses both instinct and emotion together, as the instinct of flight and the emotion of fear.

Although, in a mature human being, habits are looked upon by MacDougall as springs of action, they do not equal instincts in importance, since they are necessarily secondary to instincts. That is, the original action must be instinctive and since without the original action there could be no building up of habits by repetition, habits " are formed only in the service of instincts."

The most important emphasis to be derived from MacDougall's discussion of instincts is to be found in his insistence that the presence of a natural environmental stimulus to a given instinctive action is not enough to release the impulse. A suitable condition of the organism is even more essential. A natural love stimulus awakens no erotic response in the immature organism ; or the impulse to flight may, at a time when the organism is in an apprehensive or

nervously irritable state, outweigh curiosity, and at another
time the sometime coward may be sufficiently balanced to
investigate before leaving. In any event the activity is the
resultant of two forces, first the present organic condition
of the body, second, the incoming environmental stimulus.
A complete explanation of our fundamental activities must
take account of both.

Reaction Tendencies

In the case of the Libido and the instincts, the two types
of fundamental activity lie within the self. The environmental
stimulus although necessary, is not primary. The impulsive
act will not occur unless there is an adequate stimulus. The
stimulus is only adequate after the inner activity has already
been set up and it may occur many times before the inner
activity had been set up or after it has died down without
arousing the characteristic response. The inner impulse
springs into being regardless of environment and any number
of stimuli may be adequate to give it outlet. With the rise
of behaviourism and the rigid stimulus-response psychology,
the idea of self-activity was abandoned along with sensation,
conation, will, purpose and all other behaviour that might
be stigmatized as a subjective state rather than an overt
response. Purpose, interests, sensation, will, imagination,
however, were too potent factors in human conduct to be
ignored. It was one thing to deny a philosophical hypothesis
of self-activity but quite another to ignore these vital everyday
experiences. At the same time every one could see the value
of the objective focus of the stimulus-response psychology.
To bridge this gap R. S. Woodworth put forth his doctrine
of reaction tendencies. Woodworth maintained that reactions
apparently predetermined by the " set " of the organism are
in themselves responses to stimuli which have not yet found
motor outlet, which responses are released by coincidental
reactions to environmental stimuli. They are in the final
analysis action tendencies or action determiners, characterized
by being inner activities, by persistence over a long period
of time, and by a certain purposive aspect which predisposed
the organism toward a certain line of conduct. A tendency
is actual kinetic energy bottled up in a nerve centre and striving
to find an outlet. As long as it is blocked, this bottled-up
energy makes the individual restless. If the end-result

does not occur immediately, the bottled-up energy may be partially released by environmental stimuli associated with the principal one of a series of preparatory reactions which finally bring the organism into contact with the goal it has been seeking.

The hungry man, for instance, cannot immediately begin eating. He must first find food, in order to attain his goal of eating a good meal. To do this he responds to all likely stimuli at hand which may bring him in contact with food. If he is in the woods by a stream he goes fishing or hunts a rabbit. If at home he raids the larder. The inner state persists and continues to keep active until he commences eating.

These tendencies to action exist on three different levels. The lowest is the organic level where the inner state is largely some chemical state, like muscle fatigue, which predisposes the individual toward a slower response. The next higher level is more neural than chemical; the individual is set toward accomplishing a certain end. The hunter on the scent, the homing pigeon, are classical examples. The third level is the highly conscious level where a man knows what he wants and gets it. Action tendencies may be native or acquired. Emotions, impulses to notice and to pay attention, interests, and aptitudes may be native. Recognition of the meaning of sensations, ideas, conceptions, memories, will, and imagination are acquired. These represent modifications of the original native tendency forced upon the individual by his environment.

Instincts are the most important group of action tendencies. They belong to the second level since they are native tendencies which drive toward a certain goal. In a well organized instinct, the preparatory responses are closely linked with the main reaction tendency, so that the instinctive action occurs without undue delay. Birds set about immediately and mechanically gathering string and straw for their nests when the nesting season is on. In a loosely organized instinct, however, there are no well-proved neural preparatory reactions. The individual is restless and engages in random activities until the final goal is reached. Here learning enters in, for it is only gradually that the individual learns what activities will most likely bring about the desired end. As a result, what was in the beginning a loosely built instinct becomes a closely knit habit.

Native tendencies are a result of the original nature of the individual. The fertilized ovum contains the determiners for native activity nine months before the baby is born. This is to be interpreted as meaning that the original constitution sets the limits and range of activities, determines what activities are possible, not what will actually occur. Though the organism be ever so ready for flying, this activity will not occur until the proper stimulus, internal or external, sets proper nerve centres into activity. If the birds have been caged until maturity a toss into the air will set them flying. This shift of emphasis from the inner condition to the outer stimulus is the differentiating mark between Woodworth and the Instinctivists. He admits the necessity of an environmental stimulus as a primary part of the activity process, making action tendencies dependent upon environment for their operation if not for their existence.

Biological Action Tendencies

Closely allied to Woodworth's concept of inherited action tendencies is the premise of the biologists that living organisms have but one fundamental type of activity. This is the tendency to secure or maintain the best living conditions in its environment. This set is made up of as many fundamental activities as the animal has action mechanisms. This idea, like Woodworth's, contains two essential elements—1. Action tendencies, their nature completely undefined, somehow inherent in the protoplasm and its structural organization. 2. Environmental stimuli antagonistic to the natural action tendencies and so tending to produce unfavourable living conditions for the animal or human. This concept is not so advanced as Woodworth's in one particular; that is, Woodworth has worked out a concrete plausible mechanism for activity, a stored potential energy released by impact with the environment in the case of simple reactions and reflex responses, and in the case of action tendencies, a centrally dammed-up kinetic energy, operative over a long period of time and seeking outlet through the lower centres. The biological concept, however, is more advanced in dealing more definitely with the environmental stimulus. It defines the specific nature of all adequate environmental stimuli as antagonism to the organism's natural activities.

In general terms the biological conception reduces to the

idea of an organism, its environment, and the interactions between the two. These interactions consist primarily of the organism being stimulated to action by the environment ; that is, the initiation of the responses is chiefly attributed to the environmental factors. Psychology is mainly concerned with the organism ; if we could know what stimuli have caused an organism to behave as it has, and what other stimuli will cause it to behave in a new and predictable way, we would have, from this point of view, a complete science of psychology.

Properly speaking, the biological approach includes both the concept of the prepotent reflex as laid down by Allport and the theory of Behaviourism in its strictest sense. While the biological approach is objective and stresses the dependence of function upon structure it is not necessarily committed to the mechanistic explanation of man's activities. The biologist is willing enough to accept consciousness or even a soul if such functions can be demonstrated. In this his attitude is more flexible than that of the psychological behaviourist and allows for greater lattitude for venturing upon new lines of research ; it is therefore more acceptable to many psychologists.

Prepotent Reflexes

The prepotent reflex is a concept which has been taken over from neurology and used by some social psychologists as the fundamental element in human behaviour. The concept has three essential elements : a simple stimulus-response neural mechanism ready to be set off by environment : a prepotency attaching to certain of these mechanisms : and appropriate environmental stimuli. The new element over and above the ordinary stimulus-response doctrine is the utilization of the neurological law that some reflexes take precedence over others in the control of the motor outlets. The cause for this precedence is not known. It may be due to structural differences in the two arcs involving variations in the chemicalization or energizing of the synapses, or junctions, in the number and type of neurones involved, or in the length of arc. The knee-jerk, for instance, involves comparatively few neurones and these are connected through the centres of the spinal cord, while the most simple thought reflex involves the more complexly-pathed associative centres of the brain and very complex masses of neurones.

Neurologists say that there are two types of reflexes which usually take ascendency over all others : those loaded with pleasant affective tone and those producing an unpleasant affect. If either type occurs it will take precedence over all indifferent bodily reflexes. There is no particular law as to whether the pleasant shall be superior to the unpleasant, or vice versa. In the dog whose spinal cord has been cut at the base of the brain so that only the spinal reflexes are functioning, a prick on the sole of the foot causes the withdrawal of the foot. Tickling the shoulder results in scratching. If the two stimuli are given simultaneously, the withdrawal occurs but the scratching is inhibited. In other words, as between these two the pain reflex is supreme. Of the reflexes with a strong pleasant affective tone, it may be said that the sex embrace of a frog is so powerful that it persists even though transections are made above and below the shoulders. In every case, the prepotency of an individual reflex must be experimentally determined.

Unless the neurologist's classification is interpreted in terms of the neurological explanation of pleasantness and unpleasantness, it is subject to criticism on the ground that affective tone is subjective and " unpleasantness " and " pleasantness " merely verbal symbols for unknown phenomena. A strictly neurological description of pleasantness and unpleasantness is as follows : unpleasantness is looked upon as an antagonism of reflexes resulting in a damming-up, or stasis, of other reflexes simultaneously stimulated ; pleasantness is the facilitation of reflexes occurring simultaneously. Thus from the neurological point of view, a reflex may attain ascendance either because it is inherently strong enough to block off all other reflexes or because they facilitate its control over the final common path.

Allport, the first psychologist to discuss at length the importance of the prepotent reflex to psychology, postulates six hypothetical classes of prepotent reflexes ; these are starting and withdrawing ; rejecting ; struggling ; hunger reactions ; sensitive zone reactions ; sex reactions. Allport's classification is not based upon specific neurological laws such as those mentioned above, governing pleasantness and unpleasantness. If the word instinct were taken to mean native co-ordinated reflex behaviour, Allport's classes are more in the nature of six instincts. They are what Allport calls "broad unvarying types of response." They are not simple reflexes ; rather, each class involves many reflexes co-ordinated to bring about a certain type of response. Each class involves many movements and has many appropriate natural stimuli. In each instance all three types of effectors, the somatic, the skeletal, and the visceral, are involved. The prepotent reflexes are highly protective and adaptive and from this fact they derive their supremacy in some undefined manner. The most completely efficient reflexes from this point of view are supreme at any given moment. Most of these responses are present at birth, although reactions of the erogenous zones do not occur until soon after birth and sex reactions are delayed until the organism has matured. Together, they constitute our original native equipment. All the behaviour we later evolve is based upon and consists in part of one of these fundamental responses. From their initial appearance, however, these reflexes are subject to modification. They therefore expand into habits, skilled motor responses, and higher thought processes. Prepotent reflexes may be modified on the afferent side through the law of the conditioned reflex until the range and number and complexity of the stimuli arousing the response, are very great.

Thus a baby is not naturally startled by darkness. He does respond by starting to a sudden loud noise. If a door slams while he is asleep in the dark, the starting response may thereupon be conditioned to darkness so strongly that it will persist throughout life. The prepotent reflex may also be modified on the effector side by a greater refinement and specialization of response, as when sucking combines with biting and chewing, and finally the adult human of this particular civilization is eating with knife, fork and spoon.

Allport states frankly that the prepotent reflexes he has selected as fundamental are not simple reflexes at all but involve many reflexes and many movements. He wishes to avoid the term instinct, however, because it is so frequently used to include responses which to Allport are habitual and therefore not native. Since all native behaviour is reflex when analyzed to its simplest elements, Allport feels justified in using the term prepotent reflex to cover our fundamental, spontaneous responses. In this he would be criticized by many because he is not only using reflex to designate a complex

D

integration of reflexes but is also including within each class some reflexes that are prepotent and some that are not. Nevertheless such a handling of the fundamental activities places our behaviour on a clear-cut stimulus-response basis and avoids the necessity of any centrally stored dynamic impetus from within the organism. It also permits a sharper line to be drawn between native behaviour and habit than is drawn in the explanations of MacDougall, James and Woodworth. Flight, concealment, providing clothing and shelter, modesty, are " concealment in advance ". Flight and cleanliness are derived from the rejecting reactions. The approaching reflexes of hunger evolve into curiosity, hunting, hoarding and constructiveness. Allport has avoided some of the behaviouristic limitations by insisting upon the importance of these six native co-ordinated types of response. His stress is on native structure rather than upon environmental stimuli, a reversal of the usual behaviouristic emphasis.

But it is not at all clear where the " prepotency " springs from, according to Allport's theory. Perhaps, after all, the six " prepotent reflexes " must be thought of as deriving their prepotency from some inherent, dammed-up energy in appropriate nerve centres, as suggested by Woodworth's theory. In that case, Allport is more of an instinctivist than a behaviourist.

Reflexes

To the strict behaviourist, life in its fundamentals consists of reflexes ; in its higher, more complex moments, of conditioned reflexes. Reflex arcs furnish the structure for elementary behaviour like sneezing, winking, squirming, starting, loving, relaxing, stiffening, fearing, raging. But the reflex needs to be modified through the principle of the conditioned reflex to furnish a structure for most of our loving, raging, fearing, and for such more complicated activities as tennis playing and verbalizing. Reflexes provide the fundamental structure and the elementary, native behaviour. The reflex is intact at birth and awaits only the proper environmental stimulus to set it off. Like any other machine, it must be started by someone or something outside itself. Once the proper button is pushed, its operation is purely mechanical ; no release of inner energy or operation of a superior soul is required to set it in action. If this were the whole story, structure would be dominant and our life history predetermined by the number and type of reflex arcs present at birth. Fortunately or otherwise, the central synapses of any reflex arc can be connected under the proper conditions with those of other reflex arc circuits. Such connections are entirely determined by environmental stimuli. If a bell rings every time we approach a table laden with a hot, savory dinner, very soon our mouths will water at the sound of that particular bell whether the table is ready or not. Whether the artificial stimulus is a bell, a gong, or a woman in a blue gingham dress depends upon the country we live in, the social status of the family, the customs of our particular group, and a great many other factors, not one of which are in any way related to heredity, instinct or original native equipment. So, although he admits the existence of certain elementary native responses due to structure, the behaviourist places all his stake on environmental influence, saying that he can make a street-car conductor or a musical genius out of any man with a normal body by controlling the outside influences to which he is subjected.

The elementary activities which exist at birth in great number can be divided into three classes; First are the somatic reflexes like the eye wink, knee jerk, swallowing, coughing; the second are skeletal reflexes and consist of random sporadic movements of the body and limbs. Each such movement is a response to a specific stimulus. Usually the stimulus is from within the body and usually it cannot be named except in such instances as those of pain and hunger. The third class is made up largely of visceral reflexes or, as Watson terms them, " gut responses ". These gut responses occur in response to specific external stimuli. In them the reflexes are co-ordinated and, according to Watson's experiments with infants, are fairly well unified into three definite patterns to which Watson gives the names of fear, rage, and love. The fear consists of " checking the breath, jump or start of the whole body, crying, often defaecation and urination."[1] It is naturally aroused by two stimuli only, one is loss of support, the other is a loud noise. All previous conclusions that we are naturally afraid of snakes, furry animals, the dark, high places and so on, have been definitely proven to be false and can be set aside along with the doctrine of vestigial traces which was called upon to explain these fears.

[1] *Behaviorism*, John B. Watson, 1925, p. 124.

The only adequate stimulus to rage is restraint of movement induced either by holding the infant's arms close to his sides, holding the legs firmly together, holding the head so that it cannot move. The characteristic reactions going to make up the rage pattern are, "stiffening of the whole body, screaming, temporary cessation of breathing, reddening of the face changing to blueness. It is obvious that while these are the general overt responses, the greatest concentration of movement is in the visceral field. Blood tests of infants so man-handled show that there is an increase of blood sugar."

Love reactions are naturally aroused by stroking the erogenous regions, tickling, patting, rocking, dandling and so forth. The response to such stimuli includes cessation of crying, gurgling and cooing. "That visceral factors predominate is shown by changes in circulation, in respiration, in the erection of the penis, etc."

The reactions outlined above, that is, love, rage, and fear, comprise the sum total of our native equipment. They are the original unlearned responses and everything that comes later is developed from these by means of the interpolation of artificial stimuli on the conditioned reflex principle. Conduct consists of bodily changes and movements that can be seen and measured. When enough objective measures have been made, we shall be able to predict the response of any nameable stimulus.

This experimental limitation upon the number of demonstrable, unmodified, and unlearned human activities is now generally accepted by the majority of psychologists. The behaviourists' stress upon the all-importance of environmental stimuli and his confidence in the principle of the conditioned reflex is not so generally acceded to. The response patterns as described by Watson have never been shown to be specific and exactly the same for all infants, as they would be if the stimuli alone were the dominant factor rather than the condition of the organism at the time the stimulus is introduced. This is true even in the case of the most simple reflexes where mechanical perfection might be expected if it were ever to be found in human conduct. Variations occur in the gut patterns. Not all babies respond with "rage" to restraint of movement. Sometimes behaviour more like the love pattern occurs, that is general relaxation of the body, and sometimes if he has just been fed, the baby falls asleep.

From these two instances it will be seen that there are two possible variations ; typical movements may be differently combined and differently integrated, or a completely typical pattern may be set up due to reactions already going on at the time the stimulus is introduced.

Behaviourism represents an over-simplification of fundamental activities, in an effort to make their purely mechanical basis apparent. Behaviourism is correct in ascribing all movements and activities to mechanisms of " reflex " nature. But it is not correct in omitting all description of the constant, spontaneous activities originating within the organism itself. The integration or combination of these with activities initiated environmentally, in fact brings about a type of response very different from the simple reflex emphasized by behaviourism.

Unit Responses

The variations not accounted for by behaviouristic theory indicate that there are other factors in elementary human behaviour besides simple and conditioned reflexes. There are certainly two very important factors left out of the behaviouristic account. There are the constant interior activities originating within the organism itself, of which an example is the constant tonic motor discharge to the musculature of the organism ; most of these activities go on within the organism from before birth until three days after death. There is also the integrative principle of synaptic conduction which is similarly operative from the time the neural paths are complete until the final falling-apart of the synapses.

Moreover these two factors are simultaneously operative. As a result, from the very beginnings of life, the organism produces not merely hundreds of individual reflex activities but also ever changing patterns of self-activity. Body temperature, heart beat, changes due to growth of tissue, rate of bodily metabolism, tonus of the muscles that keep the body from collapsing, activities due to the presence of hormones in the blood, enzyme activity, all illustrate internal activity going on before the baby is born. After birth, hunger, excretory activity and respiration appear. It is only gradually that the outstanding environment is allowed to impinge upon the individual and to a noticeable extent modify his total unit repsonse. This unit response consists in the unique combination brought about by phasic (transitory) stimuli upon the existing stream of self-activities already progressing within the organism in question.

The importance of the integrative mechanisms in this connection can scarcely be over-emphasized and all responses within the psychological field must be studied with the integrative mechanism clearly in mind. The unit response has as much an individuality of its own as any single one of its constituents. This principle is readily demonstrated in the field of chemistry. We grant immediately that one atom of oxygen will not change unless tampered with. We feel the same to be true about hydrogen but let one atom of hydrogen and two atoms of oxygen combine, and we call the result water. In other words an entirely new entity with qualities and reactions peculiar to itself results from the coming together of these two elements in this particular way. Why should it be any different with the single reflex reactions which, joined together, constitute human behaviour ? Sensations from a jazz band when we are happy, successful and well fed unite with the responses already going on within us to form gaiety, hilarity and a desire to step out for the evening. To listen to the same band when we are suffering from suspense or anxiety causes a conflict which is so unbearable that we wish to annihilate the band in order to avoid suffering extreme discomfort until we are out of hearing. In other words, to explain our fundamental activities only unit responses of the organism can be considered.

If the internal responses are necessarily integrated into a unit response it is certainly impossible for an outside stimulus to have its own way regardless of internal activities. Any reflex set up from the outside must combine with the internal activities with a consequent resulting change in both.

There are four possible types of change. First, the stimulus may be either allied or antagonistic ; second, the self activities may be either increased or decreased. If the reflexes set up by the environmental stimulus are antagonistic to the self and the self activity increases, then the stimulus will be destroyed either in whole or in part. If, under these conditions, the self activity is decreased, the self will be destroyed either in whole or in part. If, however, reflexes set up by the environmental stimulus are allied to the self and the self-activity increases, the power of the organism increases because it adds to itself the strength of its ally.   If under these conditions the self-activity is decreased, the power of the ally is relatively increased.   This self-decrease, however, is not destructive as long as there is complete alliance.

In each instance the combination of the internally initiated activities with those aroused by the environment results in a new unit response which has its own unique characteristics quite apart from those of its constituents.

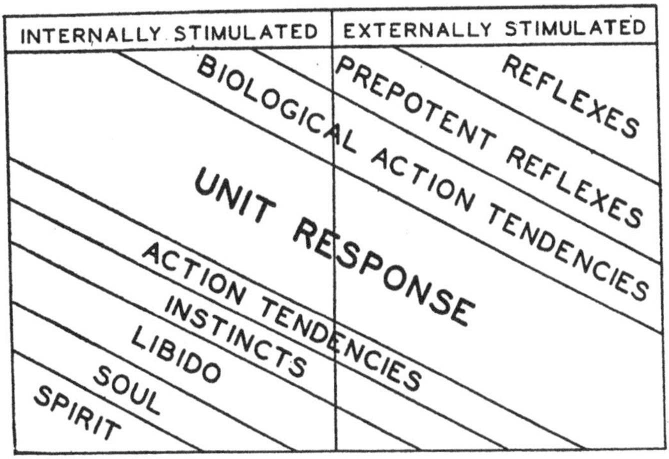

FIGURE I

Different Theories of Fundamental Activities

Chart indicates a graphic analysis of the external and internal stimulation elements responsible for fundamental activities as postulated by various theories described in the text.

Summary

Originally all human activities were considered expressions of the human soul.   This soul was identified by the primitive man with spirit or breath because, when the breath departed, the body activity ceased.   The scientist looked upon the soul as a non-material entity whose activities are paralleled by those of the body.   To-day psychology is divided between those who still stress an inner source of energy which finds expression through the body mechanisms and those who are content to describe our activities in terms of overt behaviour.

Psychologists of the first type, which we have called the Dynamic group, stress the psychic aspects of behaviour. They say that the inner life energy is constantly striving toward some definite goal or purpose. The body mechanisms it uses are the instincts. The foremost exponents of this line of thought are the psychoanalysts, Freud, Jung and Adler, and the instinctivists James, MacDougall and Woodworth. The psychoanalysts in particular are very much concerned with psychic activity and very little concerned with body mechanisms. They call the life energy the Libido. The Libido is continually fighting an antagonistic environment for self-expression. According to Freud, the Libido is chiefly sex energy and finds its outlet through sexual channels. The environment is particularly antagonistic to sex expression so that most of this energy is held in the Unconscious in the form of unfulfilled desires or wishes. Jung does not agree with Freud in this emphasis on sex but maintains that the Libido finds expression through egoistic channels quite as much as it does through sexual. The individual Unconscious is not alone in its influence on our conduct. We are equally under the sway of the collective Unconscious, which contains the racial archetypes or tendencies to thought and feeling which are our racial inheritance. Adler holds that we are all striving for the consummation and perfection of our ego. If, at any time we feel our superiority jeopardized we take refuge in compensatory conduct. Usually these compensations are more or less successful. When they fail, the individual degenerates, becoming either neurotic, criminal, or sexually perverted.

The Instinctivists start from the same hormic foundation or inner urge that the psychoanalysts postulate but instead of confining the outlets for activity to one or two instincts, the men in this group describe a great many instinctive mechanisms which the inner energy may use as outlets. Instincts are not stereotyped, cut-and-dried responses, but are merely native dispositions to certain types of behaviour. They determine the end and the mode of action, but the specific act depends on circumstance. James lists a great many instinctive impulses to action and maintains that human beings have just as many instincts, if not more, than animals do. MacDougall lists only thirteen instincts but holds that each instinct is accompanied by an emotion on the one hand and a thought-process or a recognition of a situation on the other. To bridge the gap between the dynamic group and the behaviourists, Woodworth puts forth the concept of reaction tendencies. Reaction tendencies are themselves responses to certain stimuli which have not yet found motor outlet. The tendency to action represents blocked-up energy. If the natural motor outlet is not opened immediately, the tendency itself acts as a stimulus to a series of preparatory reactions which finally result in fulfilment of the initial impulse.

Biologists, after the manner of Woodworth, maintain that the organism has but one type of activity and that is an action tendency to maintain the best living conditions in its environment. The biological concept lays great stress upon the environmental stimulus and upon the natural antagonism between an organism and its surroundings.

The prepotent reflex theory as given out by the neurologists ascribes the dominance of some reflexes over others to the pleasant or unpleasant affective tone accompanying the dominant impulse. Prepotency arising from such a cause still retains a tinge of the dynamic attitude. Allport, in taking over this concept into psychology, gets pretty far away from the original reflex idea. He maintains that the elements of behaviour consist of six prepotent types of activity. He names these types of activity prepotent reflexes, saying that because of their high protective and adaptive value they take precedence over all other types of activity as to control of the final common path.

The behaviourists on the other hand see no need for stressing this factor of prepotency. The elements of behaviour are reflexes. They are modified by experience through the principle of the conditioned reflex. The modification is continuous and immediate, so that the environment becomes more important in shaping the individual than any inherited mechanism.

This emphasis upon the parts of the mechanism and parts of the response rather than upon the integrative factor and the unit response, results in an incomplete picture. The unit response theory holds that the key factor to human behaviour is the constant activity set up within the organism day and night by neural and chemical processes within the body. Each incoming nervous excitation has to be reconciled one way or another with the activity already going on. This is made possible by the integrative mechanism of the human nervous system. The resulting response does not consist merely of the algebraic sum of all activities going on at the moment. It is in fact a Unit Response with characters derived from its unity and not shared with any of its constituents.

CHAPTER III

ELEMENTARY UNIT RESPONSES

The Organism as a Reacting Unit

THE human organism, apart from its environment, presents a unit action pattern determined by the structure and maturity of the organism itself. Beginning before birth and lasting until death, our bodies are a vast whirlpool of activity springing from the life process continuously operative within the organism, that is, from the activities of the heart, the lungs, the stomach, the intestines, the endocrines, the blood stream and other liquids, and from the activity of the smooth and skeletal muscles.

The normal baby is already in action when he comes into the world. His heart is beating, there is considerable tension in the skeletal muscles, and his bowels and digestive tract are also tense and active. His body temperature is established. Soon after birth the child begins to make a large number of spontaneous random movements with arms, legs, head and trunk. These random spontaneous movements have no reference to his environment. They occur no matter whether he is in his bed, on the table, or in the arms of his nurse. These activities constitute the original unit pattern and are maintained as long as the body continues to live.

The original pattern is, however, modified by the growth process, which brings about changes in cell structure, in endocrine activity or in the integrative mechanism itself. The sex glands, when they mature at puberty, give excess activity throughout the entire organism for a period of years. Sometimes these developmental activities become permanent parts of the spontaneous action pattern as when certain endocrine glands coming into action compel a rearrangement of the functioning of all the endocrine glands. In this case, the whole integrated unit pattern of activity shifts permanently or for the good part of a lifetime.

The unit pattern can also be modified by external objects

permanently attached to the body, or kept attached for long periods of time, like clothes, artificial limbs, and teeth.   Also permanent environmental influences like gravitation, air pressure, oxygen content in the air, temperature limits, and climate have a similar effect.

All these developmental and fixed environmental stimuli when they first appear, evoke some appropriate unit reaction from the previously existing unit or organism activities. Then, gradually, *the bodily tissues affected by the stimulus become permanently changed*.   The muscles become stretched, tightened, enlarged, or the glands become adjusted at a new level of activity, the blood formula is chemically changed, or the receptive threshold raised in the tissue.   Then, of course, the activity unit has really changed, in that degree, and its unit responses will change correspondingly ; not in *type* or *nature* but only in degree, or in increased or decreased responsiveness· to certain sorts of stimuli. *The integrated reaction unit always remains fixed and determined solely by the organism itself.*

The spontaneous action unit presents a force which any new environmental stimulus must either successfully oppose or successfully ally with before it can modify conduct.   It introduces a barrier which makes it impossible for any external stimulus to find a free and independent outlet through the motor channels.   The baby soon after birth engages in a series of activities which originate in the environment rather than within the organism.   He sucks at the breast or bottle, swallows, and digests food, then expels the waste.   He draws his foot up and pushes a hand off his other leg ; he spreads out his toes when his foot is tickled.   He cries when bathed, or when his feet are snapped with nurse's finger or when handled in certain ways apparently unpleasant to himself. He starts at loud sounds, clings to a finger, relaxes when petted.   These movements and actions do not occur except when some object comes near him or touches him.

In these instances, a baby reacts, not with a separate, new movement, but rather with a *re-alignment and modification of his spontaneous movements*.   In the case of sucking, breathing, crying, trying to move his feet and hands when they are restrained, and of digesting food, the stimulus objects bring increased energy to the parts already energized and make more active the previous activity.   Petting and startling cause decrease of energy in many parts previously energized ; crying, wriggling, and the spontaneous body movements cease. Food in his stomach stops many of the random movements of his body and limbs also, while starting new movements in the alimentary canal, salivary glands, and the blood vessels of the interior of the body. The reactions in *all* instances involve the entire unit activity of the body ; there is a shift, an increase of some activities, and a decrease of others. Thus the final response will depend on the nature of the change made in the already existing activity.

Every phasic activity, no matter how simple or involuntary or separate it may seem to be, follows this law. In the adult organism not a single reflex reaction, no matter how seemingly simple and separate from all other activities, can actually take place without being in part or whole a unit response of the whole organism. The knee-jerk, for example, differs in extent when the subject is hungry, after he has eaten, and after his food is digested. It can be " voluntarily " suppressed altogether with some practice. The wink reflex, and the pupillary reflex vary greatly according to the general condition of the organism and other activities going on. None of these simple reflexes can take place without some redistribution of many other activities in the total unit. So even these supposedly separate reactions actually take their place as unitary responses of the organism.

The " higher ", or more " conscious " activities involve unitary action of much greater portions of the whole organism. A reaction is regarded as " conscious ", in fact, in proportion as it involves more and more complete and extensive reaction of the central integrating mechanism of the organism, the central nervous system, and consequently involves more of the organism in its unitary response. The response is always unitary. But unitary responses are sometimes made with a finger, sometimes with a toe, sometimes with a single trio of reflex nerves ; while at other times, unitary responses require arms, hands, head, and body.

The child's spontaneous original activities do not spring from thin air ; nor from any unknown source of unspecified character. His original activities spring from thousands of different internal influences exercised upon the receiving organs attached to his nervous system. These impulses are conducted into the complicated system of " nerve centres " in the brain and spinal cord, where all the thousands of impulses simultaneously received are sorted out and brought together in a pattern dictated by the shape and arrangement of the child's body and by the nature of the nerve centres and their inter-connections. Once this pattern of actions becomes a single integrated unit, it must react as a unit to any fresh activity put into it.

This unit energy pattern is precisely what pioneers of psychology were trying to explain with their various theories of fundamental activities fully described in chapter two. All the early concepts of fundamental activities contained a mysterious, vaguely described, dynamic factor which expressed itself for still vaguer reasons in particular predetermined inherited types of behaviour. The Libido is a mysterious concept of this class which assumes an inner, unknown driving force compelling the individual in the general, predetermined direction of sexual activities. The concept of instinct similarly assumes an inner driving force which caused the organism to behave in various predetermined ways towards various types of environmental objects. The action tendency concept assumes the same two general factors, attempting to explain the dynamic drive in terms of neurological summation and stasis.

The idea of the biological tendency similarly included a spontaneous drive of mysterious character which made the animal seek a favourable environment and which ceased to operate when such an environment was attained.

All these theories neglected entirely the two fundamental facts upon which the concept of unit response is based. First, the constant pattern of self activity spontaneously initiated and maintained through the mediation of the central nervous system in human beings and in higher animals. This constitutes the dynamic, spontaneous driving factor of the earlier concepts. The second factor ignored by the earlier concepts is the laws of integrative activity which determine how environmental objects shall be treated by the already acting organism. These rules of integrative combination constitute the element of predetermined form of the activity which the earlier concepts found inherent in the nature of the organism.

Adequate Stimuli to Unit Responses

The adequate stimulus to a response of the unit organism

may be a simple object, like a blanket that gets over the baby's face. It may be a person, like the baby's mother or nurse. On the other hand, it may be a situation such as the child's being shut into a room for misbehaviour ; or the mother's commanding the child not to do something, or to do something that he doesn't want to do. It may be a single force, like a loud sound, or gravitation causing baby to topple off his bed. What, then, is the essential characteristic that makes for " adequacy " of any thing, person, situation, or force in evoking some unit response from a naïve baby ?

The " adequacy " of any environmental stimulus depends *upon its ability to influence the unit pattern of activities* in some way. There are many stimuli to which the human body is at all times completely indifferent, infra-red and ultra violet rays for instance, sounds above and below a certain pitch. But within the range of normal sensibility there are periods, such as infancy and old age, when certain receptors are either not functioning at all or at best have only a limited receptivity. At birth the human infant is most responsive to touch, internal pressure, and pain. He curls the fingers of his hand when the hand is touched, spreads his toes, draws up his leg if his foot is tickled, and lies relaxed if he is stroked or petted. Inside the baby's digestive track, pressures and pains from food and from the contractions of the stomach during hunger pangs register effectively very soon after birth. The new-born infant also responds to temperature and probably to taste and smell. Normally the infant when hungry will turn toward the breast, attracted by the smell of the milk. But it is said that if a strong smelling medicant is put upon the breast the infant will not take it.

Vision and hearing are least developed at birth. The pupils of the new-born will contract to light but the child does not follow the light with its eyes until the third or fourth day, and several months pass before he can discriminate colour. Hearing at birth is impossible because the middle ear is filled with amniotic fluid which may be partially replaced in a few hours, but the usual time is three or four days.

These experimental conclusions as to the functioning of the infant's receptors at birth are confirmed by the neuro-anatomists who have demonstrated that the nerve tracts from the various receptors are in varying conditions of maturity at birth. Those from the touch receptors are best developed, and those from the inner ear are least developed. Given this condition of the organism, it follows that there are many stimuli to which the baby must remain oblivious. These stimuli, since they cannot register on the child's organism, will not influence in any way the child's unit pattern activities.

The first criterion of adequacy, then, will be that the stimulus must first of all be adapted to stimulate effectively some sense organ which has " come in ", functionally, and has begun to work at the time the stimulus is applied.

Stimulus Must Compete Successfully with Other Stimuli

Many a stimulus may be suitable to register upon its appropriate receptor organ ; and it may actually register on the organ itself. But still no unit response of the infant or adult organism need occur, *unless the action impulse set up is strong enough, and of the right kind, to compete successfully* with other stimuli from without, and with the natural, spontaneous activities forming part of the unit action pattern itself.

" See, baby ! " says the mother, and dangles a dull, dark object before baby's eyes. No response. Does the dangling object register on the child's eyes ? Probably, assuming the baby is of sufficient age. But a bright ray of sunlight, reflected from a mirror is wandering across the wall, and baby's eyes follow it. The light ray competes successfully ; the dark object does not. Baby responds to the ray, and not to the other.

The baby is crying. The nurse shakes his rattle which, a moment before, he had grasped eagerly and shaken with apparent delight. No response, now. Why ? A sudden hunger pang has seized his stomach in its grip. The pang is a stimulus that can compete successfully with the rattle, so that the baby no longer responds to the rattle.

An adequate stimulus, then must not only register on some sense receptor : it must also register so strongly, or so deftly as to compete successfully with the other stimuli and activities simultaneously going forward.

Stimulus Must Change Unit Pattern of Activities

This is not the same as competing successfully with other stimuli. The situation is analogous to Weber's law of sensory discrimination which states that we cannot discriminate, or notice a difference in sensation (that is, respond to a difference in the intensity of a stimulus) unless the existing stimulus is increased by a certain fraction of itself. If there is scarcely any light in the room, you can notice a marked increase of light when a candle is brought in ; but if the room is in broad daylight, the candle light would not increase the light enough to make a perceptible difference. It would take a large electric light, or spot light, perhaps, to increase the illumination enough to be detected.

Now the same thing holds true in the matter of unit responses. If a baby has his fingers very tightly closed, as a part of his unit response pattern, a slight pull directed toward opening the fingers will not produce any result. A stronger pull at the fingers will bring a quick tightening, in opposition to the pull. The stimulus pull had to be sufficient to upset, or change, the existing activity. A little more water in a river will not change its course, but a flood of millions of gallons upsets its present action altogether, and requires a new and larger outlet. The stimulus must *appreciably increase or decrease* the existing stream of unit activity.

Stimulus Must Oppose or Ally Itself with the Activity Pattern

The same holds true, at the other extreme, if the baby's hand is relaxed completely, but for another reason. You can open his fingers up wide and pull the hand out flat, without calling forth any reaction at all. Now pull the fingers a little farther back, so that the relaxed muscles are stretched sufficiently to hurt, in spite of the lack of tension in them to begin with. The baby suddenly grasps his fingers together, and tries spasmodically to close his hand in opposition to your pressure upon it. There was no activity in the nerves and muscles of the hand, to start with, that was tending to keep it shut. The opening of the hand, therefore, had no effect of opposing an existing unit response of the organism's established pattern. In other words, if the child is not " trying " to keep his hand shut, you cannot evoke any sort of unit response by opening it. There must be *opposition*

E

to an existing activity, to evoke a response of *opposition* from the unit organism to the stimulus.

Or, on the other hand, try to evoke a reaction of alliance when the child is not active in the way you try to make him active. Let the mother, for instance, pick a child up from his play with blocks, on the floor, and begin to caress him. At other times, the baby will smile, and coo, and snuggle delightedly closer to the mother. But now, those activities going on in the child are not the ones that mother has chosen to stimulate. The baby may begin to cry, and to struggle to get down upon the floor again with his toys. In this case, the mother's caresses are felt as actual opponents to the baby's activities, and he responds with opposition. On the other hand, especially if he is somewhat tired, he may merely remain inert, and unresponsive to loving. When released, he may have forgotten all about his toys. That is, his former activities may have ceased. But until he " wants ", as we say in every-day language, " until he *wants* to be kissed and petted ", he will remain indifferent to the petting and caressing. He will not respond with allied activities. If the mother helps him with his play by bringing fresh toys, or by throwing his ball back to him, then he laughs, and manifests every sign of delight and friendliness toward the mother as playfellow. In that case, she has allied herself with activities already going on. There must be *alliance* to an existing activity, to evoke a response of alliance with the stimulus from the unit organism.

Summary

Any stimulus, whether thing, person, situation, or force, in order to be an adequate stimulus to evoke unit organism responses, must possess the following characteristics :

1. Stimulus must register effectively upon some working receptor organ of the nervous system.

2. Stimulus must compete successfully with other stimuli simultaneously operating.

3. Stimulus must increase or decrease existing activities of the organism sufficiently to change present pattern.

4. Stimulus must oppose itself to, or ally itself with, existing activities of the unit organism.

Responses of the Unit Organism

If a stimulus succeeds in modifying the unit activity pattern two general classes of response are observable.

First, a stimulus opposed to the activity of the organism calls forth a response of opposition ; and a stimulus allied to the organism's activity calls forth a response of alliance.

Second, a stimulus which injects *greater* activity into an active part of the central nervous system than the activity already going on there, calls forth a *decrease* in activity of the unit self ; and a stimulus which injects *weaker* activity than that already present, evokes an *increase* in activity of the self.

Since increase and decrease of unit pattern activity may occur under conditions of opposition as well as under conditions of alliance, four fundamental types of unit response are possible.

Responses of Opposition.
    1. Opposition and increase of activity.
    2. Opposition and decrease of activity.

Responses of Alliance.
    3. Alliance and increase of activity.
    4. Alliance and decrease of activity.

Responses of Opposition

Whenever any incoming phasic activity interrupts or inter-feres with the main unit pattern, the new activity will be found to oppose the unit pattern. Under these conditions, if the incoming activity is much stronger than that already going on, the latter will be decreased to make room for the new set of activities. If, however, the new stimulus injects a weaker set of activities into those already well established, the new activities will soon be overcome and thrown out. If you pry open a baby's fingers gently, just enough to let him grasp them shut over your opposition, he will *increase* his energy in grasping each time. If you tear his grip loose altogether, however, his hand relaxes, at least for a moment, and he makes no further effort against your superior force. In the first case, you injected *inferior*, weaker activity than that going on ; in the second case, you injected stronger, greater activity than his own.

Opposition Increase

When you flick a baby's feet he becomes more active all over. The nurse does this, primarily, to make him suck at the mother's breast more energetically. It is effective. He always attacks the nipple with more vigour ; he also whimpers, and squirms all over, and perhaps doubles both fists hard, and kicks a little. The same thing happens when the baby is bathed, particularly if a shower is used, so that he gets hundreds of little blows all over his body. He throws his arms and legs about, and screams with all his might. Also, if the baby's arms are held to his sides or his head is restrained from movement, the child will get red in the face from his violent effort to move.

In the case of snapping the child's feet, or holding the baby's head or limbs when he is making random movements with them, it is clear that the stimulus is *opposed* to the unit organism's existing activities ; opposed, in fact, to the normal unit pattern of activities, as integrated by the organism's central nervous system. Nor can there be any doubt that the kicking, screaming and pushing involve a great increase in the child's general activity.

It should be further noted that the stimulus activity, although opposed to that of the responding organism, is nevertheless much weaker than the total unit pattern. The smart of the flicked foot, the prickle of the needle shower, and even the pressure of the restraining hands are not over-whelming, although the latter might reach the point if continued long enough under sufficient pressure.

Opposition Decrease

One of the most interesting situations illustrating the most extreme decrease of the tonic self by an overwhelming incoming activity occurs when the organism is startled by some sudden violent explosive stimulus. Watson's experiments with infants show that loud sounds " almost invariably produced a marked reaction in infants from the very moment of birth. For example, the striking of a steel bar with a hammer will call out a jump, a start, a respiratory pause followed by more rapid breathing with marked vasomotor changes, sudden closure of the eye, clutching of the hands, puckering of the lips. Then occur, depending upon the age of the infant, crying, falling down, crawling, running or walking away."[1]

In terms of unit response, sharp, abnormally intense stimuli cause a sharp positive inhibition of some or nearly all activities for a fraction of a second. The incoming activity is so much larger than the normal unit energy pattern that the latter is completely overwhelmed. In the case of Watson's steel bar, the loud noise near the baby's head injects *more* activity into the integrative activity centres of the brain than that already there, and practically all activity decreases for a moment including even the heart action. The opposition to this type of stimulus is evidenced by the baby's desire to get away from it if possible by crying, falling over, or crawling away.

Another, less extreme, example of the opposition-decrease situation occurs during the digestion of food. The baby under the influence of hunger pangs is very active and noisy. He is whimpering, crying spasmodically, throwing his legs and arms about, and turning his head. When the mother gives him his bottle, his previous activity stops almost at once. He becomes concentrated on sucking the bottle, and perhaps pushing downward with his feet each time he pulls at the nipple. He also doubles his fists hard, or tries to grasp the bottle.

As the milk gets down inside his stomach, he becomes less and less active. *No activity is inhibited outright* as in the previous case ; they all continue, only much less energetically and tensely. His hands relax, his legs also. His body becomes comparatively limp. He moves his eyes rather than his head to follow passing lights or objects. He becomes *relaxed ;* all his movements are gentler and calmer. His *unit activity* at least the visible part of it, has decreased.

Food in the stomach, because of the arrangement of the nerves it stimulates, is able to inject more powerful activity into brain centres than the activity it " inhibits ". As a result there is an increase of activity in the digestive and intestinal tracts, an increase of blood supply to the stomach, and an increased flow of gastric and salivary juices. Energy is withdrawn from the skeletal muscles, the blood supply to the periphery of the body is decreased, and the precipitation of adrenin, glycogen, and other energy supplies to the muscles

[1] Watson, J. B., *op. cit.*, p. 121.

are also decreased. In other words, there is a decrease of all activities which constitute the normal, evenly balanced pattern of the organism. Sometimes pressure of food in the stomach decreases activity all over the body to the extent of putting a person to sleep if he has eaten too much and yet avoided indigestion.

In the same way that the food opposes the organic activities and overcomes the hunger pangs, the body in turn opposes the food. The opposition of the food evokes a counter pressure with the stomach and intestines and the secretion of chemicals calculated to destroy and dissolve the food. These activities are not nearly so energetic as the natural ones of the regular pattern, so that all these reactions constitute a decrease of total unit response under conditions of opposition to an antagonistic stimulus of greater volume and strength.

Alliance Responses

Not all stimuli evoke a response of opposition. Our social structure is based upon the fact that our contacts with other people are for the most part of an allied nature. Certainly our set is in that direction, otherwise we should hardly let ourselves be persuaded by salesmen, ministers, teachers and parents. In general, we are allied to organisms whose activities most resemble our own. Our own family, our own townsmen, and people of our own race come closest to complete alliance, while foreigners and members of other races are least allied.

Alliance-increase

One special type of very close alliance is found between the mother and the very young child. The child has been but lately an integral part of the mother's organism itself and still continues to be as far as mental focus and emotional attitude are concerned. Usually the mother, as a stimulus, sets up greater activity in the child's organism than that already functioning. She brings food, warmth, shelter, comfort, security, and the baby decreases its own activity in order to receive what its mother has to give.

Nevertheless, as the child grows older there are many situations where the child increases his activity in response to this very closely allied stimulus. If the mother returns to the playroom after several hours absence and simply stands quietly waiting for the child to see her she is injecting an inferior allied activity into his central nervous system, and as soon as the child sees her he responds by increasing his allied activity.   He may run to her and put his arms around her, hugging and kissing her, he may pull at her skirt, and try to climb into her arms.   Sometimes this over-activity takes the form of becoming very busy with slides, box climbing, or running, all in order to win the mother's attention and love. The response is one of increased activity on the part of the unit integrated energy pattern to an allied stimulus which sets up activity inferior to the self.

Alliance-decrease

When the child's mother takes him up in her arms, and holds him in a comfortable position, she thereby immediately allies herself with his natural unit response pattern which has to hold him in that position against gravitation.   Only this being held by the mother is still more comfortable. Also, her body heat is just like his and enhances his own, stimulating his organism in accordance with its pattern. When she kisses him the pressure of her lips on his is totally unlike the food contact ; the food gives taste and smell ; the lips give only pressure, soft, like the child's own lips, and affecting his action pattern in just the same way.   It is a perfect alliance.   Since the mother is doing part of the work of his own bodily activities for him, he has less work to do to maintain the unit response pattern in its natural condition.

If the mother hugs the child tight, and caresses it with lips and hands, so that a superior volume of allied energy is injected into the child's central nervous system, he will calm down, and yield himself happily to her caresses.   His energy decreases in intensity and in the total amount of movement in alliance with the greater activity evoked by the mother.

The same situation arouses a similar response in adults. Petting and caressing, causing love passion, make women limp all over, and at its extreme, the systolic blood pressure drops sharply, showing the heart too has decreased its pumping activity greatly.

Four Elementary Unit Responses

We are now in a position to describe definitely, the elementary unit responses, and to give them names.

Dominance

When the responses of *increase* of activity, and *opposition* to the stimulus combine in a single unit response, a good name for this behaviour is *dominance*. This is the most primitive, and the most frequently occurring elementary unit response, especially in infancy, childhood and youth. It is the action often referred to as *aggressiveness*, on the one hand when the subject takes the initiative ; and *resistance* when the subject merely hangs on to something or persists in some line of action against environmental opposition.

When the baby grasps a rod tighter to resist its being pulled away from him until he suspends his whole weight from the grasp of one hand, this is *passive dominance*, or resistance. When animals and children chase anything that runs away from them, this is *active dominance*. Running away makes the stimulus activity *inferior*.

In the case of adults, fighting, whether with the fists, guns, or by verbal combat, is the most primitive instance of active dominance ; but winning a college degree, succeeding in a profession, or success in sports, all involve active dominance exercised over a long period of time.

Compliance

When the response of *opposition* to the stimulus and *decrease* of activity combine in a single unit response, it makes an elementary unit response called *compliance*. The adequate stimulus to compliance is an *opponent stronger* than the subject. This is the response erroneously called " fear " in many instances, and which often forms the basis for fear ; fear is not compliance, but compliance defeating dominance.

Compliance is the most important of all unit reactions in preserving the organism from injury and destruction in the struggle for existence against stronger and antagonistic forces and animals. Moving in a circuitous path around a dangerous object, or handling food or some tool carefully to preserve it for use are *active* compliance.

Giving up something without a struggle, or stopping some activity when the opposition becomes too strong and dangerous, is *passive* compliance. A baby's decrease of crying when you cry at him louder is *passive* compliance. Passive compliance is a mere cessation of the activity which is opposed by a stronger antagonist.

Active compliance is engaging in whatever new, and different activity is necessary to oppose a stronger antagonist successfully.

Submission

When the reactions of *alliance* with the stimulus, and *decrease* of activity combine in a single response, the elementary unit response may be called *submission*. The adequate stimulus to submission is an *allied* human being, *stronger* than the subject. Submission is the active, willing obedience to the commands or stimulations of another person. If this surrender of the self to another's control consists mainly of giving up activities commanded, it may be called *passive* submission. If it consists of doing something active, however gentle or slight the movements required, it is *active* submission.

The child, when obeying its mother, is responding with active submission, but when it rests quietly in its mother's arms this is passive submission. With adults a favour done another person is usually active submission, lending a friend ten guineas, posting a letter, and the like. Standing aside to avoid running down a child or a pet animal is passive submission.

Inducement

When the reactions of *alliance* with the stimulus, and *increase* of activity combine into a single response, this elementary unit reaction is called *inducement*. The adequate stimulus to inducement is an *allied* human being, *weaker* than the subject in some respect that appeals.

When a person merely offers himself as a stimulus to which another may or may not respond as he chooses, this offering of the self is *passive inducement*. The mere sight of a helpless infant will induce the majority of women to submit to its needs. Beautiful show girls who merely stand around in the chorus are modern examples of the same passive inducement that the chained and garlanded slave girls of former days were trained to exercise. Their innate beauty sets up in the beholder an extremely pleasant allied activity of greater volume than his own unit self. He decreases his self activity in order that he may gaze upon the beautiful woman and further ally himself with the activities such a stimulus arouses.

The coquette, on the other hand, is a very good example of active inducement. Her vivacious manner, sparkling eyes, tossing head, witty speech and alluring body movements set up in the subject of her conquest an activity which overwhelms his own integrative pattern and persuades him to succumb to her power.

Persuading a customer to buy a line of goods is largely active inducement. So is good teaching or child training, and so are all situations where one person gains leadership over another through persuasion rather than force.

Circular Series of Elementary Unit Responses

The four elementary unit responses just described are obviously not all the possible combinations of the two simple reaction elements, increase or decrease of activity, and alliance or opposition to the stimulus.

It is obviously possible, and probable, that many intermediate gradations of both elements occur, in combination with similar gradations of the other element. The organism need not be diametrically opposed to the stimulus, but only moderately opposed, or slightly opposed. It may be slightly allied with the stimulus, or considerably in alliance with it, or strongly in alliance with it.

In the same way, the organism need not increase its activity very greatly, as a response to a given stimulus ; or the increase may be marked, or to the entire capacity of the organism. It may decrease, in the same way, in varying degrees of its full capacity.

There must be, and actually are nodal points, in each series, that represent the maximum and minimum of each reaction. Increase of activity, for instance, must reach a maximum in certain types of reactions, and then lessen, by perceptible steps, until its minimum is reached. Then, when this point is passed, the reaction, if it takes place at all, is one of decrease. The decrease in turn grows more and more pronounced, until it reaches its maximum ; then diminishes again and finally turns into an increase. Just how many steps are distinguishable in this increase-decrease series, we do not as yet know. But there are probably a definitely ascertainable number of distinguishable gradations, as there are in the colour series.

We may represent the two halves of this series graphically by means of a circle, on the circumference of which the nodal points, both maximum and minimum for each type of change, are marked off.

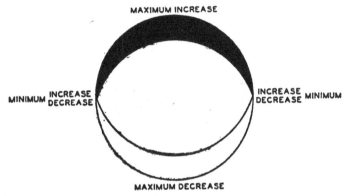

FIGURE 2
Increase-Decrease Response Circle

In the same way, we may represent the two reaction elements in the alliance-opposition series on a similar circular figure, with maximum and minimum for each element in the series.

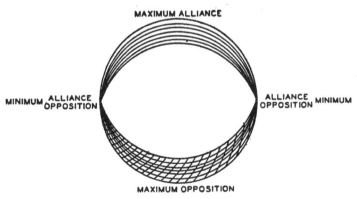

FIGURE 3
Alliance-Opposition Response Circle

Then, since we never find either series separate, but always find the two actually combined in the organism's simplest, or most elementary unit responses, we must put the nodal points for the two series together, making one complete series, with two sets of variables. The nodal demarcation points of this combined elementary unit response circle series coincide in such a way as to divide the circle into four equal segments. Each segment will consist of a type of combination between alliance or opposition and increase or decrease which will be unique for that segment and will not occur in any other

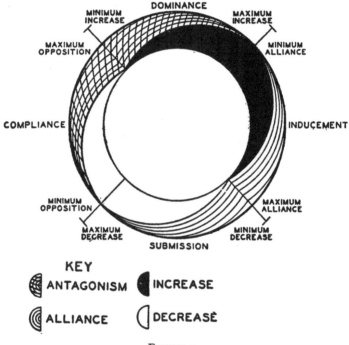

FIGURE 4

Complete Unit Response Circle

segment of the circle. Thus, the four segments will represent the four possible homogeneous combinations which we have named dominance, compliance, submission and inducement as defined in the last section. Within each segment the relative proportions of alliance or opposition and increase or decrease will vary progressively from one end of the segment to the other as shown graphically in Figure 4. Thus, it may be seen that a response of dominance may contain a great deal of opposition and a very little increase of self-activity and, on the other hand, it may contain very little opposition and a very great increase of self-activity. The half-way point in each segment will of course show an admixture of equal increments of the two elements combined in that segment. Thus, the half-way point in the dominance segment will show a response of dominance which simultaneously combines equal parts of opposition and increase of self-activity.

The summary and analysis of the four nodal demarcation points separating the primary types of elementary unit responses would then be as follows:

DOMINANCE—Simultaneous *opposition* and *increase*

Begins at:
{Maximum of opposition
Minimum of increase

Ends at:
{Minimum of opposition
Maximum of increase

INDUCEMENT—Simultaneous *alliance* and *increase*

Begins at:
{Minimum of alliance
Maximum of increase

Ends at:
{Maximum of alliance
Minimum of increase

SUBMISSION—Simultaneous *alliance* and *decrease*

Begins at:
{Maximum of alliance
Minimum of decrease

Ends at:
{Minimum of alliance
Maximum of decrease

COMPLIANCE—Simultaneous *opposition* and *decrease*

Begins at:
{Minimum of opposition
Maximum of decrease

Ends at:
{Maximum of opposition
Minimum of decrease

Each type (D.I.S.C.) represents a series of graded amounts of variables.

In conclusion, therefore, we may sum the matter up in the statement that the human organism responds fundamentally to environmental stimuli, not by separate part-reactions but by integrated unit responses which are the resulting combinations of the external stimuli and the already existing internal operations of the organism itself. Such combinations are brought about by the mediation of the central nervous system, the integrative part of the organism, and are of four primary types. These types we decided to call Dominance, Compliance, Submission, Inducement. They are the fundamental ways in which the organism responds to environment, and in their mutual combinations, gradations, and conflicts are to be discovered all of the behaviours of the human being as we find him.

CHAPTER IV

THE HIDDEN MACHINERY

Introductory

UNIT responses of Dominance, Compliance, Submission, and Inducement, may be compared to the end results of a mass of machinery, the internal workings of which are hidden from view by a heavy casing, the body.

If you go into the Automat, and put two coins in the slot marked " rice pudding ", nothing happens for quite a while, as far as you can observe. Perhaps you begin to think that you have lost your money. At last, however, you see the whole food carrier, inside the glass window, begin to turn. Then it turns back, and you notice, suddenly, that the door is open, and your rice pudding is forthwith presented to you. The final, observable response of the Automat machinery was the eventual appearance of the rice pudding. What went on between the moment when you dropped your coins into the slot and the final reaction of the machine, you have no means of knowing, unless you are a specialist in Automat machinery.

The same with human reactions. You tell your acquaintance, Jack, to mind his own business and shut up, or you'll find the means to make him. He shuts up, as ordered, and you soon resume conversation about other matters. You think nothing more is going to happen. You have dropped your coins into the slot, and heard them click. You believe the reaction of the human machine, Jack, is all completed. But not so ! Jack's machinery has gone on working, inside his nervous system, and you are going to be presented with the final result of its operations a little later. Next day, perhaps, Jack calls you up on the telephone. " I'm sorry ", he says, politely, " but I'll have to ask you to return that money I loaned you the other day. I want it by to-night or I'll have to take measures to collect it." Your mind flashes back to the scene of yesterday, when you threatened

Jack and told him to shut up ; and you realize, suddenly, that this demand for repayment is the final reaction of Jack's machinery, the rice pudding which your coins have bought.

Now it is part of psychology's task to get inside the casing of the human body, and reveal the workings of the hidden human machinery which produces the unit responses already described as its final results. When this is done it will be found that the integrative machine, just like any other machine, consists of many parts each with a characteristic function. It will also be found that certain of these parts function together as units within the larger machine, just as a carbureter in a petrol engine or a transmitter in a telephone consists of many parts arranged for a specific function which is unitary when considered by itself, but it is only a part reaction from the point of view of the operation of the motor or the successful functioning of the telephone. It will finally be found that the whole integrative machine in operation has certain unit motions characteristic of the machine itself as distinguished from the reactions of its parts. Our general plan then, will be to discuss the five most important parts of the integrative machine, then describe the various part reactions essential to every unit response, and finally give a bird's-eye view of the hidden machinery in motion, that is, a view of the fundamental unit responses.

The Parts of the Hidden Machine and Their Relation to Each Other

We have said that in our dealing with the Automat we are aware of but two factors, the coin placed in the slot and the final revolution of the machine which gives us our rice pudding. The same is true of our dealing with human beings. Without the aid of specialized instruments we see only the gross aspects of behaviour. We recognize the stimulus and the gross structure upon which it registers : the eye, ear, nose, tongue, skin, or what not. These, however, as discriminating mechanisms, are about as specific as the slot into which the coin passes. Also we see the gross movement of arm, hand, leg, or body ; the flush of the skin or its pallor just as we see the rice pudding swing toward us on its standard. We do not see that the real receptors are modified epithelial cells hidden well within the gross outer structure, nor do we recognize that the real movers are the muscles and glands equally hidden from view. Moreover, connecting these terminals are thousands of nerves and nerve tracts. A single set of nerve connections is made up of many parts. Essentially it consists of a chain of neurones connected end on end. Between any two neurones is a surface of separation which is known as a synapse. The synapse, as we shall see later, is probably more important to the functioning of the integrative machine than any other single part. Thus the important parts of the hidden machinery are the receptors, the neurones, the synapses, and the effectors. This chapter will discuss the structure and function of these parts in the order given.

A. RECEPTORS

General Classes and Types of Receptors

A receptor receives energy from outside the body and thus initiates the nerve impulse which traverses the nerve path until it finally excites the muscles and glands. Receptors are not usually part of the nervous system, but consist of highly modified epithelial (skin) cells.

There are receptors on the outside of our body, the inner linings of the body, and also in the muscles, tendons, joints, the semi-circular canals in the head. The receptors on the outside are called extero-ceptors, those on the inside are called intero-ceptors, while those of the third group are called proprio-ceptors.

The outside receptors or extero-ceptors are again of two types, distance receptors and contact receptors. The eye, the ear, and the nose are distance receptors. They sense a thing from afar off and thus give the body time to react before any contact takes place ; a very convenient arrangement when beneath a falling ladder, below a roaring avalanche, or within a burning building. On the other hand, things that are warm or cold, sweet or sour, heavy or light, smooth or rough, cannot be sensed unless direct contact is made with the receptors of the tongue and the skin.

Proprio-ceptors are sense organs in the muscles, the joints, and the semi-circular canals. These receptors furnish impulses which later in the central nervous system become regulatory in function ; these functions are brought about by reason of the fact that the proprio-ceptor impulses combine with the extero-ceptor impulses in ways which either compensate for

F

or reinforce the influences exerted by the latter.   For example, it is due to this type of excitation that it is possible for us to maintain an upright position in spite of gravity.

The intero-ceptors, which are located in the smooth walls of the viscera, are also known as visceral receptors.   Their location makes experimentation difficult so that we have much less information concerning them than we have of the extero-ceptors and the proprio-ceptors.   There have been cases where an artificial entrance through the body wall permits direct experimental stimulation of intero-ceptors, however, and from these cases we have discovered that there are comparatively few intero-ceptors.

The popular idea that we have but five senses, or receptors, sight, sound, taste, smell, touch, has become so firmly rooted that it can be found even in the medical dictionary.   As a matter of fact there are a great many more than five and some of those included within the popular list are complex.

The skin, in addition to touch organs, contains receptors for warmth, coolness, deep pressure, and pain, and some neurologists claim a chemical sense as evidenced by certain reactions to acids.

The ear has three receptors, those for hearing, balance and position.

Our taste receptors are of four sorts, sweet, sour, bitter, and salt.

There are sense organs in the muscles, tendons, and joints.

Neurologists think it probable that there are special receptors for hunger, thirst, nausea, and abdominal pain.

Thus the original five are extended to fourteen that we are sure of and six more that are probable, making a total of twenty.

Reception versus Sensation

Seeing, hearing, tasting, smelling, and all our other sensory experiences are not functions of the receptors.   These experiences occur only after the nerve impulse from the receptor has safely reached the sensory areas of the brain. If the nerve connecting the receptor and brain is cut leaving the receptor intact, no sensation will occur when the receptor is stimulated.   An experiment by Head and Rivers[1] illustrates

[1] Head, Rivers, and Sherren, *The Afferent Nervous System from a New Aspect*, Brain, 1905, xxviii, pp. 99-115.

this point. Head acted as subject. After carefully testing the normal sensitivity of the left forearm and hand the ulnar nerve was cut near the elbow. As a result all cutaneous sensitivity disappeared from quite an extensive area of the skin. The nerve was tied together, and as it healed, the sensations gradually came back. The first to be restored was deep pressure ; then the sensations of extreme cold and warmth and medium intensities of touch and pain. The receptors all the while were intact but had no means of communicating with the central synapses. As long as these remained inactive awareness of sensation was not possible.

This difference between reception and sensation has never been stressed. American text books of psychology, in recent years, have explained reception at length, sometimes using the term as if it were synonomous with sensation. For the most part sensation has gone out of fashion chiefly because of the refusal of the behaviourists to recognize any inaccessible factor like consciousness or sensation and the fear of the non-behaviourists that they will be dubbed old-fashioned or behind the times if they do not fall in line.

We believe that it is necessary to discuss reception in order to understand the mechanics of human action and reaction. On the other hand it would be impossible to understand the unit response of the organism if so important a part as sensation were left out. It is our purpose therefore to give the physiology and neurology of reception at this point, leaving for a later chapter all the important psychological phenomena included in sensory part-reactions, or sensations.

Skin Receptors

The receptors of the skin, besides being of varying types, are also unevenly distributed throughout the skin. If a hollow pointed brass tube filled with warm water is passed over the surface of the forearm with an even pressure, it will contact some spots which give a sensation of warmth, others which arouse only a slight pressure and others where there is no response at all. If the rod is filled with cold water, then cold sensations will occasionally appear and the warm sensations will drop out. In other words the skin is not evenly sensitive to the various sensations assigned to it. Only certain minute points scattered here and there respond to mechanical and thermal excitations and among these spots there is further differentiation in that a spot excited by warmth will be impervious to other types of stimuli and vice versa.

Touch and Pressure.

Contact sensibility is usually divided into two types, light contact or touch, heavy contact or pressure.

1. Pressure : The Pacinian corpuscles are thought to be the receptors for deep pressure. These organs consist of a free nerve ending heavily sheathed in a bulb of connective tissue and are found in all the subcutaneous tissues throughout the body. Any mechanical pressure from within or without, sufficiently great to cause a deformation of the tissue in the area immediately surrounding the end-organ, is an adequate stimulus. The Pacinian corpuscles found in the skin very closely resemble the sensory receptors found in the smooth inner walls of the body and in the muscles, tendons, and joints, and probably share also a similarity of function. These pressure corpuscles of the skin are primarily extero-ceptive but insofar as they are excited by changes in muscular position, contraction and dilation of the blood vessels, and other internal stimuli, they also function as proprio-ceptors. It is safe to say that they are continuously excited from within by these agencies as well as continuously excited from without by changes in atmospheric pressure. Through these avenues they take their place as part of the great action system of the body.

2. Touch : The receptors for light touch are found in the dermis and underlying tissues. There are several recognizable types, a fact which makes more readily understandable the wide variation in thresholds of sensibility in various parts of the body. The lips and finger tips are very sensitive to light touch. The middle of the back is comparatively

FIGURE 5—continued.

A. Pacinian Corpuscle with finely branched central fibre surrounded by connective tissue.
B. Meissner's tactile corpuscle with thin connective tissue capsule and elaborate skein of free nerve endings.
C. Merkel's Corpuscles, with the nerve ending in a disc attached a modified cell of the epidermic.
D. Nerve endings around the root of a hair with horizontal branches encircling the hair and ascending branches running parallel.
E. Free nerve endings in the dentin of a fish's tooth.
F. End bulb of Krause with thin delicate connective tissue capsule and globular skein of nerve endings.

CUTANEOUS RECEPTORS

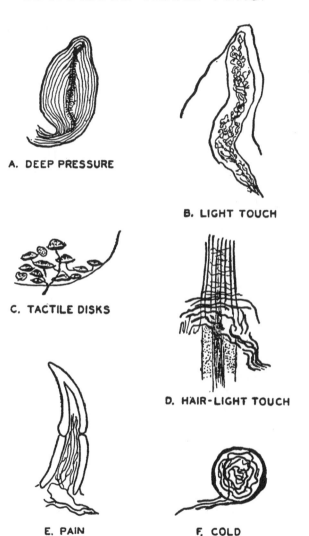

A. DEEP PRESSURE

B. LIGHT TOUCH

C. TACTILE DISKS

D. HAIR-LIGHT TOUCH

E. PAIN

F. COLD

FIGURE 5

Cutaneous Receptors

A schematic arrangement of cutaneous receptors showing the essential
characters of each. (See continuation of legend on p. 68, opposite)

impervious. The variation in number per square centimeter is also significant in this connection, provided summation of many stimuli be taken as a factor in intensity. It has been estimated that, excluding the head, the rest of the body is supplied with 500,000 touch spots. The average number of touch spots per square centimetre is 25 but the number sometimes falls as low as seven and sometimes rises as high as 300.[1] Where the touch spots are most numerous they are usually of one type, namely the corpuscles of Meissner, such as on the finger tips and lips. If within a given area, threshold variations occur, several different types of receptors are found.

There are two main types of touch receptors. Those found at the roots of the myriads of hairs which cover the body and those found in the hairless intervals. The nerve endings of touch receptors at the roots of hairs sometimes follow parallel to the hair but more frequently twine around it. They are stimulated by any movement of the hair or by direct contact on the skin at the side of the hair. The receptors for light touch in the hairless regions are thought to be Meissner's corpuscles and Merkel's corpuscles.

Meissner's corpuscles are most definitely identified with touch. These end-organs consist of an elongated skein-like mass of nerve tissue sometimes surrounded by connective tissue.

Merkel's corpuscles, which are supposed to take care of a different intensity of touch, consist of an end-plate attached to the sensitive cell at the end of each arborization of the nerve. The light touch spots in the skin are smaller and more numerous than the thermal receptors.

It is estimated that there are about 500,000 touch spots on the body.

Thermal Receptors

Physiological experimentation has shown that if the surface of the skin is explored with a stimulus slightly warmer or slightly cooler than body temperature, certain spots will be found which react to the warm stimulus and certain others react to the cool. A stimulus at the same temperature as the body, that is, somewhere around 30 degrees C., will not stimulate these spots at all. This temperature is therefore known as the physiological zero.

[1] *Physiology*, W. H. Howell, 1913, p. 278.

Extreme cold will excite the cold and pain spots ; extreme heat usually excites the warmth and pain spots, but will also arouse a sensation of cold in the cold spots if the stimulus contacts them. This may be why we shiver after a bad sunburn or are covered with gooseflesh when we first step into a hot bath. The stimulation of the cold spots in this manner is known as " paradoxical cold ". The true nature of the end-organs of temperature is not known.

The end bulbs of Krause have been designated as cold receptors principally because they are so numerous in those areas which are sensitive only to cold or at most to cold and pain. There are many more cold spots than there are warm spots. Some authorities put the ratio as 13 to 2. It is argued by some neurologists that, because there is a longer reaction time for warmth, the warmth receptors are deeper than the other skin receptors. On this basis, some neurologists have designated the corpuscles of Ruffini as warmth end-organs.

Thermal receptors belong to both the intero- and extero-ceptive systems. Direct contact is not necessary for stimulation. Radiation from any object near or far, within or without, is adequate if sufficiently intense. The continuous stimulation going on from within is of particular interest to us in understanding unit responses and part-reactions. The normal bodily temperature is due to many factors, such as circulation, respiration, growth of tissue, and other continuous long-run internal activities. The physiological zero pro-bably represents an adaptation of the receptors to all these factors.

In addition we experience continuous stimulation from within and without. A summer in northern Canada will subject us to continuous stimulation from the surrounding atmosphere far different from that we receive in southern California. Our physiological zero will be about the same for both places. In addition, we adapt in one locality to a cool summer, in the other to a warm or hot one. In either place, we are still subject to temperature changes of a phasic sort due to eating, sleeping, loving, running, fearing, malarial fever, sunstroke, and a great many other temporary internal activities. At the same time we are subject to stimulation from the outside, icebergs, hot springs, desert sands, and the like. On the whole, the internal activities are quite as much responsible for our thermal experiences as are the environmental stimuli.

There are supposed to be about 30,000 warm spots, and 500,000 cold spots on the human body.

Pain

Although pain receptors are located throughout all the membranes of the body we have very little knowledge of any save those to be found in the skin. The method of punctiform stimulation demonstrates that pain spots exist in great numbers all over the surface of the body. Some areas, such as the corner of the eye, are sensitive to pain only. Other areas like the tips of the fingers are more sensitive to touch than to pain. But certain inner organs and tissues like the intestines and brain are not sensitive to pain at all.

It is pretty well established that the receptors for pain are the free nerve endings to be found in the skin. In the first place the pain spots are found in great numbers and the only receptors existing in equal quantity are the free nerve endings. The central part of the cornea, the tympanic membrane, and the dentin and pulp of the teeth, areas sensitive only to pain, are profusely supplied with free nerve endings. The finger-tips which are rich in touch spots with comparatively few pain spots, have many Meissner corpuscles and few free nerve endings. Finally there is greater sensitivity to pain where there are many free nerve endings than in the deeper tissues where free nerve endings are rare.

Experimenters estimate that there are a total of between 2,000,000 and 4,000,000 pain spots on the body.

Pain may also be aroused by over-stimulation of other sensory receptors. It has been shown for instance that the tactile nerve impulses from the face under ordinary stimulation pass to the higher nerve centres and thence to the tactile centres of the brain. If the receptors are over-stimulated, the impulse also descends to a lower nerve centre in the chord and thence to the pain centres, the stimulating impulse for both sensations passing over a single afferent path up to the point of bifurcation. Herrick says " there is an overflow from one path to another of higher internal resistance ".

Chemical Sensibility

The existence of a general chemical sense in man is mostly

conjectural. It is thought that general chemical sensibility may exist in the moist membranes of the mouth and nose. There are no modified epithelium cells acting as receptors for this sense but the impulse is carried by free nerve endings quite deeply imbedded in the tissue. The threshold is much higher for general chemical sensibility than for taste and smell, both of which are chemical receptors. The receptors of general chemical sensibility are excited by acids, by an electric current, by alcohol, menthol, and other stimuli of this type.

Vision

The eyeball and the retinal receptors constitute the gross structure of the organ of vision. The eyeball is a slightly flattened sphere containing a liquid called aqueous humor. It has three coats, an outer fibrous coat called the sclerotic coat, a second vascular layer called the choroid coat, and a third innermost layer called the retina.

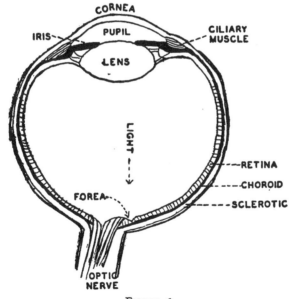

FIGURE 6

The Eye

The retina contains the rods and cones, which are the true receptors for vision. The other parts of the eyeball function as auxiliary structures to soften the intensity of light as it strikes the retina and to control the size of the image. The functions of these parts, that is, the pupil, the lens, and the ciliary muscles, have been worked out in great detail and may be studied by consulting any good physiology.

The retina lines the entire eyeball but only the cupshaped portion farthest away from the light is receptive to light. It is made up of three functional layers, an outer layer containing the rods and cones, an inner layer of bipolar cells, and a third layer of ganglion cells that connect with the optic nerve. There are also some horizontal neurones in each layer and its supporting tissue. This arrangement is modified at the fovea centralis which is made up for the most part of cones with a few of the pigmented cells which lie between the layer of rods and cones and the choroid coat. The fovea lies at the posterior portion of the retina near the exit of the

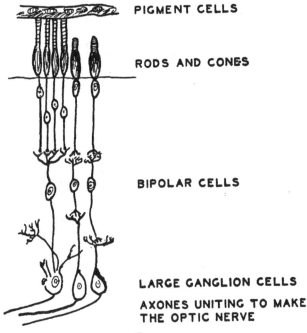

PIGMENT CELLS

RODS AND CONES

BIPOLAR CELLS

LARGE GANGLION CELLS

AXONES UNITING TO MAKE THE OPTIC NERVE

FIGURE 7
The Retina

The diagram shows the three major layers of the retina. The characteristic features of rods and cones are emphasized.

optic tract. It is susceptible to colour only. There is no sensitized tissue at the point where the optic nerve leaves the retina and the area is therefore blind. Normally the blind spot is filled in centrally from experience or is covered by excitation of the opposite retina.

The visual cells themselves are notable because of their red and cone-like appendages which are apparently directly photochemically sensitive to light. The rod cells are made up of the rods, the rod fibre, and the nucleus. The rod consists of an outer portion which contains the visual purple and an inner granular portion. It joins the rod fibre which leads to the nucleus. The nuclei of the rod cells occur at different levels and the fibre continuing from the nucleus ends in a nodule, instead of an arborization, which connects with the afferent bipolar cells.

The cone cells have much the same gross structure except that the cone is shorter and broader than the rod and does not contain visual purple. The fibres are short and tapering, with the cell body coming at approximately the same interval for each cell, that is, just below the margin of the outer limiting membrane. The cone cells have terminal arborizations and can therefore connect with more than one bipolar cell. Apparently the cones are more complex in structure and function than the rods.

The rods and cones are not evenly distributed throughout the retina. At the fovea there are only cones. Gradually the number of rods increase until at the periphery of the retina there are only rods to be found.

The retina is sensitive to light rays within the range of 397mm. to 760mm. It is thought that shorter rays are absorbed by the lens and fluid before they reach the retina. Visual discrimination of from 150 to 230 pure spectral tints has been demonstrated. Since these tints can blend with each other and with black and white, it is estimated that it is possible for the human eye to discriminate from 500,000 to 600,000 light values.

The retina is also stimulated by impulses from the cerebral cortex. Such stimulation is made possible by the presence of nerves originating in the central parts of the head and among the rods and cones of the retina. Impulses over these motor nerves would account for the presence of ideo-retinal light, for electrical stimulation of the eye, for hallucinations and all other instances where the rods and cones are apparently responding even though no corresponding light values are objectively present.

Hearing

The ear is a complex structure containing many parts which serve a purely auxiliary function. The outer ear consists of the auricle and the tube terminating at the ear drum, or tympanum.

Beyond the outer ear is an air-filled cavity containing three irregular-shaped bones (malleus, incus and stapes) and the Eustachian tube which leads into the throat. This is

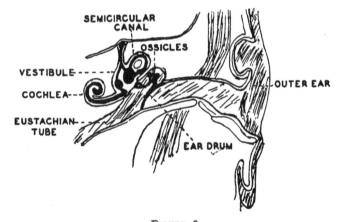

FIGURE 8

The Ear

The diagram shows the three parts of the ear ; the outer ear, the middle ear and the inner ear.

ordinarily termed the middle ear. The middle ear connects at the fenestra ovalis with the inner ear, a complex bony labyrinth encasing a similarly shaped membranous labyrinth which contains the several sensory receptors of the inner ear. These outer structures serve to condense air waves, intensify them, and transmit them to the liquids of the inner ear.

The inner ear contains the ventricles, the saccule, the semi-circular canals, and the cochlea, each of which contain characteristic and functionally separate sensory receptors. The receptors for hearing are found in the organ of Corti, a strip of sensory epithelium running the length of the ductus cochlearis. The ductus cochlearis is a membranous cavity within the cochlea, triangular-shaped in cross section. Along the base of the triangle runs the basilar membrane which supports the organ of Corti. Above this membrane rest supporting cells so arranged that they are separated at the base to form the arches of Corti. Through the aperture thus formed, fibres from the auditory nerve which penetrates the soft inner boney structure of the cochlea, pass to the auditory hair cells. These cells are arranged on either side of the tunnel of Corti, one cell on one side and four on the other side.

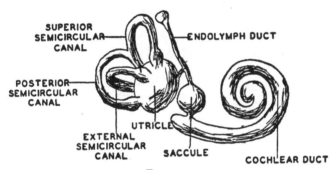

FIGURE 9
Labyrinth of the Inner Ear

The diagram shows the relationship of each part to all the others; the semi-circular canals set on three divergent planes, the vestibule and the cochlea.

Strong bristles project from the auditory cells through the enclosing reticulum into the endolymph. Projecting from the membranous side-wall into the endolymph well over the organ of Corti is the tectorial membrane now supposed to be very important in imparting sound waves to the cells of Corti. This membrane is gelatinous in character and is supposed to pick up the vibrations of the endolymph sympathetically and transmit them to the auditory receptors with which they are in contact.

According to some accounts the tectorial membrane floats freely in the endolymph and can therefore make only a chance contact with the receptors since its position is such that it is not subject to the pull of gravity. It is generally agreed that the basilar membrane is structurally incapable of playing the role assigned to it by the Helmholtz theory of hearing.

Air waves transmitted via the tympanum, auditory ossicles, and fluids of the inner ear to the cells of Corti are the adequate stimulus for audition. Vibration of the bones of the head, and variations in the air pressure of the middle ear, violent contact or internal bodily conditions which cause the bony structures or liquids of the ear to vibrate, will also stimulate the auditory receptors. In the neurological accounts no mention is made of efferent nerves in the organ of Corti which

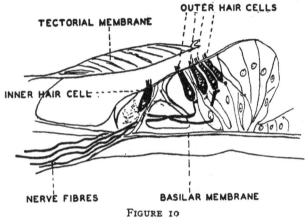

FIGURE 10

The Organ of Corti

would permit central stimulation of the auditory receptors.

The ear responds to both periodic and aperiodic air waves. The first are called tones and the second noises. The range of sensitivity runs from 30 frequencies per second to 30,000. Some cases range from 12 to 50,000. Titchener sets the number of pitch qualities capable of differentiation at 11,000.

Smell

The olfactory receptors are located in a small patch of sensitive epithelium in the top and side of the upper nasal passages. The total area does not exceed five square centimetres. This area is not in the direct line of the respiratory passage but is so situated that gaseous particles from the main stream have access to the receptors. The true receptors are the olfactory vesicles which penetrate the membrane. Five or six minute hairs extend from each vesicle. From the vesicle a process leads to the olfactory cell which is directly connected with the olfactory nerve. The olfactory receptors are the only receptors united in this way with the nerve connecting the receptor with its corresponding centre in the brain. Gaseous particles in direct contact with the olfactory vesicles are the recognized adequate stimulus for smell. There is some

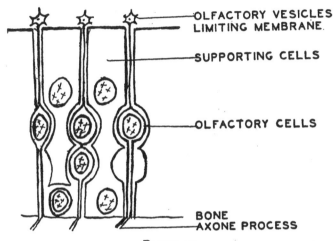

FIGURE 11

Olfactory Receptors

Diagram shows axone processes piercing the bone. These axones connect directly with synapses in the brain stem.

question as to whether or not the receptors are sensitive to liquids. Experiments on this point are difficult because it is almost impossible to entirely exclude air from the liquid, at the time of stimulation. The exact number of recognizable odours is not known although nine classes are usually cited.

Taste

The receptors for taste are found on the tip, sides, and edges of the tongue, on the palate epiglottis and fauces, and in portions of the pharynx and larynx. They are more numerous in children than in adults. In the tongue, the taste buds centre around the circumvallate and fungiform papillae. As many as 400 taste buds have been found around a single circumvallate papilla. A single taste bud is made up of sensitive cells and supporting cells. The sensitive cells are elongated and from the end of each a hair projects through a pore-like opening in the taste bud so that it is in direct contact with the stimulus.

The taste buds cannot respond to a dry substance. To solutions or sapid substances there are four primary responses, salt, sour, sweet, and bitter. Various areas of the tongue are

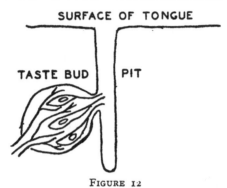

FIGURE 12

Taste Receptor
Liquid retained in the pit contacts the taste bud and stimulates the sensory nerve endings.

found to be more responsive to one of these stimuli than to the others. The mid-dorsal region has no taste buds.

Muscular Sensitivity

Every time a muscle contracts, afferent sensory impulses corresponding to the degree of muscular activity are sent to the cortex. The receptors for these impulses are found in the nerve endings from the sensory nerve which wind around the muscle spindles. These sensory fibres vary in size from 18mm. to 2mm. or less and as many as 12 have been found in contact with a single muscle spindle. The stimulus is mechanical and results from changes in the form and tension of the spindle.

Tendon receptors

The surface of a muscle tendon reveals a rich arborization of nerve endings which run through the thickness of the tendon and sometimes spread 500 mm. along the tendon bundle. These receptors are known as the organs of Golgi. The tendons also show modified Pacinian corpuscles and true Pacinian corpuscles. The latter are particularly adapted for stimulation by compression, and are located in parts of the tendon and neighbouring tissue where such deformation is most likely to occur.

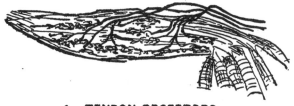

A. TENDON RECEPTORS

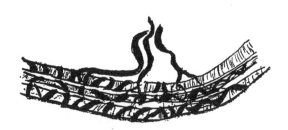

B. MUSCULAR RECEPTORS

FIGURE 13

Muscle and Tendon Receptors
A. The endings of the sensory nerve are spread over the surface of the tendon.
B. Shows three muscle fibres and three sensory nerve fibres which enter the muscle spindle and wind spirally throughout its members.

Joint Receptors

The Pacinian corpuscles are presumed to be the joint receptors. The bending of the joint operates as stimulus.

The impulses from the muscles, tendons and joints together go to make up kinæsthetic sensibility. The continuous stimulation of a certain number of these receptors in all three categories is involved in maintaining the passive attitude of the body. These tonic attitudes are necessary to combat the

G

force of gravity, atmospheric pressure, and to maintain an upright attitude. Summation is a factor in instituting changes in the tonic set, as are also the various phasic activities voluntarily assumed.

Balance and Equilibrium

The semi-circular canals, the utricle, and saccule of the inner ear each contain patches of sensitized tissue wherein are found the receptors for balance and equilibrium. There are three semi-circular canals which are set so as to correspond roughly to the three planes of space. Each canal before it reaches the utricle ends in an extension, or ampulla, which contains a patch of sensitized cells. Hairs project from these cells into the liquid which fills the canals. They do not float freely but are matted by a sort of mucous. It is thought that when the head is moved the pressure of the liquid on these hairs is changed and that it acts as a constant stimulus to the end-organs. The movement has to be sufficient to disturb the capulla or mucous which holds the hairs together. Similar receptors are found in the saccule and utricle. These hairs are finer and more closely matted. Small particles called cristae float in the lymph of the utricle and saccule. It is thought that these two structures work to keep the line of the body within the centre of gravitation. When balance is disturbed, the cristae are displaced and settle down in response to gravity, they then arouse the hair cells which communicate to the nervous system the degree of displacement.

Any disturbance of the receptors of the semi-circular canals, utricle, or saccule, is transmitted via the vestibular nerve to the cerebellum and thence to the muscles all over the body. The eyes and the stomach are particularly sensitive to disturbances in the semi-circular canals with the result that loss of balance is often accompanied by nystagmus and nausea. Since there is constant pressure of the liquids of the inner ear upon these receptors, the excitation to the brain and muscles is also constant, making the inner ear the most important single source of tonic innervation.

The Visceral Receptors : Hunger

Experimentation by Cannon, Washburn, and Carlson has demonstrated that hunger sensations occur concomitantly with violent contractions of the stomach. This would make hunger a variety of muscle sense. The objection has been raised that the contractions occur also during digestion but it seems evident that the tensions, distortions, and pressures occurring in the tissue while the stomach is full of food will be duller, more diffuse, and much less intense than when the stomach is empty and the movement completely unrestricted. It does not seem necessary to postulate greater irritability of the sensitive cells during hunger.

Thirst

When the water content of the body falls below a certain minimum, nerve fibres in the pharyngeal membrane are stimulated and are perceived as thirst. It is supposed that there is a special end-organ because local dryness due to a salt or similar stimulation induces thirst. A mouthful of water will relieve the thirst without the necessity of taking any of the water into the system. On the other hand, if the local stimulus is intense and constant, no amount of water taken into the system will relieve the thirst.

Abdominal Pain

Since so much of the mucous membrane of the viscera is insensible to pain, the presence of pain during colic, gall-stones, and other irregularities, is difficult to account for. Some neurologists have suggested that summation is a factor but others say that muscular tension and not cutting, pricking, etc., is the cause of abdominal pain. There are free nerve endings present in the smooth muscles which could act as receptors of this sort.

Other Visceral Receptors

It is generally conceded that there are several other types of receptors present in the viscera. Circulatory and respiratory systems give rise to certain characteristic sensations. Internal secretions arouse the sex receptors, and anti-peristalsis results in nausea ; pressure due to distension of the stomach, rectum, and bladder arouses sensations from these sources. The sensory receptors for the viscera have no specially developed auxiliary apparatus. Except for the Pacinian corpuscles which we have discussed elsewhere, there are two main types of receptors. One type consists of terminals in the muscles and the other type is found in the free nerve endings in or under mucous surfaces.

B. NEURONS

General Structure of the Neuron

The next part of the integrative machine set in motion after the receptors, consists of the cells composing the nerves.

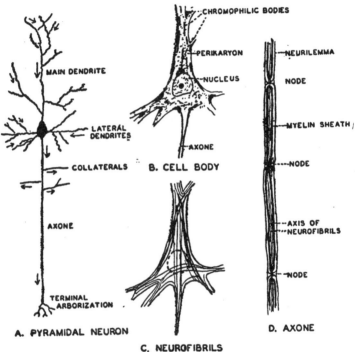

FIGURE 14

Analysis of a Neuron

Analysis of a pyramidal cell of the cerebral cortex and its processes.
A. The neuron as a unit shows the dendrites with gemmules and a very much shortened axone.
B. The cell body shows the nucleus of the triangular chromophilic bodies in the crotch of the dendrites and the axone process devoid of chromophilic bodies.
C. Cell body showing neurofibrils connecting one dendrite with another and passing through the cell.
D. The axone process showing the axis of neuro-fibrils surrounded by the myelin sheath and neurilemma.

These cells are called neurons. The neuron is the structural, functional, and nutritive unit of the nervous system. It consists of a nerve cell and all its processes. Although neurons vary greatly in size and outward appearance, their structure throughout the nervous system is fundamentally the same. There are three main parts, the *dendrites*, the *cell body*, and the *axone* with its terminal arborization.

The *dendrites*, as the name indicates, consist of many tapering, unsheathed, branch-like processes of the same plasmic substance as the *cell-body* with which they are continuous. They are broadest where they leave the *cell-body* and terminate only a short distance away. The gross structure is such that the *dendrite* and *cell-body* together are able to tap a large area for nutritive purposes and also, by presenting a large sensitive area of contact for the *axones* of other *neurons*, increase the receptive power of both elements.

The *cell-body* consists of a nucleus, which is thought to be the centre of the neuron, surrounded by a structureless protoplasmic substance known as the perikaryon. Throughout this substance are found the *nissl bodies*, and the *neuro-fibrils*. There are also present some other structures not of particular interest to us at this time.

The *neuro-fibrils* are thought to be the pathway along which the nerve impulse travels in passing through the neuron. They are continuous throughout the neuron. Beginning with the *dendrites*, they enter the cell body, where they can be seen connecting the *dendrites* with each other, inter-lacing and passing in great numbers through all parts of the perikaryon except the nucleus which they do not penetrate. They traverse the *axone* in long parallel lines and are the only structures present in the plasm of that process. Some neurologists maintain that the *neuro-fibrils* are continuous from neuron to neuron but this is not the majority opinion, which holds that the *neuro-fibrils* terminate at the synaptic membranes in the terminal arborization of the *axone*.

The *nissl bodies* are of particular interest to us in our study of the part reactions which go to make up the unit response. The *nissl bodies*, or nigroid bodies as they are sometimes called, appear, after staining, in the *cell bodies* and *dendrites* of all large neurons and in the *cell bodies* alone of the smaller neurons. It is thought that they may be artefacts, that is, coagulation due to staining or post mortem conditions, representing a substance which permeates the protoplasm of the live neuron giving it a darkened appearance. It has been found that neurons of like function show *nissl bodies* of similar size, texture, and arrangement. Thus, in the motor cells of the spinal cord, they are large and wedge-shaped with a coarse granular structure. In the sensory cells the *nissl bodies* are smaller, of an even size, finer grained, and arranged symetrically parallel to the surface of the *cell body*. It has been possible to delineate certain functional areas of the cortex by marking off the boundaries of those cells having a similar arrangement and distribution of *nissl bodies*.

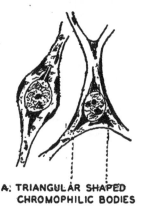
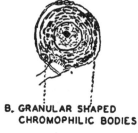

A: TRIANGULAR SHAPED CHROMOPHILIC BODIES

B. GRANULAR SHAPED CHROMOPHILIC BODIES

FIGURE 15

Nissl Bodies

The diagram illustrates the two major types of chromophilic bodies.
A. Shows bodies of motor cells from the spinal cord of a kitten with chromphilic bodies and nuclei. On the left is a fusiform cell and on the right is a triangular cell with points of the chromophilic bodies directed toward the dendrites (After Cajal).
B. Shows a sensory ganglion cell from the spinal cord of a rabbit with the cytoplasm of the cell thickly strewn with chromophilic Nissl bodies (After Cajal).

It is thought that the chromophilic substance, which contains acid and iron, provides substance for the electrical and chemical changes involved in the propagation of nerve impulses. This fact, if true, would account for the disappearance of the chromophil upon over-fatigue of the neuron and would also give a functional basis for the *nissl body* arrangement among neurons. The large motor nerves which send strong impulses over long distances could utilize the greater quantity and strength of substance.

The *axone* is a long whitish process of even diameter, which comes out of the *cell body* by way of the *axone hillock*. At its termination it spreads out in a fan-like arrangement of processes known as the terminal arborization, or "end-brush". The *axone* is sheathed throughout its length by a white fatty substance known as the myelin sheath. Outside the myelin or medullary sheath is a structureless membrane known as the neurillemma.

Within the medullary sheath is a filament of protoplasm which carries the *neuro-fibrils* and is spoken of as the axis cylinder. The sheath is broken at intervals. The nodules formed by this break are known as the nodes of Ranvier. It is thought by some neurologists that only the *neuro-fibrils* protected by the neurilemma are present at the nodes.

The *axone* generally has one or two collaterals which branch at right angles not far from the axone hillock. This structure of the *axone* is particularly fitted to the function of transmitting and distributing nerve impulses. The protective sheath prevents diffusion of neural energy and excitation from the outside, provides nutriment and probably auxiliary material needed in the propagation of nerve impulses, leaving the axis cylinder free of all bodies except the *neuro-fibrils*.

Axones vary in length from very minute structures like the olfactory neurons to several feet in the spinal motor neurons. A single fibre runs from the sacral division of the spine to the toe. A single *axone* is spoken of as a nerve fibre. The long white thread-like tracts which we call nerves are made up of many *axones*. Large insulated bundles of fibres are called nerve tracts.

Nerve Trunk Conduction

The excitation of a neuron at any point spreads equally in all directions throughout the structure. Since, however, the neuron is merely a link in a chain of nerve cells, a specific direction of transmission is forced upon it by its synaptic connections with adjacent cells.

Impulses are received by the *dendrites* and the *cell body*. These processes are unsheathed and sensitive to excitation from surrounding neurons either by direct contact or by diffusion. It is thought that the *cell body* may also integrate as well as receive the impulses. Upon reception, the impulse is transmitted from the *dendrite* through the *cell body* over the *axone* to the terminal arborization, whence it is distributed to other neurons. If a structural analogy may be permitted, it is as if the *dendrites* were the tributaries at the source of the river receiving neural energy from all sides and carrying it thence to the reservoir of the *cell body*, whence it is concerted into the main axonic stream which it traverses to the delta-like terminal aborizations.

The direction of the neural impulse can never be reversed. For this reason it would seem best to use the word *dendrite* for the receiving processes of the bipolar and unipolar neurons which are axone-like in structure but dendritic in function. Such processes are found in the sensory ganglionic neurons. The *cell bodies* of these neurons lie just outside the spinal cord, which means that excitation received at the periphery of the body has a long way to travel, with the result that their axone-like structure is necessary. If, however, our definitions are based upon functional polarization and the direction of conduction with reference to the *cell body*, then this process should be called a *dendrite*.

It has been demonstrated experimentally that the all-or-none law applies to the passage of a nerve impulse. After anæsthetizing a portion of a nerve fibre, varying intensities of stimulation were applied. It was found that if the impulse passed over the dormant portion at all, it passed *in toto* without any diminution of intensity.

There is reason to suppose that there are rhythmic variations in neuronic impulses. The speed of transmission varies with different types of organisms. The rate in the myelinated fibres of a normal human being is from 120 to 125 meters per second. This will be found to vary with different nerves and with differing physiological conditions in the same nerve.

Very little is known about the exact nature of the nerve impulse. Electrical changes occurring concurrently with the passage of a nerve impulse have been demonstrated. The amount of CO_2 given off during the passage of an impulse is greater than when the neuron is resting. The consensus of opinion seems to be that the propagation is electro-chemical and at the same time explosive in character ; that is, the impulse travels by means of energy liberated from within the cell itself. Nerve impulses are technically termed " propagated disturbances."

A very plausible theory of nerve trunk conduction has been proposed by L. T. Troland.[1] The interior of the nerve cell is in a liquid condition and thus its chemical components are in solution, with the result that many ions are present within the cell body. The effect of a solution is to separate its components into ions, that is, the atoms composing the solution are split up into particles bearing positive and negative charges of electricity. These ions are smaller than atoms, since they are parts of atoms, and because the walls of the cell bodies must be composed of atoms, these walls must therefore be porous, as regards the ions. The result is that the positively charged ions within the cell bodies, being smaller than the negatively charged ions, will penetrate the cell walls, to a greater degree than the negatively charged ions. Thus a layer of positive ions will exist along the outside of the nerve sheath and a layer of negative ions along the inside. This constitutes an electrical double layer and the nerve sheath will be in a polarized condition.

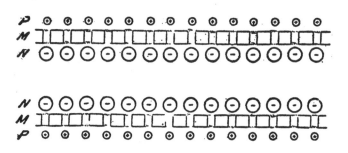

FIGURE 16

Diagram of Unexcited Nerve Fibre

This drawing is taken from L. T. Troland's *Mystery of Mind*, D. van Nostrand and Co., New York, and is intended to represent the polarization layer according to Troland's theory. P. shows the outer layer of smaller positive ions ; M. the porous membrane ; and N. the layer of large negative ions.

It is now supposed that the effect of stimulating the nerve is to render the cell bodies of the neurons more porous. When this occurs the negative ions on the interior of the sheath will

[1] L. T. Troland, *The Mystery of Mind*, 1926, p. 184.

be permitted to pass through, and so to neutralize the positive layer of electricity on the outside. Having passed through, however, they will not only neutralize the positive ions immediately opposite their point of exit, but will also spread to some extent along the sheath, thus neutralizing some of the positive ions adjacent to their point of exit. The result will be to render the sheath more porous at these adjacent points also, more negative ions will pass through from the interior, and will fully neutralize this portion ; the process will be repeated until it reaches the end of the nerve. After the impulse has passed along the nerve in this fashion, the chemical processes within the nerve cells will successively restore the former state of porosity of the sheath. The negative ions will no longer be permitted to penetrate and neutralize the outside layer of negative ions, and the nerve will be ready for further excitation.

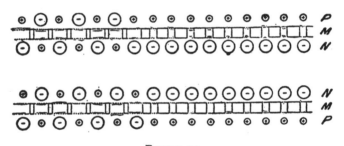

FIGURE 17

Diagram of Excited Nerve Fibre

This drawing also is from Troland and is intended to show the holes in the membrane being enlarged so that the negative particles can pass through, thus neutralizing the polarization layer during the exicted state of the nerve fibre.

It is obvious that porosity and excitability will vary inversely, and until the usual state of porosity is re-established, it will be impossible to re-excite the nerve for the reason that, when the outside electrical layer along the sheath is fully neutralized, it will be impossible to neutralize it further. Thus there will be a very short refractory period, during which the positive ions that have neutralized the outside layer, are passing back into the interior of the cells again, and during this time the nerve will be non-excitable.

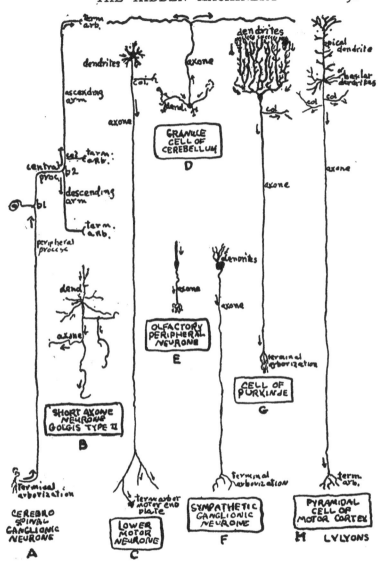

FIGURE 18
Some Common Forms of Neurons

Except in B, the axones in the diagram are much shorter in proportion to size of body and dentrites than they actually are in the nervous system. Arrows show direction of conduction. *Col.* means collateral branch ; *Proc.* means process ; *Term. arb.* means terminal arborization. (From Strang and Elwyn's *Text-Book of Histology,* William Wood and Co., New York City).

Size and Function of Neurons

The accompanying figure gives a few standard illustrations of the great variety to be found in the sizes and shapes of the neurons. There appears to be a close correlation between size and function. It must be remembered that while the function of neurons in general is conduction and distribution of nervous impulses, the function of any one particular neuron is the conduction of a particular type of impulse from one definite point to another definite point under very specific conditions.

We have spoken already of the sensory neurons from the periphery of the body, which have a medulated dendrite suitable for transmission over a long distance.

Another interesting type are the Purkinje cells of the cerebellar cortex. These cells are characterized by a flask-shaped cell body with heavy, profusely branching dendrites, collaterals, and an end-brush with many terminals permitting widespread contact with other Purkinje cells and also the cells of the granular layer. Such intimate contact is quite in conformity with our knowledge of the functions of the cerebellar cortex. This is the great proprio-ceptive correlation centre of the brain. It is connected with all the bodily receptors, especially those of the striped and smooth muscles. Efferent fibres also pass to the motor centres giving the cerebellum an important part in the maintenance of muscular tone. The carrying out of such a function involves the simultaneous discharge of whole groups of neurons, a correlation which the Purkinje cells are structurally well adapted for. Other parallels between function and form might be drawn but it is well to realize that the description cannot be carried out in full because of our limited knowledge of neuronic function. We know in many instances, sources and terminals, shape and size, length, and the general function of any one centre, but we do not know the nature of a nerve impulse or what the variations between impulses may be, whether of rhythm, intensity or what not ; nor do we know the steps within a given centre whereby the main function of that centre is attained, so that while the main thesis that neuronic shape and size are correlated with function seems clear, it is impossible to substantiate this hypothesis in detail.

C. Synapses

Structure of the Synapse

If a ring the shape of a doughnut is cut from a jellyfish and the enclosed nerve-net stimulated electrically, the ensuing nerve impulse has been known to run round and round the circle without stopping during eleven days for a total distance of 457 miles. Its final cessation, even then, is not due to fatigue of the nerve itself, but to counter-impulses set up by the regenerating tissue. The continuation of the nerve impulse over so long a period is possible because the nerve filament of the jellyfish is unbroken. It is like a net with the cell bodies at the points of intersection, so that an impulse, once started spreads equally in all directions.

The human nervous system is quite different. It is not a continuous circuit like a simple nerve-net, but is made up of thousands of individual neuron elements, each with a definite beginning and a definite ending. The total juncture where the end of one neuron contacts the beginning of another is called a *synapse*. The presence of synapses has so many important effects on the conduction of a nervous impulse that nervous systems of this type are in a class by themselves.

No one knows exactly what structures go to make up the synapse. There are two theories. One is that the tiny nerve filaments that carry the nerve impulse are continuous and pass without break through the cell wall of one neuron, across the interval between the neurons, and through the cell wall of the other neuron. Such inter-cellular filaments, or neuro-fibrils, are much smaller in diameter than any parts of the cells that they connect. Several neurologists claim to have seen the filaments thus unbroken, under experimental conditions.

The majority assert, however, that what seem to be neuro-fibrils in the stained segment of a synapse, are merely artefacts ; that is, they are not present in the living organism, but represent an effect of the solution used to stain the tissue so that it can be put upon a slide and examined under the microscope.

The contact theory is felt by most neurologists to be more in accord with the known facts than the continuity theory just outlined. Barthelmess, examining under the microscope the giant Mauthner cells of the eighth cranial nerve, demonstrated the presence of a surface of separation at the synapse.

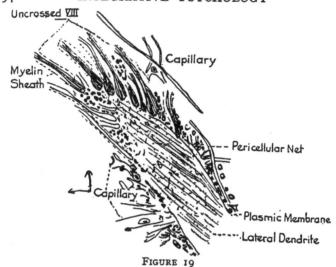

FIGURE 19
The Synapse
(From Bartelmez, *Jour. of Comp. Neurol.*)
PART A.—" The detail of the VIIIth nerve endings, and pericellular net of the lateral dendrite of Mauthner's cell, drawn from a single section of an adult Ameiurus brain fixed in osmic-Zenker and strained with iron hemotaxylin . . . The section passes obliquely through the base of the lateral dendrite, and shows the bulb-like endings of the VIIIth root fibres, and the fine meshed neuropil of the pericellular net on its surface."

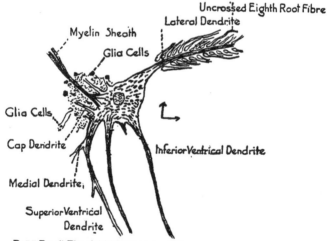

PART B.—" The right Mauthner's cell from a young Ameiurus male, fixed in a formol-osmic-Zenker and stained with iron hematoxylin. A semidiagrammatic reconstruction of ten sections, 5u thick, magnified 250 diameters, to show the relation of dendrites and axone to the cell body and the two striking synapses of the cell, viz., the endings of the VIIIth root fibres (Uncrossed VIII) upon the lateral dendrite, and the axone cap covering the medial surface of the cell. Only four of the cap dendrites are shown."

When the terminals of axone and dendrite come together, each is surrounded by a plasmic membrane, so that no direct continuity is possible. Structural separation of neurons is further evidenced by the fact that degeneration of one neuron can never traverse the synapse and thus contaminate contacting neurons.

These two different theories as to the actual structure of the synapse lead to two different explanations of the way in which the nervous impulse passes across the synapse in its journey from neuron to neuron. We may term these two the " tungsten filament " and the " sheet electrode " theories.

In the continuity, or tungsten-filament, theory the minute fibres supposed to conduct the impulse across the synapse would bear the same relation to the nerve trunk that the small filament in a tungsten lamp bears to the rest of the electric circuit. The impulse passing through the minute fibre might then be supposed to have an effect upon its conductor similar to the incandescence brought about in the tungsten filament, although of course the effect would not actually be incandescence.

On the other hand, the contact theory leads to a view in which the separate but contacting parts of the adjacent neurons are considered to bear the relations to each other of two sheet electrodes. The impulse that passes such a juncture must penetrate the neuron coverings somewhat in the manner of the electric impulse that passes through an electrode of lower conductivity between the adjacent ends of two wires. In this case, too, the passage of the impulse will obviously affect the synaptic tissue quite differently than it affects the neurons themselves.

Points of contact between neurons may be of three types. In some cases the axone throws off a series of club feet known as pseudopodia, which contact the next neuron. In other cases the dendrites of the receiving neuron are characterized by small bud-like structures, or gemules, that contact the unsheathed ending of the axone. In still other cases axone and dendrite or axone and cell body are merely in a lateral position at the point of contact.

The surfaces of separation at the synapse should not be thought of as inserted between the neurons like dead skin ; these surfaces are probably semi-permeable and act like a valve in permitting the nerve impulse to pass in one direction only, that is, from axone to dendrite, or from axone to cell body. It is further thought that these synaptic membranes are capable of some specific and characteristic activity as yet undiscovered experimentally.

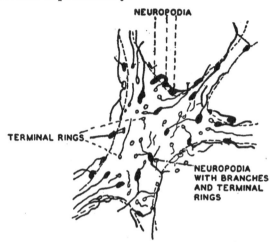

A. NEUROPODIAL SYNAPSE

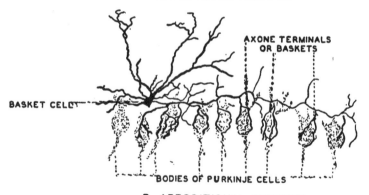

B. APPOSITIONAL SYNAPSE

FIGURE 20

Types of Synapse

A. Neuropodial Synapse, axones terminating with neuropodia or terminal bulbs upon the cell bodies and the bases of the dendrites of a motor neuron.

B. Appositional Synapse, collaterals from the axone of the basket cell descending to the bodies of Purkinje Cells and surrounding them after the fashion of a basket.

Function of the Synapse

A nerve impulse in passing from neuron to neuron across a synapse, leaves the neuro-fibrils of the sending neuron, enters the perifibrillar substance, activates the first cell membrane, traverses the inter-cellular substance, energizes the synaptic membrane of the receiving neuron, is transmitted thence through the perifibrillar substance to the receiving neuro-fibril.

Passage over the synapse has many known effects upon the conduction of the nerve impulse :

(1) It slows up the nerve impulse materially,

(2) It seems to store up the energy of the impulse and discharge it in later repetitions, much like reverberations ; this phenomenon, is known as after-discharge,

(3) It interferes with the rhythm of the nerve impulses, which, until these impulses reach a synapse, correspond to the rhythm of receptor stimulation.

(4) An impulse that fails to pass the synapse the first time, may succeed in doing so at a later time. This is because each attempt leaves a trace or an effect on the synaptic membrane. All these traces add themselves together until finally the impulse crosses the barrier ; this phenomenon is called temporal summation.

(5) There is greater fatigue effect at the synapse than is evidenced by the neurons themselves.

(6) The nerve impulse, whose intensity was originally proportional to that of the receptor stimulation, loses much of this correspondence at the synapse. This effect is similar to the loss of correspondence of rhythm mentioned above.

(7) Many impulses are inhibited entirely at the synapse.

(8) The synapse serves as a variable threshold for the passage of the nerve impulse.

(9) The synaptic tissue is more dependent than the neuronic tissue proper on blood supply, and is also more susceptible to narcotics and other drugs.

(10) Two separate nervous impulses arriving at the same synapse may there conflict with each other or facilitate and reinforce each other during their synaptic passage.

There are, perhaps, other variations in conduction, caused by the synapse, but these suffice to show that the function of this structure in the bodily economy is of high importance. This is especially so since these variations in physical transmission correspond so closely with similar variations in conscious experience that they are at the very foundation

H

of the psychonic theory of consciousness. For this reason the function of the synapse will be discussed again later on, when we come to take up the subject of consciousness in detail.

Here we will merely call to the reader's attention the obvious fact that the synaptic influences listed above, really *regulate* fundamentally the nervous conduction that takes place in the bodies of human beings and the higher vertebrates. The synapses have a greater and more diverse influence upon this conduction than any other part of the nervous system. It is plain that the kinds of action and reaction possible to any organism will depend to a great extent upon the type of nervous conduction that organism possesses ; with regard to this question the importance of the synapses is paramount.

D. EFFECTORS

General Types of Effectors

We have been taking up one by one the four important parts of the integrative machine. In every unit response of this machine the terminal part is either a muscle or a gland. There are two types of muscles and two types of glands.

The striped muscles are those that move the skeleton of the body. The two hundred bones that support us are operated upon the lever principle with the muscles acting as sources of energy supply to initiate movement. These muscles are sometimes called our " voluntary " muscles, in contrast to the smooth muscles, over which we have no voluntary control. The smooth muscles are those found in the tissues of the viscera. Their activities are slow, smooth, rhythmic, as best becomes their function of supporting the walls of the viscera and moving the visceral contents onward.

The glands are either duct glands or ductless glands. The latter, more frequently called endocrine glands, are looming large in physiology, medicine, psychiatry, and psychology, since they seem to play an important part in determining the mental, physical and intellectual development of the individual. The important duct glands include the salivary glands, the lachrymal gland, the sweat glands, the liver, the pancreas, and many others. The ductless glands are the pineal, thyroid, parathyroid, gonad, adrenal, pituitary, and thymus.

The Muscles

One of the greatest sources of constant activity to be found in the hidden machinery arises in the muscles, both smooth and striped. Neither type is ever completely relaxed, as is evidenced by the fact that if a muscle is cut, the ends will always curl up. The explanation of this constant tension is found in the presence of sensory receptors lying deep within the muscle tissue, that are innervated whenever the muscle becomes too greatly relaxed. Impulses from these proprioceptors give rise, probably via the cerebellum, to efferent impulses which contract the muscles. The result is an endless chain of impulses that keep the muscle under continuous though slight tension. Such tension is necessary for the maintenance of bodily attitude. It keeps us from collapsing under the pull of gravity, keeps our mouths closed, our heads up, our backs straight, our veins and arteries of a certain constant bore or interior diameter, and so on. This matter of tonus is the only activity common to both sets of muscles. Otherwise, they are dissimilar in structure and are differently innervated, since the skeletal muscles are excited directly by the motor nerves from the spinal cord, while the smooth muscles are connected with the cortex via the post-ganglionic fibres of the autonomic nervous system.

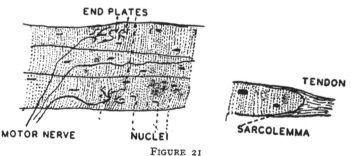

FIGURE 21
Fibres of Striped Muscles

The Striped Muscles

The striped muscles are bundles of thread-like cells that run lengthwise throughout the muscle. Each cell is known as a muscle fibre. The muscle fibre is the structural element of the muscle just as the neuron is the structural element of the nervous system. The muscle fibre, in turn, is made up of a series of fibrils also running longitudinally. These fibrils are the elastic element in the muscle and are surrounded by a semi-liquid plasm. The plasm shows numerous cross-bands, light and some dark, which vary in size according to the activity of the fibre, and give rise to the name, striped muscle. The whole fibre is covered with a limiting membrane, called the sarcolemma.

The muscle fibres of the striped muscles are excited directly by the motor nerves. The axones of the motor nerves lose their medullary sheaths upon reaching the muscles, and break up into many collaterals. Each of these passes to a muscle fibre, where it terminates in a complex structure known as the motor end-plate. Excitations from the motor nerves contact the fibrils, distend the surrounding plasm, tense the limiting membrane, and contract the muscle fibre. The contraction exerts a pull on the tendon to which the fibre is attached, and if enough fibres are activated, moves the bone.

It has been found that the all-or-none law operates in regard to muscle fibres as well as nerve fibres ; that is, if a muscle fibre is contracted at all, it contracts to capacity. The number of muscle fibres in each muscle varies from several hundred to several hundred thousand. A certain percentage of these fibres are always active. Gradation of intensity of response is obtained by increasing or decreasing the number of active fibres. If more than seventy per cent. of the muscle fibres contract, the muscle will break. After prolonged stimulation, fatigue of the end-plate occurs and certain chemical changes take place in the muscle fibre. In the maintenance of muscular tone, the muscle fibres seem to work in relays, so that no one group will be fatigued to the point of destruction.

The fineness of motor co-ordination attained in our movements is made possible by the fact that many of the skeletal muscles operate in pairs that are continually antagonistic ; every extensor has its flexor. When one is contracted, the other is relaxed, the ensuing movement being a balance of these two forces. There are over 200 pairs of muscles in the body co-operating in this way. The neural principle involved is called reciprocal innervation.

While the muscle fibres are usually activated by an efferent nerve impulse from the brain, they will also respond to a blow, an electric shock, and to chemicals. It was thought at one time that the muscle tissue itself reacted to these stimuli directly, but since, in the cases from which this deduction was drawn, the nerve endings were still left embedded in the muscle fibres, even though the nerve itself had been severed, more recent opinion maintains that these stimuli excite the nerve endings, which in turn activate the muscle tissue.

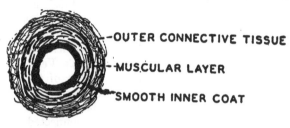

—OUTER CONNECTIVE TISSUE

—MUSCULAR LAYER

—SMOOTH INNER COAT

A. CROSS SECTION
OF
AN ARTERY

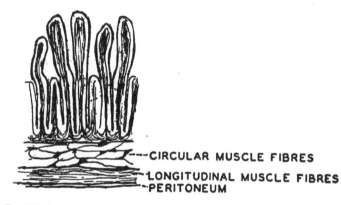

—CIRCULAR MUSCLE FIBRES

—LONGITUDINAL MUSCLE FIBRES

—PERITONEUM

B. WALL OF SMALL
INTESTINE

FIGURE 22
Smooth Muscle Tissue

The Smooth Muscles

With the exception of the heart muscle, which is striated in appearance but smooth in function, the inner cavities of the body are lined with smooth muscle. Smooth muscle tissues are found throughout the alimentary canal from the lower oesophagus to the anus. They are also found throughout the bronchii and the genital and urinary systems ; they line the blood vessels, form the iridic and ciliary muscles of the eye, and the hair-raising muscles of the skin.

The smooth muscles are made up of minute spindle-shaped cells which sometimes run parallel in a longitudinal direction and at other times form a circular band, as in the veins and arteries. In some tissues both arrangements of cells appear.

The smooth muscle cell is usually circular or hexagonal in cross-section. It contains but one nucleus. Very fine myo-fibrils can be observed running the length of the cell.

The sacroplasm fills the space between the fibrils and forms a limiting membrane at the outer boundaries. It is not known exactly how one smooth muscle cell is connected with the others. It is thought that the myo-fibrils may be contimuous or that the cells are embedded in a delicate tissue which acts as a connector. The smooth muscles are normally activated via post-ganglionic fibres from the autonomic nervous system. Contact is made by means of free nerve endings at the surface of the muscle cell. The smooth muscles are also excited directly by drugs and also by hormonic activity from the endocrines.

Glands

The second type of effectors, the glands, through their secretions, determine the growth, development, and efficient functioning of every part of the body. They promote the ingestion and digestion of food and take care of the elimination of waste products, they provide chemicals which accelerate the heart, constrict the blood vessels, speed up digestion, throw sugar into the blood for the utilization of the muscles, determine the length of the skeletal bones, control their calcium content, affect memory, speech, and general intelligence ; in other words, the glands are the most important single element which promotes the development of both the person and the personality.

The glands are made up of special epithelial gland cells, connective tissue, smooth muscle, and blood vessels. The gland cells differ from other body cells in that they have the capacity, in addition to securing nutriment from the body for their own use, of manufacturing substances which are either rejected for the use of other cells of the body or excreted as waste products. There are two types of glands, those with ducts and those without.

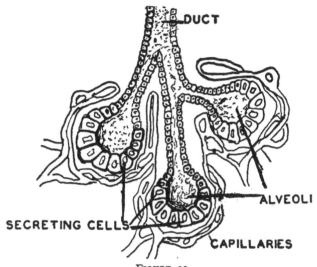

FIGURE 23
A Simple Duct Gland

The Duct Glands

The duct glands are also known as glands of external secretion. They are glands with direct openings on the various epithelial surfaces of the body, both internal and external. The most important ones are the salivary glands, the pharyngeal glands, the glands of the stomach and intestines, the sudoriferous (sweat) and sebaceous glands of the skin, the kidneys, the prostate, the lachrymal (tear), and the mammaries, the liver, and the pancreas. Structurally, the duct glands consist of a mouth or surface opening, a passage way which varies in length according to the gland, and the fundus or deep, inner part. They may be either tubular or alveolar (like a flask) in shape. The tubular gland as the name indicates has a cylindrical passageway. This may be a simple straight tube such as is found in the glands of the large intestines, or coiled as in the sudoriferous glands of the skin, or branched as in the glands of the mucous membranes of the mouth or the stomach. Other tubular gland systems are quite complex consisting of many complex branches opening into a main outlet. The salivary glands and kidneys are examples.

The alveolar type of duct glands are flask-shaped. They do not occur in simple form in the human organism. The sebaceous glands of the skin are examples of simple branched forms, while the mammary glands are alveolar structures of a complex type.

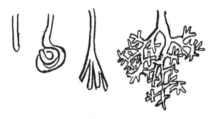

A. TUBULAR GLANDS

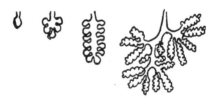

B. ALVEOLAR GLANDS

FIGURE 24

Types of Duct Glands

The Ductless Glands

The ductless glands are known as endocrine glands, or glands of internal secretion. They have no ducts or special openings through which the secretion passes out of the gland to other parts of the body. Instead, the secretion is absorbed directly by the blood which passes through the gland and is carried out by way of the circulatory system to all parts of the body.

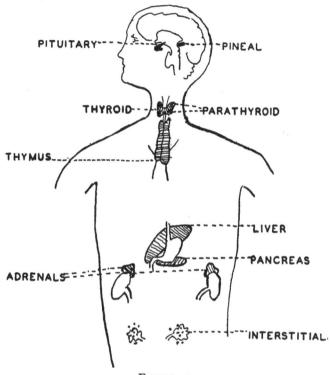

FIGURE 25
Location of Endocrine Glands

The Endocrine Glands

The endocrine glands manufacture secretions (endocrines) of great power called hormones, a word with a Greek root, meaning "stir up". The hormones are absorbed into the blood-stream, which acts as carrier, bringing them into contact with both smooth and striped muscles of the body, with other glands, with the heart, the lungs, the cerebral cortex, and all other internal organs. The effect of any single type of secretion on these structures may be either to depress or excite. The result is not always similar for all structures, as in the case of thymic activity which stimulates physical growth but checks sexual development.

The Thyroids

The thyroids are two lobes on either side of the windpipe. They are connected by a narrow strip of tissue and support the parathyroids, which are small pea-like bodies differing somewhat in function from the thyroids. The active principle of thyroid secretion has been extracted and is called thyroxin. It has been found to consist of 60 per cent. iodine. Thyroid secretion affects the basal metabolism of the body. It is thought to act as a catalyzer, that is, an agent which speeds up chemical changes without itself changing. Thyroid secretion acts in this way in precipitating the destruction of the amino-acids into lower compounds, that is, in the burning of the body's chemical fuel, and the formation of waste products.

There are many diseases of the thyroid glands, which may cause them to secrete too much or too little thyroid secretion. The glandular condition which secretes too little is known as hypo-thyroidism and an over-secretion is known as hyper-thyroidism. Each condition involves specific physiological results with accompanying personality changes.

Extreme cases of hypo-thyroidism occurring in infancy or early childhood are known as cretins. Cretins are of a dwarf-like appearance with protruding abdomen, a large head proportioned so that it appears broad and short, lack of tone in the skin, which perspires very little, coarse hair which is dry and brittle, slow sex development and low mentality. These children can be brought to normal by feeding them with thyroid extract, sometimes supplemented with other glandular extracts determined by the special case diagnosis. A similar condition in adults is known as Myxedema because it is characterized by a mucous-like substance which infiltrates the skin, causing it to thicken and to bloat.

Underactivity of the thyroids occurs in varying degrees. Even where it is slight or in some degree compensated for by the activities of other glands, such symptoms as slow respiration and heart beat, low body temperature, low blood pressure, constipation, thin hair, and so on, occur. The personality tends to be lethargic, given to over-much sleeping, mentally inactive with a very poor memory, and given to depressed sullen fits of sudden bursts of anger.

Cases of over-activity of the thyroid, or hyper-thyroidism, are equally marked. If over-extreme, other glandular activity is greatly increased. The individual is extremely active, mentally and physically. He is usually thin in spite of eating quantities of food, particularly of proteins. He perspires freely and his skin flushes readily. Exopthalmic goitre, frequently associated with hyper-thyroidism, is the result of a diseased gland which may or may not be over-active.

Hyper-thyroid people are extremely nervous, irritable, and tend to be emotionally unstable. They are given to causeless fears and suspicions. They are likely to criticize their doctor and to find fault with his treatment, whatever it may be. They are given to insomnia, and are extremely hard to get along with. There is a reference in early Sanscrit literature to " women with swollen necks," whose dispostions were said to be so bad that no man should marry them. These unfortunate women were probably hyper-thyroid cases.

Thyroid gland irregularities are most frequently caused by lack of the normal amount of iodine content in the community source of drinking water. Thus " goitre belts " have been discovered in the lake regions of Switzerland and America. The spread of goitre can be checked by adding iodine to the water supply.

Hyper-thyroidism is much more difficult to cure than hypo-thyroidism. Rest and quiet are the usual prescriptions. If the case is extreme, an operation to remove part of the thyroid gland may be undertaken.

The Parathyroids

Attached to the thyroid are four very small bodies that for a long time were thought to be part of the larger gland. These are the parathyroids. They are independent organs, closely connected with the calcium activities of the body. Removal of the parathyroids frequently results in death. Partial destruction or degeneration may be followed by tetany, that is, violent, spasmodic contractions of the muscles, which is often fatal.

The Adrenals (also called Supra-renal Glands)

These are small, flat capsules, found on either side of the body attached to the kidneys but not functionally associated with them. They consist of a cortex, surrounding a medulla. These two organs, although in juxtaposition, act independently of each other. It is thought by some scientists that their functions, although disparate, may be complementary.

Not much is known concerning the function of the adrenal cortex. Its cellular origin is similar to that of the ovaries, with which it seems to be directly associated. It has also been suggested that the activities of the adrenal cortex parallel those of the cerebral cortex. Its activities certainly differ from those of the adrenal medulla, which controls the involuntary functions of the vital organs and the blood supply to the skeletal muscles. It has been found that the adrenal cortex in man is about nine times larger than the medulla. In the lower animals, the size ratio is much smaller, and in some instances the relationship is reversed. It is argued that as the species evolves and the control of behaviour by the cerebral cortex increases, the adrenal cortex also increases in size and importance of function.

The adrenal medulla has been more extensively studied than any of the other endocrines. Its tissue is of the same origin as that of the autonomic nervous system and is quite different from that of the cortex. Its secretion has been extracted and is known as adrenin or epinephrin. It is manufactured commercially under the name of adrenalin. Adrenal secretion has precisely the same effect upon visceral effector organs as have the efferent nerve impulses of the sympathetic nervous system. It has a pressor effect upon the heart-beat, and thereby raises the blood pressure but also causes a greater flow of blood to the blood vessels of the skeletal muscles. Adrenin has the general effect of slowing up the activity of the stomach, inhibiting the gastric juices, increasing the pulse, enlarging the pupils, and arousing other symptoms that are usually associated with the excitation of the sympathetic branch of the autonomic nervous system. Adrenin also stimulates the liver and pancreas, so that sugar is released into the blood stream to provide additional nutriment for the skeletal muscles. This endocrine likewise clots the blood and is used surgically for this purpose. Cannon describes the general effect of adrenal secretion as " rapid mobilization of bodily reserves ", under conditions of violent physical exertion and muscular effort.[1]

The individual of hyper-adrenal type is full of physical

[1] W. B. Cannon, *Bodily Symptoms of Pain, Hunger, Fear and Rage*, 1920, p. 129.

aggressiveness and initiative, easily excited, optimistic, and is pervaded by a sense of well-being. But on the other hand, such persons are apt to be pugnacious and given to sudden spurts of anger.

The hypo-adrenal personality is quite the opposite. Such persons have no reserve strength. They are quickly brought to the point of exhaustion in almost any emergency situation, whether emotional or physical, and they are sometimes subject to constant fear.

The Pituitary Gland (Hypophysis)

The pituitary gland, located in the very centre of the head, is embedded in a bony cavity called the sella turcica, and is attached at one end to the infundibulum. The pituitary gland has three parts, each of different function ; the anterior lobe, which is the gland proper ; the posterior lobe ; and an intermediate part called pars intermedia, which also connects the two lobes. Removal of the pituitary usually results in death in from one to thirty days.

The hormones from the anterior lobe maintain the nutritive balance of the connective tissues, especially those of the skeleton. If these hormones are over-active in childhood, the bones of the arms and legs become very long, and gigantism results. Should this condition appear after adolescence, the bones of the face become much enlarged and the hands and feet extend to an abnormal size. This deformity is known as acromegaly. The secretions of the anterior lobe are also supposed to influence the activity of the gonads.

The posterior lobe is said to manufacture several secretions. Timme sets the number at eight ; other, more conservative estimates put the number at three to four. The best known extract from this lobe, and the one most used commercially, is pituitrin. Pituitrin, when injected intravenously, increases the activity of the smooth muscles and the contractions of the bladder. It is extensively used to stimulate the contractions of the uterus during the third stage of labour, when the walls tend to relax, with a resultant hemorrhage. Secretions from the posterior lobe are also known to increase the production and flow of the mammary glands.

The pars intermedia also has a specific secretion. Its effects have not been ascertained with certainty, but it is supposed to influence genital development and to inhibit the action of the pancreatic juice.

Abnormalities of the pituitary gland have marked effects upon both physique and personality ; the exact nature of these effects depends upon the location of the infected area within the gland. One commonly known symptom of disease of the pituitary is one-sided or pituitary headeache, which is caused by an enlargement of the gland, usually at the side, so that it presses against the bony cavity and results in severe pain at the temple. This is only one of many known effects. Psychically, the personality symptoms of over-activity of the pituitary gland can easily be confused with the characteristics of the hyper-adrenal type, while an under-active pituitary gland results in traits and attitudes superficially resembling those of the hypo-thyroid.

This gland seems to work in close connection with the other glands of internal secretion. The over-active pituitary state in childhood results in early sexual maturity, while the under-active is thought to be the cause of sexual infantilism.

The Thymus

The thymus is located in the lower part of the neck and upper part of the chest. Its glandular function has sometimes been questioned, but it is now generally accepted as established. This gland is enlarged in childhood and increases in size until it attains its maximum at puberty, after which it atrophies.

The thymus is supposed to check sexual maturity and provide elements for the all-round development of the body. If this gland fails to atrophy, with the on-coming of adolescence, the secondary sex characteristics do not appear.

Individuals of this so-called " thymic type " have a very soft, smooth, and child-like skin, the breasts are underdeveloped in the female, and there is no beard or moustache in the male. If this condition is accompanied by underactivity of the supra-renals, any emergency situation where adrenal activity is needed, results in collapse. An individual in whom the atrophy of the thymus is delayed, remains very child-like. He is self-centred, very simple in his mental processes, lacking in initiative, and seeks the protection of others.

In other cases the thymus atrophies too early. Under these

conditions the individual usually is of short stature and the secondary sex characteristics appear early. Personalities of this type are apt to show remarkable sophistication at a very early age and are sometimes called the " old-young " type. They are self-willed, independent, and given to unreasonable fits of anger when opposed.

The Pineal Gland

The pineal gland is a very small structure which is part of the brain. It was originally considered to be a vestigial eye, but the experimentation of recent years has established it as a gland of internal secretion.

Very little is known concerning its functions. It is thought to promote the general growth and strength of the body in opposition to the development of the sexual processes, in much the same manner as the thymus does, except that the pineal hormones probably inhibit the size of the genital organs, while the thymus inhibits their functional maturity. It is known that the removal of this gland results in rapid growth in the size of the genital organs of both sexes.

It is supposed that the pineal gland atrophies at about the age of thirty, since at this period a substance known as " brain sand " appears, representing a crystallization of pineal substance which could not occur while the pineal remains active.

Philosophers once believed that the pineal gland was the seat of the human soul.

The Gonads (Sex Glands)

While the ovaries and testes are the sex glands proper, other associated structures have been located whose hormones appear to be responsible for the development of the secondary sex characteristics. These are the cells of Leidig, or interstitial cells, called by Steinach the " puberty gland ". Secretions from these glands are supposed to account for those characteristics that differentiate man from woman, that is, the length and distribution of the hair, the differences in the tones and pitch of the voice, the growth of the mammary glands in woman, and the curves of the body. Interesting experiments with the transplanting of tissue containing Leidig cells show a rejuvenating effect that varies with individuals and in any event wears off in time.

It seems highly probable that the gonads give off hormones that have the effect of causing erotic excitement. We shall have occasion to consider erotic drive more fully in a later chapter.

In general,it must be remembered that all the endocrine glands interact one upon another. Also, their effects upon bodily tissues sometimes reinforce one another, and sometimes prove antagonistic. Changes in the activity of one endocrine gland, therefore, result in changes in other endocrine glands, and in changes in the entire endocrine balance of the body. The pattern, or balance, of endocrine gland functionings at any time is called hasyndrome. Only in case the entire syndrome is known and understood, can any specific knowledge of the resulting emotional or personality traits be obtained.

CHAPTER V

PART REACTIONS OF THE HIDDEN MACHINERY

Putting the Hidden Machinery Together

So far we have considered the separate parts of the hidden machinery in some detail. We have divided these parts into four classes, receptors, neurons, synapses, and effectors. This is as though we had purchased a lot of manufacturing machinery which was delivered to us, dismantled, in four crates, each crate containing all the machine parts of a certain type. In the first crate were packed all the electric buttons, switches, and automatic starting devices by which the machinery would eventually be set in motion. In the second crate was packed a huge mass of electric wires of all shapes, sizes, and lengths. In the third crate were all kinds of junction boxes, binding posts, and connecting devices to put the wires together. And in the fourth crate were several different types of motors that eventually would do our work for us when the entire lot of machinery had been connected together in just the right way.

So far, so good. On each crate was printed a list of the parts contained therein, and a general description of the structures and functions of these parts. But now we want to see the whole mass of machinery put together in the right way so that it will work. The description of each type of machine-part is bound to appear much more intelligible when we see the parts connected together so that all can actually function.

In order to put the different parts of the hidden machinery together and view it in working order, we shall be obliged first of all to learn something more about the parts and arrangements of the nervous system. The neurons with their connecting synapses constitute, as we have seen, the inner connective portion of the hidden machinery of human behaviour. We have described in some detail the individual nerve cell and the individual synapse. Now it becomes necessary to consider briefly the chief groupings of neurons and synapses as they occur in the human nervous system. In other words, when we start putting our machinery together, we must begin by drawing a blue print of the way our wires must run to different parts of the factory, together with the central grouping and connection of these wires.

The Reflex Arc

The set of nerve cells and the connections between these nerve cells which conduct impulses to action from the receptor organs to the final muscles and glands that do the acting is known as the reflex arc. The reflex arc might also be termed the unit system of reflex conduction. If we take a single, artificially simplified *reflex arc* theoretically connecting a single receptor with a single effector, we find six essential parts.

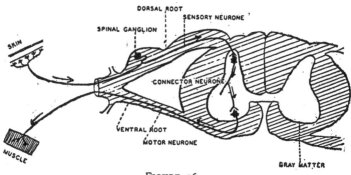

FIGURE 26

Diagram of a Simple Reflex Arc

1. An afferent, or inward bound nerve tract, leading from the receptor organs inward to spinal cord or brain.

2. A synaptic junction, connecting this afferent nerve tract with other nerves in the central nervous system.

3. A set of connector nerves, lying inside the central nervous system, and carrying the nervous excitement to whatever outward bound nerve tracts are required to bring about the unit response.

4. Various synaptic junctions between the different connector nerves. (In the artificially simplified reflex arc, diagrammed out in many text books, this set of connector synapses is eliminated, and the connector part of the arc **is**

treated as though it were a single nerve cell, lying within the central nervous system. Sherrington has proved that any reflex arc *must* include at least three neurons; but it seems very questionable whether any reflex connection, in the living organism of man and the higher vertebrates, ever actually does include *only* three. Certainly a vast majority of reflex activities excite a considerable number of connector nerve cells, with necessary interconnections, as stated here.)

  5. Synaptic junctions, connecting the connector nerves with the final motor, or efferent, nerves.

  6. Efferent, or outward bound nerve-tracts, finally effecting the connection between central nervous excitation, and the effector organs to be moved in carrying out the final unit response.

There are the cog-wheels, in human machinery that connect the receptors of stimuli, from outside, with the muscles and glands that can finally be seen responding to that stimulus. It can be seen at a glance that there are two different types of structures in the connective, or conductive mechanism : nerve cells, and junctional tissue. There are three sets of each, afferent, connector, and efferent. Since the receptor organs are also called sense organs, the afferent nerve tracts and junctional tissues are also called *sensory*. The efferent structures, leading as they do directly to movement, are called *motor*. The entire junction between two or more nerve cells, including the junctional tissue as its most vital part, is called the *synapse*. The junctional tissue within the synapse is called a *psychon*. Synapses seldom occur alone, but almost invariably are located in large groups, where many nerve tracts converge and form interconnections. These switching stations, or masses of synaptic connections, are called *nerve centres*. There are three types of nerve centres : sensory centres, connector or correlation centres, and motor centres.

The entire human nervous system is customarily divided, for convenience of description, into two parts, the central nervous system and the peripheral, or outlying, groups of neurones.

The Central Nervous System

The central nervous system is made up of the brain and the spinal cord. Both brain and cord consist of a series of centres, or intricately related groups of synapses.

The cord retains the primitive segmentation found in lower

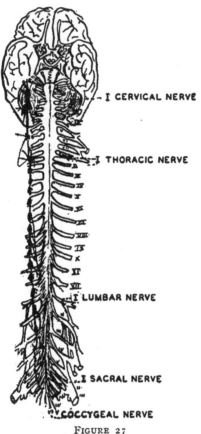

— I CERVICAL NERVE

— I THORACIC NERVE

— I LUMBAR NERVE

— I SACRAL NERVE

— I COCCYGEAL NERVE

FIGURE 27

The Human Central Nervous System

Diagram shows ventral view of Central Nervous System and also its connections with the cerebro-spinal nerves. The Autonomic Nervous System is also shown in black at the left of the diagram in correct relative position. (After Allen, Thompson and Rauber, from Morris' *Anatomy*, W. B. Saunders and Co., Philadelphia).

forms of life and controls the reflex reactions of the body. The parts of the central nervous system located in the brain have evolved at a later period in the history of man, are more complex, and control all simpler and lower centres.

The Brain

The brain itself is a large, protoplasmic mass, the weight

of which " is exceedingly variable even in a homogeneous population. The average weight of the normal, adult European male brain is commonly stated to be 1360 grammes (49 ounces) and that of the female 1250 grammes (44 ounces)."[1]

The brain floats in a liquid within the bony cavity of the skull, is grey in colour, and due to the myriads of convolutions, has a bark-like appearance that gives its outer covering the name of the cortex. This mass of grey matter is made up of unmedullated cell bodies and dendrites of the cortical neurons. It has been estimated that in the optic tract alone there are one hundred thousand separate fibres ; the number of *neurons* in the brain is believed to total nine billion, two hundred million (9,200,000,000).[2] Beneath the bark-like covering of the brain is found a large, white mass called the corpus callosum, and long, heavy, white strands connecting the various parts of the brain with each other and with the spinal cord. These strands consist of the medullated axones of afferent fibres running to the brain and of efferent fibres running to the muscles.

The brain is divided into many parts, four of which are of special interest in the study of unit response psychology. The entire mass lying nearest the top of the head and larger than the other divisions, is called the cerebrum. The smaller mass, below and at the back of the head, is the cerebellum. In the centre of the head is the thalamus. Behind and lowest of all is the medulla oblongata, which is really a swelling or expansion of the spinal cord. The grey matter is on the *outside* of the brain, and is called the cortex, or bark. The grey matter is on the *inside* of the cord. There are two equal and corresponding parts of the top of the cerebrum, called the cerebral hemispheres.

The cerebrum

Looking at the diagram of the cerebrum, see that it is divided into two hemispheres connected by the corpus callosum. In addition to its division into two halves, there is a fissure that runs from the top diagonally forward, and another that runs back from the temple, terminating just above the ear. The first fissure is known as the Fissure of Rolando and the second as the Fissure of Sylvius ; on the

---

[1] Herrick, C. J., *Introduction to Neurology*, 1918, p. 132.
[2] *Ibid*, p. 27.

back inner surface there is a third fissure called the parieto-occipital. These fissues form natural boundaries for the four lobes of the cerebrum, the frontal, temporal, occipital, and parietal. These are useful in describing the few functional areas that to date have been experimentally defined.

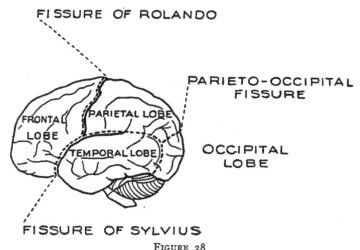

FIGURE 28

Divisions of the Cerebrum

Looking at the cerebrum from the side, the centres that control cutaneous and kinaesthetic activities are to the rear of the Fissure of Rolando, running from the top of the cortex nearly to the ear.

In front of this area is another long strip running somewhat forward, at the top of which is the motor projection centre. An unexpected discovery concerning this group of centres is that those nearest the top of the head connect with the parts of the body that are farthest away, namely with the toes and feet. Coming downward along this area, the points of motor control ascend to body, shoulder, and neck, until finally at the lowest region of all we find the points of projection for the muscles of the cheeks, jaws, and lips.

The auditory centres are located directly back of the Fissure of Sylvius, in what is known as the temporal lobe. The regions in the very back part of the head, about on the level of the eye, are the visual centres. On the inner side of the brain hemisphere right behind the nose are situated the olfactory and gustatory centres. The exact functioning of these centres is very roughly known and large areas of the cortex are as yet unaccounted for. It is thought that the majority of these have an associative function, co-ordinating sensory impulses and correlating them with the motor areas. There is no reason to believe that every functional area is the only possible point of connection between the particular sensory centres it may serve and the motor arcs. Experiments have shown that in some types of activity, the function can be renewed gradually and taken up by other centres after the natural centre has been partially destroyed.

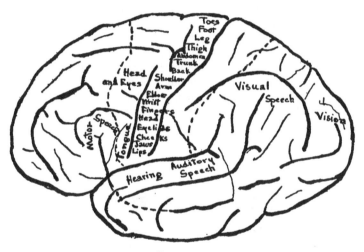

FIGURE 29
Localization of Function in the Cerebrum

The cerebral cortex controls the activities of the rest of the body. This function has evolved slowly and its development originally was necessitated by the fact that, as the animal moved forward, the head was the first portion of the body to contact environment and to be in a position to initiate preparatory and defensive measures. Through necessity distance receptors were evolved and for the same reason the organism was forced to connect these specially sensitized tissues with the action system of the body. The cerebral cortex continued to be the centre of greatest activity, a factor that confirmed its control over the simpler, less closely organized parts of the body. This functional superiority is known as head dominance.

The Cerebellum

The cerebellum, sometimes known as the pallium or old brain, although smaller than the cerebrum, has a similar gross structure. The cerebellum is remarkable for the intricate interconnections of the neurons composing it. They have heavy, interlacing dendrites and very rich terminal arborizations that permit the simultaneous stimulation of many neurons. The cerebellum is the great proprioceptive co-ordination centre of the body. It is connected with every bodily receptor and through its complexly arranged neuron system can connect the incoming sensory axones with practically every striped muscle in the body. It is therefore the great centre for the maintenance of muscular tone, and for co-ordinating and synchronizing the sending of impulses to the muscles in such a way that the balance is maintained between extensor and flexor activity.

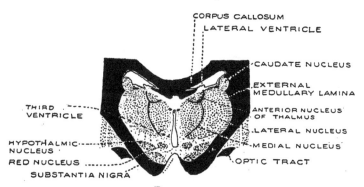

FIGURE 31

Frontal Section Through the Human Thalamus

This diagram shows a frontal section through the thalmus and the structures which immediately surround it. (Redrawn from Ranson).

The Thalamus

The thalamus is in the middle region of the whole brain mass and is a centre through which somatic, sensory nervous

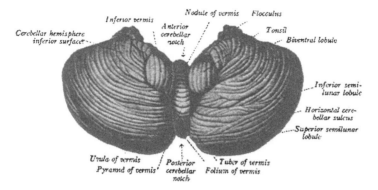

Fig. 30

THE HUMAN CEREBELLUM, VENTRAL VIEW (SOBOTTA-McMURRICH)

From " The Anatomy of the Nervous System " by S. W. Ranson. : Published by
W. B. Saunders & Co., Philadelphia

[face p. 120

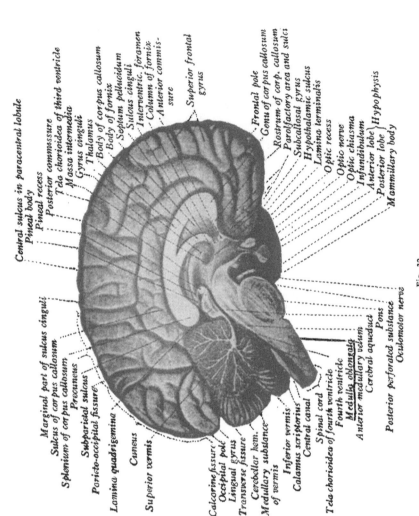

Central sulcus in paracentral lobule
Pineal body
Pineal recess
Posterior commissure
Tela chorioidea of third ventricle
Massa intermedia
Gyrus cinguli
Thalamus
Body of corpus callosum
Body of fornix
Septum pellucidum
Sulcus cinguli
Interventric. foramen
Column of fornix
Anterior commissure
Superior frontal gyrus

Marginal part of sulcus cinguli
Sulcus of corpus callosum
Splenium of corpus callosum
Precuneus
Subparietal sulcus
Parieto-occipital fissure
Lamina quadrigemina
Cuneus
Superior vermis

Frontal pole
Genu of corpus callosum
Rostrum of corp. callosum
Parolfactory area and sulci
Subcallosal gyrus
Hypothalamic sulcus
Lamina terminalis
Optic recess
Optic nerve
Optic chiasma
Infundibulum
Anterior lobe } Hypophysis
Posterior lobe
Mammillary body

Calcarine fissure
Occipital pole
Lingual gyrus
Transverse fissure
Cerebellar hem.
Medullary substance of vermis
Inferior vermis
Calamus scriptorius
Central canal
Spinal cord
Tela chorioidea of fourth ventricle
Fourth ventricle
Medulla oblongata
Anterior medullary velum
Cerebral aqueduct
Pons
Posterior perforated substance
Oculomotor nerve

Fig. 32

MEDIAL SECTION OF THE HUMAN BRAIN SHOWING THE MEDULLA OBLONGATA AND
NEIGHBOURING STRUCTURES (SOBOTTA-McMURRICH)

impulses reach the cortex.   It consists of a large, oval mass, chiefly of grey matter, separated into two main divisions : the central part contains the motor co-ordination centres ; and the dorsal part contains the sensory correlation centres. Its functions have been extensively studied by Cannon, who looks upon it as the centre for those impulses connected with emotion, because those emotions that are usually regarded as fundamental remain when other parts of the brain are eliminated (by operation or otherwise), but disappear when this particular centre is extirpated.

On the sensory side the thalamus acts as a receiving station for somaesthetic, visual, and auditory impulses.

The Medulla Oblongata

The medulla is an expansion of the spinal column, which lies in the lower portion of the brain and is known as the " bulb ".   Its function is similar to that of the cord, except that it seems to be the centre of all visceral impulse activity.

It is the terminal for the great vagus nerve, receiving via this tract, afferent impulses from the general bodily receptors and from the important visceral organs, that is, from the stomach, heart, lungs, arteries, pharynx, larynx, and oesophagus.   The visceral efferent fibres passing to these same organs from the medulla, constrict the arteries, depress the heart action, increase the contractions of the stomach, and constrict the bronchii.   Thus all the most important life functions are under the control of the medulla.

The Spinal Cord

The spinal cord runs two-thirds the length of the backbone. It lies within the vertebrae and consists of a white exterior portion surrounding a grey centre which is butterfly-shaped. Within the very middle of the grey matter is a central canal containing the spinal fluid ; this same liquid is found in the brain and is called the cerebro-spinal fluid.   When it increases abnormally in volume, it results in what is called water on the brain.   The spinal fluid is susceptible to attack by bacteria and is treated directly through hypodermics in certain cases of cerebro-spinal syphilis.

There are thirty-one pairs of spinal nerves with points of entry between the vertebrae, the sensory fibres entering via the dorsal horns, the motor fibres leaving the ventral horns. The first eight pairs of nerves compose the cranial division of the cord. The next twelve pairs make up the thoracic divisions. There are five pairs in the lumbar division, five in the sacral division, and one pair of coccygeal nerves.[1]

The centres in the spinal cord are much simpler than those in the cortex. The grey matter is made up of the cell bodies of motor neurons, and of small connecting neurons. The simplest type of centre, therefore, would consist of a sensory nerve terminal, connecting with an intermediate neuron, which in turn connects with a motor neuron. Complicated responses in the cord are made possible by the fact that both sensory and motor neurons frequently divide in the cord, one collateral going to a lower centre, the other going to a higher centre, thus arousing several centres simultaneously. Such a conduction system also relays impulses to the brain in the same way. While one branch of an afferent nerve connects immediately with the centres in the cord, the other branch ascends to the brain, connecting there with neuron chains which cross to the motor side of the arc, out to the lower centres in the cord, and thence to the muscles. This is known as the loop line and it makes possible all the complex responses in civilized man.

Peripheral Nerve Groups

We have already mentioned the extensive system of nerve processes leading from the surface of the body to the spinal cord and again from the spinal cord to the smooth muscles of the viscera. These two peripheral nerve groups are entirely different in structure and function. The first type are generally referred to as the cerebro-spinal nerves, the second as the autonomic nervous system.

The Cerebro-spinal Nerves

The cerebro-spinal nerves are characterized by long fibres axone-like in structure but dendritic in function. They lead

[1] Ransom, *The Anatomy of the Nervous System*, 1927.

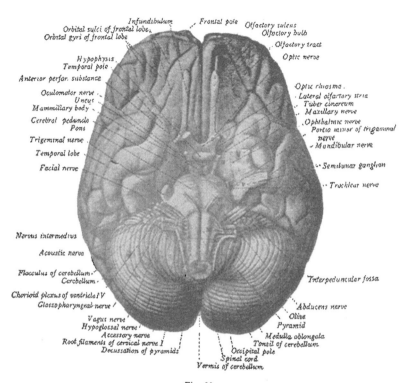

Orbital sulci of frontal lobe
Orbital gyri of frontal lobe
Infundibulum
Frontal pole
Olfactory sulcus
Olfactory bulb
Olfactory tract
Optic nerve

Hypophysis
Temporal pole
Anterior perfor. substance
Oculomotor nerve
Uncus
Mammillary body
Cerebral peduncle
Pons
Trigeminal nerve
Temporal lobe
Facial nerve

Optic chiasma
Lateral olfactory stria
Tuber cinereum
Maxillary nerve
Ophthalmic nerve
Portio minor of trigeminal nerve
Mandibular nerve
Semilunar ganglion
Trochlear nerve

Nervus intermedius
Acoustic nerve
Flocculus of cerebellum
Cerebellum
Chorioid plexus of ventricle IV
Glossopharyngeal nerve
Vagus nerve
Hypoglossal nerve
Accessory nerve
Root filaments of cervical nerve I
Decussation of pyramids

Interpeduncular fossa
Abducens nerve
Olive
Pyramid
Medulla oblongata
Tonsil of cerebellum
Occipital pole
Spinal cord
Vermis of cerebellum

Fig. 33

VENTRAL VIEW OF HUMAN BRAIN WITH SPINAL CORD EMERGING

Figure 27 above shows the full length of the spinal cord with the thirty-one pairs of cerebro
spinal nerves, while Figure 26 above shows a diagrammatic section of the spinal cord with
the butterfly pattern of its grey matter (Sobotta-McMurrich). From "The Anatomy of the
Nervous System" by S. W. Ranson. Published by W. B. Saunders & Co., Philadelphia

[face p. 122

from the somatic receptors to cell bodies that lie outside the spinal cord.

These axones are all sensory and send a second process that enters the cord and bifurcates, the lower process passing to the lower centres in the cord, the upper process ascending to the brain.

The Autonomic Nervous System

The autonomic nervous system consists of a series of ganglionic cells lying just outside the spinal cord. These ganglia are more primitive structures than the axone system of the central nervous system. They are connected with the central nervous system by means of fibres coming from the cord to the plexi of the ganglia. These fibres are called pre-ganglionic fibres. Within the ganglia impulses travel in much the same fashion as in the nerve-net systems of lower organisms. The ganglia control the activities of the smooth muscles of the body by a series of post-ganglionic fibres running to the heart, stomach, liver, intestines, and so on.

The autonomic nervous system is divided into three parts, the first and third of which are functionally antagonistic to the second. These are the cranial, the thoracico-lumbar, and the sacral divisions. The cranial and sacral co-operate in the majority of instances. The thoracico-lumbar, also called the sympathetic, division in general accelerates where the cranial and sacral inhibit, and vice versa.

The cranial division has control of the respiratory, cardiac, and alimentary functions. This means that it accelerates the muscles of the alimentary tract during the processes of ingestion and digestion, and in so doing depresses the activation of the heart, lungs, and skeletal muscles.

The sympathetic division, on the other hand, is the great emergency energizer of the body. It stirs up the glands of internal secretion, the liver, and the pancreas, and supplies the striped muscles with increased blood and sugar ; it increases heart action, but practically cuts off the innervation of the stomach. The diagram below gives in detail the functional effects of these various divisions of the autonomic system upon different visceral organs.

Ganglionic Plexi

There exist throughout the body groups of ganglionic cells, whose function is to control the activities of the local organ

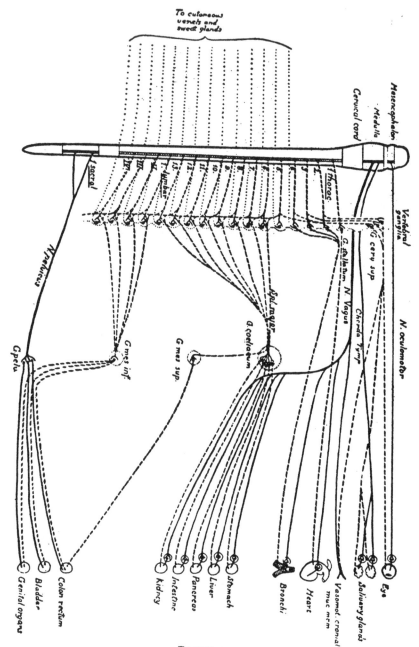

FIGURE 34

Diagram of the Autonomic Nervous System

Diagram shows, in solid lines, the cranial and sacral subdivisions of the autonomic system at top and bottom of the cord respectively. Motor discharge from these systems is reciprocally antagonistic to the thoracico-lumbar division of the autonomic system shown in dotted lines in the central portion of the cord. Table on opposite page lists the end effects of motor impulses emerging through different divisions of the autonomic nervous system. (Diagram modified by Ranson from Meyer and Gottlieb, *The Anatomy of the Nervous System.* Published by W. B. Saunders and Co., Philadelphia.)

FIGURE 35

Table Showing End Effects of Motor Discharge through the Cranial-Sacral and Sympathetic Branches of the Autonomic Nervous System (Junctions between pre- and postganglionic portions of both branches paralyzed by nicotin).

Sympathetic System	Action on the Organ	Cranio-Sacral Systems
(Nerve endings excited by adrenalin and paralyzed by ergo-toxin)	− equals inhibition +equals excitation	(Nerve endings excited by muscarin, pilocarpin and paralyzed by atropin)
Cervical Sympathetic		*Cranial Autonomic*
Inhibition (relaxation of sphincter, dilation of pupil)	− Sphincter iridis+	Excitation (contraction of sphincter, narrowing of pupil, via N.111)
Relaxation (?)	− Ciliary muscle of eye+	Excitation (contraction of muscle, increased convexity of lens, via N.111)
Excitation (Exophthalmos)	+Orbital muscle of Müller −	Relaxation (Enophthalmos)
Inhibition (?)	− Lacrymal glands+	Excitation (via N. petrosus superficialis major)
Inhibition (?)	− Lacrymal glands+	Excitation (via chorda tympani)
Excitation	+Sweat glands of the face −	Inhibition
Vasoconstriction (pallor)	+Blood vessels of the face −	Vasodilation (reddening)
Excitation	+Piloerectors of head−	Relaxation of contraction (?)
Thoracic Sympathetic		*Vagus*
Inhibition (relaxation)	− Bronchial muscles+	Excitation (contraction)
Excitation (acceleration)	+ Heart beat −	Inhibition (slowing))
Inhibition (dilation)	− Oesophagus+	Excitation (contraction '
Superior Splanchnic (Th. 6—9)		*Vagus*
Inhibition of peristalsis (Vasoconstriction)	− Gastric musculature and glands+	Excitation of peristalsis (Vasodilation)
Inhibition (?)	− Pancreas+	Excitation of secretion
Inhibition (Vasoconstriction)	− Small intestine+	Excitation (Vasodilation ?)
Inhibition of secretion of urine (Vasoconstriction)	− Kidney+	Excitation of secretion of urine
Excitation of secretion of adrenalin (Vasodilation)	+Adrenal −	Inhibition of excretion of adrenalin (?)
Inferior Splanchnic (Th. 10—12)		*Sacral Autonomic, Pelvic Nerve*
Inhibition (Vasconstriction)	Descending colon, Sigmoid. − flexure, Rectum+	Excitation (contraction and peristalsis, vasodilation, via N. pelvicus).

Hypogastric Plexus (upper lumbar)	Action on the Organ	Pelvic Nerve (lower sacral)
Inhibition of detrusor, excitation of sphincter (retention of urine)	− Bladder+	Excitation of detrusor (via N. pelvicus), relaxation of sphincter (emptying of bladder)
Vasoconstriction. Ejaculation	+Male genitalia −	Vasodilation of penis (via the N. pelvicus or erigens). (Erection)
Vasoconstriction. Excitation of contractions of uterus	+Female genitalia −	Vasodilation of clitoris (via N. pelvicus) Inhibition of movements of uterus
Ventral Thoracic and Lumbar Roots		Dorsal Thoracic and Lumbar Roots
Vasoconstriction	+Blood vessels of trunk and extremities−	Vasodilation
Excitation (sweating)	+Sweat glands of trunk and extremities−	Inhibition
Excitation (goose flesh) Excitation	+Pilomotor muscles— +Smooth muscle of scrotum −	Inhibition Inhibition

(Modified by Strong & Elwyn from L. R. Muller; Published by William Wood & Co., New York City.)

to which they are connected. The most important of these ganglionic plexi are found in the cortex, in the pharynx, and in the bronchii. They are the superior cervical ganglia, the pharyngial plexus, the bronchial plexus, the cardiac plexus, the superior mesenteric plexus, the hypogastric plexus, and the sacral plexus. The neurons of this peripheral autonomic nervous system are the most primitive to be found in the human organism. They are thought to have been retained from the original nerve-net type of system, because the organs with which they are connected are so complex that it is not possible to control their activities from the central nervous system.

The Simple Reflex and the Total Response

We may differentiate at this point for our own convenience between those fragmentary portions of the entire unit response which are the reactions actually designated by the term " simple reflex ", and which are found constantly recurring in psychological and physiological text books ; and the total, integrated response of the whole organism, which is customarily termed the " total pattern " of reflex response.

The patellar reflex may serve as an example of a " simple reflex ". The receptor organs are the pressure bulbs in the patellar tendon of the knee. A sharp, light blow is delivered upon this tendon, in such a way that the receptors are stimulated. The afferent nerve trunk connecting these organs is aroused to action. It conducts a battery of nerve impulses into the spinal centre. There a tiny connector nerve cell is energized. It communicates the energy to the efferent nerve trunk which conducts a battery of impulses along a number of its-own nerve fibres simultaneously to the leg muscles. A number of muscle fibres in these muscles shorten or contract, and the lower leg is jerked outward and upward, " extended ", using the knee joint as its hinge. This whole knee-jerk reaction occurs with great promptness, and probably it is nearly completed before any other portion of the entire unit response, or pattern of reflex response gets under way. It gives the superficial appearance, therefore, of being a single, isolated " simple " reflex action, which can be regarded all by itself as the inevitable, machine-like result of a blow on the patellar tendon.

Such is far from being the case however. The response is neither simple, fixed, nor isolated. In this so-called simple reflex, as in all others of its kind, a receptor, or sense organ always receives the energy from some extrinsic source, the stimulus. A muscle, smooth or striped, or a gland, with or without ducts, always performs the final action of the organism. As a matter of actuality, no single sense organ is ever stimulated by itself, without many others receiving stimulation at the same time, except under artificial laboratory conditions. And no single muscle or gland ever moves all by itself, without the simultaneous movement of other muscles and glands, unless the muscle fibre or secreting organ and the connecting nerves are dissected out of the animal's body, and lie thus artificially isolated on the laboratory table. Many receptor organs of similar kind and lying in the same general area of the body, are connected by thousands of nerves and hundreds of thousands of nerve junctions, with all the effector organs, muscles and glands of the entire body.

The receptors are usually *most directly connected*, through many nerve cells and junctions, with the muscles and glands in the same general area of the body where the sense organs themselves lie. But this is not always true, by any means. The directness of nervous connection varies vastly, under different conditions of the organism's spontaneous activity. It also depends, in principle, upon the *function* of both receptors and effectors in the life or the organism, rather than upon the structural facilities for conducting energy from one to the other. The eye, for example, may be most directly connected, for action purposes, with any part of the body which is needed to carry out the unit responses of the moment. Leg muscles already tensed, and set to go, as at the start of a race, may become most intimately connected with eye or ear which receives the starting signal. The pressure and pain receptors at the back of a child's knee, seem inherently most directly connected through the nervous system with the muscles of the other leg and foot, which serve to bend the leg and push away the pinching hand. The same is true of the " scratch reflex " in animals, and particularly the " crossed scratch reflex ".

Many receptors, then, simultaneously stimulated, are connected through a great mass of nerve cells and junctions, with all the muscles and glands of the body ; but they are most closely connected with those muscles and glands best adapted to carry out the organism's unit response toward the sort of stimulus adequate and usual to the receptors stimulated.

The foregoing discussion indicates that no reflex response is really " simple ". We may further assert that no natural reflex response is fixed, or invariable. The patellar reflex, or knee jerk, as we have already noted, is frequently cited in the text books as an example of reflex reaction which is practically uniform on all occasions. But merely because one part of the total patellar reflex response pattern, viz., the knee jerk, occurs first and is relatively fixed and constant (though its variability is actually used as a measure of hunger pangs[1] and of emotional excitement), we still have no logical reason to consider it separately from all the rest. True, we cannot describe the rest of the unit response in specific, invariable terms. Sometimes the rest of the response might consist of pushing away the thing that hit us ; sometimes of increase in heart beat ; sometimes we might " feel " the blow that caused the knee jerk and exclaim " ow ! " The particular unit response would depend upon the relation of the stimulus to the organism. But we can describe the reflex mechanics of the rest of the unit response fairly well. In the spinal

[1] Carlson, A. J., *The Control of Hunger in Health and Disease*, 1916, p. 86.

cord are numerous connections, afferent nerve tracts, that lead
upward to other spinal nerve centres and to the brain.   These
nerves are excited simultaneously with the excitement of the
short connector neurone in the spinal centre which sent the
impulse over to the efferent tracts leading to leg muscles.
So, the larger pattern of reflex response actually does begin
at the same time the minor detail, or part reaction, which
is usually termed a " simple reflex response," begins.

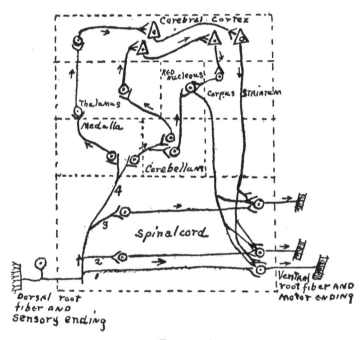

FIGURE 36

Diagram representing some of the Conduction Paths through the
Central Nervous System.   (Redrawn from Ranson).

The afferent nerves conduct their impulses to brain centres.
There innumerable nerve tracts are set into activity.   Some
or all of these connector tracts excite, in turn, other afferent
nerve tracts.   The efferents conduct a new, and much larger
battery of impulses outward, to arms, heart, trunk or vocal
cords, as may be.   Then the major part of the unit reflex
response becomes evident.   The subject is seen to push away

K

the object that struck him, his pulse increases its rate, or he may be heard to ejaculate " Ow ! ' "

Says Herrick[1] " Our picture of the reflex act in a higher animal will, then, include a view of the whole nervous system in a state of neural tension. The stimulus disturbs the equilibrium at a definite point (the receptor), and the wave of nervous discharge thus set up irradiates through the complex lines determined by the neural connections of the receptor." If the stimulus is weak. " the neural equilibrium will be only locally disturbed ". Under other conditions, " almost the whole nervous system may participate in the reaction, a part focal and sharply defined, and the rest marginal, diffuse, and exercising more or less inhibitory or reinforcing control on the final reaction ". This is an excellent description of *unit* reflex response as we have tried to explain it. The part of the entire unit response which is most immediate and obvious is never to be thought of as a truly " simple " reflex, but only as the most central part of the total unit reflex re-action which, because of its central position in the entire neural reaction pattern, is most " focal and sharply defined ", as Herrick puts it. Often it is not even that ; it may be only the most obvious portion of the " sharply defined " part of the unit response.

Classes of Part-Reactions

We have used the words " response " and " reaction " very broadly up to the present to include everything that happens to the organism as a result of stimulation. It now becomes necessary to differentiate, somewhat, between different portions of the total unit response, because some unit responses have more of one element than another in their composition. Separable portions of any total unit response may conveniently be termed part-reactions. There are three classes of part reactions, differentiated according to the class of living tissue within which they occur. These three kinds of part-reactions are bodily reactions, nervous reactions, and psychonic reactions.

First, it is convenient to draw a rough line of distinction between what may be termed *bodily reactions* and *nervous reactions*.

[1] Herrick, C. J., *op. cit.*, p. 70.

Bodily reactions consist first, of the changes in tissues caused by the stimulus (temperature, etc.), and, second, of the physiological-chemical reactions of the sense organs in or near these tissues when the stimulus is received. Then the unit response passes into the nervous system, as it were, and does not emerge again into bodily response until the effector organs are finally moved. Thus the third element of bodily reaction includes shortening of muscle fibres, or relaxation of same ; increased secretion of glands, or decreased action of same. The fourth element of bodily reaction is the movements of bodily parts, organs, and tissues as a result of changes in muscles and glands. Entire legs or arms are extended or flexed ; the heart pumps more or less blood through the arteries ; or the adrenin potency of the blood stream is increased. This fourth section of bodily reactions is not truthfully describable merely as a collection of all the muscular and glandular movements assigned to the third group of bodily reactions. For, if the arms or legs are tied down, then the muscles may shorten until they break without moving the limbs ; and if there is some endocrine antidote in the blood stream, the increased adrenin poured into the blood may not actually result in giving the blood stream hyper-adrenal potencies.

Nervous reactions consist of the release of nervous energy within whatever nerve cells may be excited as a result of stimulation of receptor organs. The nervous reactions of any particular group of neurones may, or may not, conduct the train of excitations to their synapses with adjacent nerve cells with sufficient force to insure a crossing of the synapse, and completion of a reflex circuit. The energy which determines the strength and spread of reflex conduction is energy which finds its source within the protoplasm of the neurons themselves. Each neuron is to be thought of as an electro-chemical reservoir of potential conduction energy. Each neuronic reservoir is tapped, and its energy released in the form of a nerve impulse, if the neuron is sufficiently excited by the psychon or synaptic tissue joining it to another neuron which is already excited.

There are three types of neurons necessary to the completion of any reflex circuit, as we have seen. They are the afferent, the connector, and the efferent neurons. Therefore, we may say, for convenience, that there are three types of nervous reactions ; sensory, connector, and motor reactions. It is not clear that the connector neurons are essentially different in structure from either the sensory or the motor, though they undoubtedly differ in organization and arrangement in the nervous system. It is clear that sensory neurons differ in these characteristics from motor neurons ; and also differ with regard to structure, as already noted. Because of these differences, it is well to regard each type, or element, of the nervous reactions as intrinsically different from the other types of nervous reactions. For every nerve impulse, as we have seen, consists simply of energy already stored within the cell ; and if the cells differ essentially one from the other in structure and organization, the energy released during their excitation must similarly differ. The motor nerve conduction, for example, is much more rapid, and less subject to synaptic interference than is sensory nerve conduction ; while connector nerve conduction is most diffuse, and most of all subject to synaptic modification. It is enough, however, as far as psychology goes, to realize that these differences exist. It is for neurology to trace out the exact character and meanings of these differences.

Psychonic Reactions

The precise nature of the reaction of the synaptic tissue, or psychon, is not known. It depends of course upon what ultimately turns out to be the structure of the synapse. If the psychon really consists of minute threads of protoplasm, as the continuity theory maintains, then the release of energy within each synaptic neurofibril, or psychon, must resemble in nature the release of conductive energy within the individual neurons which are joined by the synapse. If, on the other hand, the contact theory of synaptic juncture is correct, a totally different type of reaction may occur at the psychon. If the cell membranes are the essential elements of the psychon, then psychonic conduction may resemble more nearly the excitation of an electrode by an electric current. The energy released from the psychon may be comparable to the setting up of a magnetic field. It is too early, as yet, to state any theory of the psychonic reaction with definiteness or assurance. We must await further evidence.

It is very clear, however, that three groups of psychonic reactions must take place whenever any reflex circuit is completed. The sensory centres are first excited. The degree and pattern of this excitation determines the lines of connector nervous reactions to follow. Then the connector centres must receive the excitation and react in kind. This set of psychonic reactions in the connector centres, in turn, will determine the ultimate connector paths to the motor centres. Here a third group of psychonic reactions must occur, leading to the final efferent nerve reactions, which eventually instigate bodily reactions in the effector organs. It would seem that the order in which these three types of psychonic reactions occur is more or less strictly determined by the structure and organization of the central nervous system. The sensory psychonic reactions always occur first ; the connector psychonic reactions second ; and the psychonic motor reactions third.

It will be made clear in a later chapter (that on Consciousness) that the total phenomena which comprise or accompany the three types of psychonic reaction seem quite radically different, one from the other. Suffice it to say, at this point, that the sensory psychonic reactions appear to determine the quantity and pattern of sensory stimuli which are to determine the entire unit response to follow. If any stimulus, or any portion of a stimulus situation fails to find representation in the ultimate pattern of nervous conduction impulses sent forward by the sensory centres, then the portion of the stimulus left out, has no part in determining the balance of the nervous and bodily responses to follow.

The connector psychonic reactions appear to determine which relationships between the incoming stimulus pattern and the already existing sensory pattern of psychonic excitations, and which relationships between different parts of the incoming stimuli, registering upon different types of sense organs in different regions of the body, shall play a determining role in fixing the pattern of motor part-reactions to follow. This is a long, complex statement. But the idea of the psychonic connector reactions' function is really simple If it were possible, for example, for reflex excitement to pass over directly from the sensory centres to the motor centres, then the sensory pattern would come into immediate *action* relationship with the constant bodily activities already going on. The sensory excitement caused by the new stimulus would tend to arouse certain new activities, and these new actions would have to fight it out with the ones already going on in the motor centres. The relationship between the new sensory excitations would have no opportunity for playing a part in determining the final unit response. It might be, for instance, that the sight of a train rushing down the track toward you, when you were walking on another track, would cause sensory excitement which would in itself overwhelm the motor activity of walking, which was already going on. But suppose the sensory excitement caused by the onrushing train is first correlated, or connected with, the previous sensory picture of the two tracks, and the distance between the track over which the train is rushing and the track you are walking on. Then that relationship between the two sets of sensory data itself plays a determining part in your unit response, before your motor centres or existing reactions are effected in the least by the new stimulus.

If the relationship between train-track and walking-track can be fairly represented by the word " safety ", then your unit response to the train may result in no more change of bodily movement than a raising of your head to look at the train as it roars past you. If the connector part of the unit reaction had been dropped out, you would probably have leaped off the track with all your might and would, perhaps, have emitted a " startled " yell. The unit response that psychology is interested in, remember, includes the sensory train-excitement, the comparison or correlation of this with the sensory walking-track excitement, and the final motor element in the response resulting from the first two elements of psychonic reactions.

It may, apparently, happen sometimes that the connector centre element of psychonic response is minimized or dropped out altogether. Herrick tells us of mid-brain neurons which send dendrites to connect with both visual and auditory centres. If these be excited simultaneously, therefore, the resolution of impulses takes place within the single neuron, and a simple facilitation of one or the other sensory group only, can thus be effected. The neuron then communicates its total sensory excitement directly to the motor centre in which its axone terminates. The motor centre must then change its activity in accordance with the direct relation between this new element of motor excitement, and that previously going on in the centre. This type of unit response is obviously less efficient and less complete than the type containing psychonic connector reactions.

The motor psychonic reactions appear to determine how the constant, or " self " pattern of activity natural to the organism, is going to be modified to meet the incoming pattern of stimulus excitement. Here we begin to get close to the final bodily reactions which we can see and measure. But still we must remember that the psychonic reactions within the motor centres must *precede* and *predetermine* the final bodily reactions. A good part of the motor excitement which played a leading role in the psychonic motor reactions may be defeated and inhibited within the motor centres. That part of the psychonic reaction, therefore, will find no direct representation whatsoever in the final bodily reactions. During a dominance response of the baby's hand, for example, the previously existing motor centre energy which was expressing itself in a grasping tension of the fingers is *increased* to combat the new motor energy forced into these centres by the stimulus of trying to force open the infant's hand. The motor psychonic reactions in the motor centres include both increments of motor energy and a conflict between them. But the final bodily reactions consist simply of a tightening of the fingers, i.e. an increase of the previous activity. The conflicting element in the psychonic response has been eliminated before it reached the bodily response mechanisms at all, and the bodily reactions only show some traces of the motor energy increase whereby this result was accomplished. In " mental " struggles and decisions of adults, it may frequently happen that not even this increase of natural activity shows in the final bodily responses. The adult may smile calmly, or keep a perfectly straight face, and only minor visceral, " involuntary " leakages of the increased self activity may seep through into the final bodily reactions.

In summary, then, we have three types of psychonic reaction participating in completed unit responses of the reacting organism. First comes the psychonic reaction of the sensory centres ; then the psychonic reactions of the correlation centres ; and, finally, the psychonic reactions of the motor centres. Can one of these psychonic reactions occur in the absence of the other two ? Very possibly sensory centre psychonic reactions may occur without any connector or motor centre activity to follow. It seems probable, also, as above suggested, that sensory centre activity may be followed immediately by motor centre response, without connector centre excitation intervening. It does not appear possible, however, that motor centre response could occur, under natural conditions, without sensory centre reactions preceding, because otherwise there is no natural method of communicating neural excitement to the motor centres. There exists, in short, a causal and time sequence imposed upon the three types of psychonic reaction by the very structure of the central nervous system. The sensory reactions must occur first, the connector centre reactions next, and the motor psychonic reaction is causally dependent upon its predecessor.

We must not think of a given sensory centre reaction as being invariably followed by the *same* correlation centre or motor centre excitations, however. Different types of unit responses require different connections between different individual centres. Sensory centre A might be connected with correlation centre B and motor centre C, during a certain unit response ; while upon another occasion, sensory centre A might be followed by reactions in correlation centre X and motor centre Y. This is still another reason why it is not safe to think of simple, structurally determined, reflex arcs existing as fixed units out of which the whole nervous system is composed by combination of the simple units. Only the outlying portions of each unit response are in the least degree kept constant, in this fashion, by the structure of the nervous system. The pupillary reflex, wink reflex, knee jerk, etc., may occur as minor parts of various unit responses without varying very greatly. The outlying reflex connections, upon which these reflexes depend, possess very little, if any, flexibility. The same outlying afferent synapse must always excite the same outlying efferent synapse, whatever else it does. But the major portion of the unit responses which include these inflexible units are exceedingly variable, and are almost never twice connected through the higher centres of the brain in just the same way.

Referring back to our automat illustration, again, we may explain the matter thus. Suppose, when you dropped the proper number of coins in any machine a little signal light immediately showed itself. Then nothing more seemed to happen for a while, though the internal, hidden machinery was grinding away. Then, at last, the pudding machine lifted up its food-containing cylinder, whirled around, dropped into place again, and opened its door to present you with a rice pudding. The sandwich machine, simply unlatched its door and dropped a sandwich within reach. The coffee machine let flow exactly a cupful of coffee, and so on. The final observable responses of these machines turned out to be very different. And, of course, the operations of the inner, hidden machinery whereby these final responses were produced must have been different too. But, in each case, an identical signal light flashed on, the moment you shot your coin into the slot. Would you think it logical to suppose that the internal workings of these machines were just as simple, and just as similar as the signal light response common to all? No, the hidden machinery must have been quite different, in each case, to produce different results. All the machines were connected up with the same signal light and this light informed you that the inner reactions of each different machine were under way.

Now in just the same way, the total unit responses of the human organism are quite different, one from another. These differences begin *after* the outermost reflex reactions have taken place. The simple, fixed responses like the signal light, are always the same. But the inner, hidden reactions, and the final results of all the reactions combined in a unit are very different indeed. In the human machine, the internal differences are achieved, not by physically different machines, as in the automat, but rather by a single machine, not fixed in its internal workings, but capable of switching itself about inside, and so working sometimes as a coffee-giving machine, sometimes as a pudding-giving machine, and so on. This internal self-switching mechanism is radically different, in principle, from the simple relatively fixed machine connections that produce the outlying reactions, or signal lights, which are the least important parts of the whole unit performance. The signal-light reflexes, with a minimum of synaptic connections, are the only portions of the total unit response which are relatively fixed and invariable.

Summary

Let us take a completed unit response, and list in order of their occurrence all the different varieties of reaction which compose it.   It is well to have in mind a very concrete picture of just what goes on between environmental stimulus and final bodily responses.

For illustration, let us take the sun shining on the subject's face as a stimulus, and follow the chain of reactions which result.

Subject : A girl sitting on the beach, talking to a man, her hat in her lap.
Stimulus : The sun shines upon the subject's forhead.

1. Bodily Reaction, Class A.	The skin temperature rises, oxidation (burning) begins, the skin tightens and dries.
2. Bodily Reaction, Class B.	The rising temperature causes physiological changes in the warmth receptors in the skin ; the tightening causes changes in the pressure receptors in the skin ; the burning and drying causes changes in the pain receptors of the skin.
3. Nervous Reaction, Class A.	The afferent neurons connected with warmth, pressure, and pain receptors of the forehead become excited. A stream of nerve impulses begins to travel inward along these neurons, starting in the dendrites, passing to the cell bodies, and then along the axone fibres.
4. Psychonic Reaction, Class A.	The sensory centres in the brain for warmth, pressure, and pain become simultaneously excited as soon as a sufficient number and intensity of afferent nerve impulses impinge upon the psychons which connect these centres with connector neurons travelling still further into the brain. The new excitations are compounded with excitations going on as part of the total activity pattern.
5. Nervous Reaction, Class B.	The connector neurons, leading from the three sensory centres already excited to various correlation centres, become excited. Nerve impulses begin to travel along these connector neurons, toward the correlation centres.

6. Psychonic Reactions, Class B.	One or more (probably several) correlation centres of different lobes of the brain become active. Probably many thousands of synapses in all, are excited, the psychon in each synapse making new connections between the nerve impulses which impinge upon it, and other neurons not yet excited. New excitations are compounded with those going on before new connections are made.
7. Nervous Reactions, Class C.	More connector neurons which are in contact with the correlation psychons, give rise to nervous impulses. These neurons conduct their impulses toward the motor centres.
8. Psychonic Reactions, Class C.	The psychons in one or several motor centres of the brain become excited as the nerve impulses from the correlation centres impinge upon them. New excitations are compounded (integratively)˙ with excitement already going on as part of natural constant action pattern of the organism before final connections are made with outward bound neurons.
9. Nervous Reactions, Class D.	A number of outgoing, or efferent nerve trunks each containing a large number of individual motor neurons, receive excitations from the motor centres with which they connect. These motor nerve trunks carry their batteries of nerve impulses outward, away from the central nervous system toward the muscles of the girl's arm and shoulder.
10. Bodily Reactions, Class C.	The biceps, triceps, and other appropriate muscle fibres in the girl's right arm and shoulder shorten, exerting certain delicately adjusted and correlated leverages upon her fingers, wrist, forearm, upper arm and shoulder.
11. Bodily Reactions, Class D.	The girl's fingers grasp her hat, lying in her lap, turn it right side front, and then her hand moves upward

and her fingers adjust her hat on her
head at such an angle that her fore-
head is protected from the hot sun.

All this complex mass of reactions is absolutely necessary
to complete the single, though compound, unit response of
dominating the opposition stimulus, sun's rays. (This unit
response is compound because it contains simultaneous
compliance response toward the hat as we shall have occasion
to note in a later chapter.)

One other point about this series of reactions may be noted
in summary. The final unit response of putting the hat on
the head represents the resultant of the excitations evoked
in the organism by the stimulus, and the excitations already
going on in the organism evoked by the body itself and its
constant stimuli setting up the self-action pattern. This
resolution of the self and the stimulus activities does not take
place in the nervous reactions as far as we can tell because
different neurons are probably excited by the stimulus than
those already conducting impulses in the self-action pattern.
Moreover, if the same neurons are used, facilitation and interference occur in the synapses. The resolution takes place
in the synapses in the course of the three classes of psychonic
reactions, sensory, correlative, and motor.

These three types of psychonic reaction, then, are the
reaction elements in the whole series that are most important.
They decide not only how the excitations aroused by the
stimulus shall be related one to the other, but also they decide
how these new excitations shall be related to (integrated with)
self activity. The psychonic reactions are the deciding factors
in the entire unit response. The psychonic reactions are the
ones, therefore, to which psychology is compelled to pay
attention.

CHAPTER VI

ACTIONS AND REACTIONS OF THE HIDDEN MACHINERY

IN the first three chapters of this book we looked at the human organism from the outside, and studied its fundamental modes of behaviour which we then termed elementary unit responses. We noted that despite the multifarious forms which specific reactions to environment might take, all these different responses might be analyzed into four elementary types called dominance, compliance, submission and inducement. Two of these elementary types of response, dominance and compliance, occurred whenever the environmental stimulus impressed itself upon the organism as antagonistic ; and the organism's responses of dominance and compliance in turn tended to move the organism in ways antagonistic to the stimulus. The other two elementary responses, submission and inducement, occurred when the stimulus was allied with the organism, and tended to move the subject into closer alliance with the object.

Dividing the four elementary responses another way, we discovered that dominance and inducement occurred when the stimulus appeared to be weaker than the organism ; and these responses further tended to increase the organism's own activity which was directed toward asserting superiority over the stimulus. The other two elementary types of response, compliance and submission, were evoked, we observed, by stimuli perceptibly stronger than the organism ; and these responses decreased the organism's activity in such a way as to enable the stimulus to control it more effectively.

So much for the unit behaviour of the human organism looked at from the outside, with no insight as to how these final behaviour results were brought about by the various interacting mechanisms inside the organism. These inside mechanisms, hidden from the casual observer's view within the body, we termed the hidden machinery. In Chapters IV and V

141

we attempted to describe the hidden machinery of the human organism and to list in order its inter-communicating cog-wheels or part reactions. We have now to put this hidden machinery together, as it were, and observe its various parts in harmonious motion. We already know from our outside observations of the human organism's elementary unit responses that the hidden machinery must bring about these responses when it is operating normally.

When we looked at human behaviour from the outside we noted two distinct elements : actions of the organism, and reactions of the organism. In other words, we noted that the organism is spontaneously active entirely regardless of the environmental influences which may happen to be playing upon it at any given moment. This spontaneous activity of the organism may be termed its *action*. We also noted that environmental influences caused certain changes in the action of the organism. These changes we call *reactions* or *responses*. The four elementary types of change in the organism's activity brought about by environmental influences we called the *elementary unit responses*.

It now concerns us to discover : first, the source of power which brings about the actions of the hidden machinery, and second, the elementary unit reactions of the organism which occur when environmental stimuli influence the actions of the hidden machinery.

A. Actions of the Hidden Machinery.

The " Self " and Its Role in the Unit Response.
In the preceding chapater we described in detail the structures which participate in reflex conduction and which may be thought of as the hidden machinery of unit response. We have set forth, in order, the different classes of reaction that must occur within the organism in order to complete a single unit response by means of this hidden, reflex, conduction machinery. We call attention once more to the fact that the reflex excitations caused directly by the stimulus to any unit response must meet and become integrated with the more or less uniform and constant reflex excitations set up by various inherent, spontaneously operating stimulus mechanisms within the organism itself. We have referred to this spontaneous, natural activity as " self-activity ", or the " self pattern of

action ". It may prove more convenient, in the long run, to term this factor in unit response simply the " self ".

There is some danger in reviving a term like " self " that readers will misunderstand the sense in which the word is used. For many generations, in fact from the very beginning of introspective psychology and philosphy, the term " self " was used to indicate some sort of ultra-physical entity, thought of as the soul or inner immaterial being of the human individual. Of course we intend no such connotation. The " self " as we shall use it, and as one of the present writers has already used the term in a previous volume,[1] means simply the constant inescapable increment of reflex activity which characterizes all human beings and animals in which psychology is interested.

This " self " is a dynamic, automatically regulated pattern, or organized flow of reflexly conducted energy, which makes the organism move spontaneously, keeps it constantly active no matter what environment it may happen to be in, and forms the background or reservoir into which further reflex activities are poured by innumerable environmental stimuli. The pressure of this self reservoir of activity seems to determine, for the most part, the ultimate form and pattern of unit responses. When such is not the case, when the environmentally instigated activity overwhelms the self activity, and assumes arbitrary control of the unit response, then we find conflict, and internal breakdowns of the reflex machinery with inefficient and incomplete unit responses.

The reflexly conducted activity constituting the " self " as we propose to use the term, is initiated and carried forward in precisely the same way that the reflex activity initiated by environmental activity is carried on. The self activity is initiated by physiological and physical influences of the various bodily tissues, organs, and secretions upon sense receptors and their surrounding tissues, causing Bodily Reactions, Class A, as detailed above. Afferent, connector, and efferent reflex excitations follow, as we have already noted, and finally the effectors are moved, and the bodily parts correspondingly affected. There is no difference whatsoever in the reflex mechanism from start to finish between the self activities and the environmentally initiated activities.

How, then, can we differentiate self activities from the others ? By one criterion only. *Reflex activities composing*

[1] Marston, W. M., *Emotions of Normal People*, New York, 1928, p. 93.

the self originate from stimuli manufactured exclusively by the subject organism, without reference to its state of adjustment or adaptation to environment. For instance, the constant tension or tonicity of the muscles of stomach and intestines is part of the self, because there is a reflex activity which originates in the actions of certain hormones (see endocrine glands) upon the tissues of the alimentary canal, and so upon the sense organs contained therein. But the much stronger, peristaltic (caterpillar) movements of stomach and intestines during digestion are not part of the self, since these movements are reflexly instigated by pressure of food within the canal. The digestive movements are unit responses, representing the composite integrations of self and food-initiated activities.

It will readily be seen that the self is not fixed or invariable by any means. We have referred to the self activities as " constant ", but we must amend that idea by saying " relatively constant ". The organism varies its own condition from time to time, and it possesses certain periodic activities like hunger and erotic activities, that are present only at certain times and not at others. Moreover, the organism passes through a predetermined life cycle, developing new structures and tissues up to a certain point, called maturity, regenerating its tissues at varying rates for a number of years thereafter, and then starting down hill again in its physiological functioning during senility. The self, or background of spontaneous activity, then, may be expected to change partially at frequent periods during each day and month. It may be expected to change very radically at different developmental milestones in the organisms' life cycle ; babyhood, childhood, adolescence, maturity, old age.

Let us attempt at this point to put together a rough review of some of the most characteristic spontaneously initiated activities that go to make up the psychological " self ", as we propose to term it.

Genetic Stimulus Mechanisms and the Reflex Activities They Cause.

The intrinsic energy of the adult organism can be said to be generated even before conception. The parent cell, that is, the spermatozoa in the male and the ova in the female, are part of a continuing stream of living protoplasm which has persisted generation after generation, presumably antedating even the appearance of man as such. These living tissues are so highly energized that their activities continue both in the perpetuation of their own type of cell structure in the new organism, and in the development of other specialized tissues which go to make up the more transient individual life processes. Of these two classes of cell differentiation, the sex cells are continuous to the next generation, and even the other cells do not escape the original impetus initiated by the parent cells until they have attained complete maturity. This means that within the organism there is always a constant source of activity of genetic origin. It should be understood that this activity maintains a constancy of rate or kind. Some of the cells, as they develop, have a far higher energy value than others. Thus the muscles and glands are more active actually and potentially than the connective tissue which sustains them. The connective tissues in turn are energy centres of a higher rate of activity than the bone structure.

We have said that the energy value of living cells increases up to maturity. This is best illustrated by the development of the nerve cells. In about the third month of uterine life the primitive nerve cells, known as neuroblasts, develop. These neuroblasts show a cell body with embryonic processes, but the total structure is more simple than that of the mature neuron with its branching dendrites and long sheathed axones. The neuroblasts are not able to contact each other. It is said that when the uterine period is half over the number of nerve cells is complete although very few cells have attained their mature form at this time.

A few months later, at birth, many systems of neurons have developed sufficiently to permit the integration of the vegetative functions and certain gross muscular co-ordinations. The cells of these systems are by no means mature. They can still grow in length and in girth and by increasing the number of connections with other cells. This leaves millions of other neurons still to be accounted for. Some of these cells begin their time of growth immediately. Others, as far as we know, are never mature in some respects since sufficient modification at the synapse to permit contact with other neurons does not take place. In general, the energy arising from cell development and its consequent effect upon the activities and potentialities of the individual is due to changes in size of the neuron, the elongation of fibres and the development of sheathes, the approximation of one neuron to another, and the modification of synaptic resistance.

The genetic influence on reflex activity is widespread. The infant does not sit up until his leg and back muscles are sufficiently co-ordinated to support his weight and impulses from the semi-circular canals are sufficiently correlated with muscular tensions to keep him from falling over. The same applies to walking. The child is not functionally ready to support his own weight, stand upright, balance, keep the soles of his feet on the ground, keep his legs close together,. flex the knees at just the right angle, until he is about eleven months old. Even then the skill comes gradually with the development of the bodily structures. Handedness is not definitely defined until the infant is about a year old. Skills and aptitudes, when very marked, may be evidenced by excellent motor co-ordination at a very young age. But the special outlet is usually not sought until the child is about seven or eight years old. Other activities, particularly the reflexes and conditioned reflexes going to make up sexual behaviour, do not begin to make their appearance until puberty, while the final pattern is not completed until the early twenties.

On the negative side certain activities of childhood are cut off as the body matures. This is particularly so in the case of certain endocrine activities. The thymus gland, for instance functions until puberty, growing gradually larger until it reaches a maximum at adolescence, after which time it atrophies. This gland is supposed to hold in check the differentiation of sex characteristics until physical maturity has been attained. If it continues to function for longer than a normal period, the individual retains many of the physical characteristics of childhood. A similar atrophy occurs in the case of the pineal gland when the individual reaches the approximate age of thirty.

The maturing of the organism obliterates certain reflexes which are present at birth. The fan-like spreading of the toes tends to disappear when the infant is about a year old. The so-called grasping reflex is superseded at about the age of four months. Dribbling subsides at about the end of the ninth month, a fact which indicates the attainment of proprioceptive control over the jaw muscles by the cerebellum. There are known variations in the receptor thresholds which have a genetic origin. There are, for instance, many more taste receptors in the tongue and mouth of a young child than there are in that of an adult. Thermal sensitivity also seems to be more acute during childhood. Many other examples could be cited, but these are sufficient to demonstrate the effect of various developing structures upon the reflex activities of the individual.

Mechanical and Physical Stimulus Mechanisms Resulting in Reflex Activity

If it were possible so to regulate the environment that it stimulated the body evenly; that is, if sound were at a minimum, if pressure were even at all points in the body, if odors and all noxious stimuli were eliminated, if the mouth were tasteless—if all these and similar external factors could be maintained so that no change from the environment would interrupt the constant tonic flow and register sensory impressions, it is nevertheless a fact that very nearly every type of receptor would still be stimulated by the physical changes going on within the organism itself.

The body is a hollow filled with fluids. It has weight, and so must oppose the forces of gravity. Its muscles contract and expand. Tension occurs in its tissues. The liquid contents press outward on the walls of the various organs and institute pressures. The bodily functions result in the creation of heat. In short, practically every known force familiar to the physicist is at work *within the body* stimulating the internal receptors. The activities arising from these stimulations constitute the greater part of the basic self activity which either gives in to or conquers phasic impulses from the environment. In the attempt to understand human behaviour as a series of unit responses, it is very necessary to inquire into the possibilities of this type of stimulus as a cause for constant organic activity.

Semi-Circular Canals.

It will be remembered that the semi-circular canals of the inner ear are filled with a liquid which presses upon the sensory tissues of these structures. If the pressure were the same at all times, probably no consciousness of this stimulation would be present. But it varies with the slightest movement of the head and body. The result is increased pressure at some points, decrease of pressure at others; the point of focus always determined by the pull of gravity upon the fluid involved. Because of excitations aroused by the constant change in the pressure of the fluids, we are aware of corresponding changes in the position of the body and are thus enabled to stand erect and to maintain our equilibrium whether running, walking, swimming, or what not. It will be noted that deaf mutes having these structures impaired, are not able to tell whether they are swimming down from the surface of the water or coming up for air. With the semi-circular canals intact this difficulty is not encountered.

Dilation of Blood Vessels

If one were warm, in a comfortable bed, not hungry, and asleep, it would be found that the blood pressure, although slightly below normal, would maintain about an even level. What happens, however, when we wake up ? If it is a sun-shiny morning, and we can smell the coffee percolating, hear the sausages sputtering in the pan, and receive other sensory impressions of a good breakfast in progress, under usual conditions we get up feeling moderately gay, active, and ready for a good day's work. Our blood pressure rises immediately, thereby altering the tensions in the smooth muscles which are found in the arterial tissue and arousing the sensory centres. These are so connected with the muscles and glands that the result is a feeling of bodily warmth. At the same time, if our adrenals are at all active, and we have faithfully performed our morning exercises, certain hormones are let loose in the blood stream which send greater nutriment to the skeletal muscles. We say we feel full of pep and vigour, a statement which represents an actual balance of internal activities precipitated initially by the increased tension of the dilated arteries.

Similar variations in pressure occur all during the day as a result of variations in hormone precipitation, ingestion, digestion, increase or decrease of muscular work, variations in emotional states, marked changes in external temperature and attitude, making the pressure changes in the walls of the veins and arteries a source of constant stimulation of reflex activity.

Variations in Smooth Muscle Tensions

Changes in tension of visceral muscles, either by the endocrines or automatically as a result of their own cyclic activity, stimulate a wide series of reflexes. The hunger contractions of the stomach constitute one important type. It has been experimentally determined that hunger sets up a general restlessness and a speeding up of all motor and even cerebral functions. The patellar reflex is speeded up appreciably when the individual is hungry. He tends to move his arms and legs and head and, for a while, to engage in similar undirected somatic movements. During hunger, mental processes are also quickened, speech becomes more fluent, and reaction times faster.

Tensions in the pharynx induce sensations of thirst with compensatory reflex activity. Tensions in the tissue of the intestines result in the contraction of the longitudinal and spherical muscles with subsequent movement of the intestinal contents. Activity of the cells of Leydig and the corpus luteum brings about a dilation of the tissue of the genital organs with a tensing of the muscles which set up the sexual reflexes.

Self Initiated Contractions of the Skeletal Muscles.

In our discussion of the receptors we described the end-organs to be found in the striped muscles, which are excited by changes in the contractile state of the muscle spindles. The presence of these receptors insures a constant minimum amount of tonicity in all skeletal muscles by a motor discharge back to the muscle itself, which results in further contraction. Sherrington demonstrates this self-contraction of the muscles by experiments on a decerebrate animal. If the animal is placed in a holder so that the limbs and tail receive no artificial support but maintain their attitude by means of tonic motor discharge only, forcible movement of the limbs in an opposite direction results in increased extensor contraction. When the pressure is removed the limb returns to a more extreme position than that in which it was originally held. If the afferent nerves from the rigid limbs are cut, the efferent discharge is diminished or abolished altogether, indicating that the enhanced contraction is aroused by stimulation of sensory fibres within the muscle itself.

Constant Auditory Activity

Reports are frequently received that deaf people are extremely annoyed because of the grinding noises they hear inside their heads. The possible sources of these noises are several. Vibrations may excite the auditory apparatus, working the jaw and facial muscles stimulates the muscles controlling the small bones of the inner ear which in turn relaxes the tympanum and sets up vibrations which result in hearing. The yawning reflex contracts the tympanum, and in so doing causes temporary deafness. It has also been experimentally shown that the contraction of the tympanum of one ear causes a reflex contraction of the tympanum of the other ear. Variations in the pressure of the air in the inner ear and atmospheric pressure on the outside are known to increase or decrease auditory sensibility according to the conditions present. These instances indicate that the ear is subject to a bombardment of stimulation from within as well as from without.

Regulation of Body Temperature

Body metabolism is a constant source of heat from within the organism. Some of this heat results from the digestion of food, but the largest source is that generated by the muscles in the course of their activity. The amount of heat generated is far in excess of what is needed for the efficient maintenance of body function. The unneeded increment is thrown off chiefly by the skin through evaporation and radiation, and, to some extent, by the lungs when cold air taken into the body is heated through the process of respiration. Heat is likewise lost when cold food is taken into the stomach, and when digested food is eliminated by the body.

The amazing thing about bodily temperature is that it remains normally in the neighbourhood of 98.6 degrees, Fahrenheit, in spite of the wide range of environmental temperature from the arctic regions to the equator. This constancy of temperature is found in all warm blooded animals. Cold blooded animals, like the fish, have a very high bodily temperature when they are in tropical waters, for instance, and a very low temperature when they are in cold waters. They apparently have no regulatory mechanism which keeps the body temperature at any one level. The preservation of a level of heat in warm blooded animals is due to vaso-constriction and vaso-dilation control by the central nervous system. When a warm blooded organism is taken into a very cold atmosphere, sensations of cold and pain from the skin are correlated with the vaso-motor centre which constricts the blood vessels on the surface and those just below the surface of the body. This diminishes the volume of blood exposed to the cold on the surface of the body, and increases the volume supplying the inner organs, thereby raising their temperature somewhat.

When the surrounding medium is too warm, the sensations of heat from the skin dilate the cutaneous blood vessels. The superficial circulation is increased thereby warming the skin, which gives off excess heat by radiation and evaporation of sweat. The vaso-motor centres also control the frequency and depth of respiration. In some animals, as the dog, this is an important method of lowering bodily temperature, the heated animal having from 150 to 200 respirations per minute, while the usual rate is about 28. Increase in bodily temperature is also centrally controlled by means of impulses from and to the muscles. The vaso-motor centres also activate the contractile response of the smooth muscles at the surface of the body. It has been found that if a warm blooded animal is anæsthetized, central control over body temperature is lost and he responds as a cold blooded animal does, that is, bodily temperature rises or falls according to the temperature of the surrounding environment.

Pressure of Secretions

A source of constant stimulation of a mechanical or physical sort is the pressure of internal secretions. The action of the duct glands in discharging their secretions to the organs of the body, sets up new reflexes in these organs and causes them to discharge their contents, as in the case of the stomach, intestines, and bladder. The pressure of secretions within the organs of the body must not be confused with the ductless gland secretions, since in the latter there is no physical sensation of pressure when they function. We are concerned merely with the organs which take care of the excretory functions.

Chemical Stimulus Mechanisms: The Endocrines.

There is no doubt that the ductless glands are constantly setting up a continuous stream of spontaneously initiated activity within the organism. How this reaction takes place is another question. There are two possibilities. One is that the endocrine secretions, or hormones, which circulate through the blood stream affect various tissues in precisely the same way that a motor nerve impulse of corresponding type would affect these same tissues. In the case of adrenin, for example, it is well known that this hormone produces the same effect upon viscera and muscle tissues as that produced by motor impulses discharged through the sympathetic branch of the autonomic nervous system. Some researches have tended to show that adrenin in the blood stream influences the nerve-muscle junction. The second theory assumes that the secretions absorbed by the blood stream are necessary for certain metabolic processes of the body, and that their effect is felt only in so far as they increase or decrease the efficiency of the other cells.

Thus, the thyroids are found to be necessary to nerve cell metabolism. Nerve cell metabolism has two aspects, the first involving the general health and nutriment of the cell, the second having to do with the generation of those products which are necessary to the propagation of a nerve impulse. Experiments where the thyroids have been wholly or partially removed show degeneration of the nerve tissue itself. In further support of the latter explanation it has been found that degeneration of the thyroid has a distinct effect upon the vascular system, modifying the usual reactions to temperature in such a way that the usual body temperature is not maintained but is quickly affected by the temperature of the surrounding atmosphere. It is probable that both types of endocrine influence occur. The first, that is, direct stimulation of the end organs, may be the means of insuring immediate effects to the muscles. The second probably effects the more subtle nerve tissue changes.

Taste and Smell

Under usual conditions the taste buds are always under stimulation by sapid substances, and the olfactory epithelium is with equal constancy under stimulation from the respiratory tract. If external stimulation could be completely eliminated from both types of receptors they would still continue to function ; the taste buds through excitation from saliva, and the chemicals of the mouth ; the olfactory tissue through bodily vapours coming to the nasal passage during expiration from the esophagus and mouth.

Basic Metabolism

There is also a possibility that each type of metabolism may directly stimulate afferent impulses which initiate reflex activity. Dashiell says (p. 31)[1] that " Energy is continuously being taken in with food and in other ways and it is released in activities of different sorts, especially in motions of the movable members. Spontaneous activity, then, may be primarily the expression of the metabolism of the organism ". And later, " The external agency, such as a bright light, an electric current, or a needle prick primarily effects liberation of energy stored up in nerve, muscle, gland and other tissues, and this takes the outer observable form of a bodily movement ". If these combined statements mean that an oversupply of stored potential energy is responsible for random movements, then the same may be said for every other type of activity discussed in this section on spontaneously initiated activities.

If, on the other hand, we understand that certain specific forms of metabolism result in reflex behaviour, then all genetic and chemical stimuli would fall within this class. The number could be specifically amplified beyond those already cited, as when carbon dioxide above the usual amount is generated in the lungs, and vagus afferent impulses set up reflex contraction of the bronchii; or when the chemical condition of the stomach during hunger directly arouses afferent impulses which result in hunger contractions. There is little doubt that fatigue products in the muscle reflexly induce a gradual slowing up which forces the organism to seek relief from further activity.

From this analysis it would seem that general metabolism has an underlying fundamental effect on spontaneously initiated activities and in some instances acts as the direct stimulus for releasing reflex action.

Nervous Mechanisms Especially Devoted to Self Activities

Recent neurological experiments tend to show that although the cerebellum is the great tonic centre, the brain stem and cortex also play a part in the maintenance of the constant tonic discharge which permits the human organism to function in spite of gravity, temperance, air pressure, and other forces

---

[1] N. F. Dashiell, *Fundamentals of Objective Psychology*, Cambridge, 1928.

constantly operative from within and without. The cerebellum, as we have said elsewhere, is the great "balancing brain ". "Its cortex ", says Herrick,[1] " seems to be a great reservoir of latent nervous energy which may be tapped for discharge into any neuro-motor apparatus as needed. Its stabilizing influence may be compared with the action of a gyroscope on a large steamship, insuring steady progress of the vessel in its course by compensating the buffeting of wind and waves ".

Sherrington[2] found that decerebrate rigidity, which closely resembles the normal unrestricted tonus, arises from proprioceptive afferent impulses and some cranial activity. He places this cranial activity in the bulb, since ablation of the cerebellum does not abolish the rigidity. Sherrington also says[3] that " we must admit that the cortical innervation, preeminently phasic though it may be, also is to some extent tonic ". Lashley[4] in supporting this view says " A normal function of the stimulable cortex is to supply a substratum of facilitating impulses which act in some way to render paths excitable by more finely graduated impulses ".

Importance of the Self in the Unit Response

The above description of the spontaneously initiated activities will suffice to dispel any notion that the nervous system with its receptors and terminals exists merely to provide a channel or telephone system whereby external influences may have their sway over the human organism. The many sources of spontaneous internal stimulation are constantly operative. They make up a unit of activity which any phasic impulse must either join or oppose. Since the genetic, mechanical, and chemical stimuli are about the same from one day to another, we can expect to find a constant stream of activity involving glands, muscles, tendons, joints, proprioceptive end-organs, and chemical receptors all over the body maintaining a large volume of activity which also varies but little from day to day. The effect of any phasic excitation

[1] C. J. Herrick, *Neurological Foundations of Animal Behaviour*, 1925, p. 242.
[2] C. S. Sherrington, *The Integrative Action of the Nervous System*, 1906, p. 302.
[3] C. S. Sherrington, *op. cit.*, p. 304.
[4] K. S. Lashley, " The Relation Between Cerebral Mass Learning and Retention," *Journal of Comparative Neurology*, August, 1926, vol. IV.

will therefore be the algebraic sum of all internal and external factors operative at the moment of excitation. *Thus, in psychology, as in any other science, reaction must be defined with reference to action.* And accurate description of behaviour cannot be made without due consideration of both factors.

It is not necessary to go very deeply into neurology, however, to understand that the self activities are already in more or less complete control of the reflex mechanisms when the environmental activities are superadded to them. The self, then, is the regulating, determining factor, with regard to the manner in which the new phasic activities shall be integrated into the total activity pattern. The self increases or decreases, opposes or allies itself with the phasic excitations, according to the relationship which the new activities assume toward those already in possession of the integrating centres.

Returning to our automat illustration, we may now see that the human machinery which grinds out unit responses to environmental coins dropped into it, is not a passive, inactive mechanism to begin with. It is, rather, an *already acting* machine. And a machine that is already going when you try to change its movement in some way, is a very different proposition from a machine which is not moving at all when you do something to it. The going machine is much more easily influenced in alliance with its previous motion ; but it is very much harder to influence in a direction contrary to its initial movements. There is a considerable momentum to be overcome. Moreover, new cog wheels, forced into gear with those already moving, may assume different relationships to them, and produce different final results of combined actions when the great mass of cogs with which the new ones must mesh, are already in motion.

We may now begin to understand why we get one type of unit response from a baby's organism when we forcibly hold his hand, which is already clenched, and another type of unit response when we press back his fingers when they are in a relaxed and limp condition. The same with the stomach, the intestines, and all other parts of the organism. If the tonicity (self activity) is already great, a unit response of one sort occurs ; if the tonicity is slight, a totally different type of unit response appears.

Actions of all eleven types detailed in the preceding chapter constitute the self activities. A unit response includes any new reactions, or changes of reactions of all eleven types that are caused by the environmental force impinging upon actions already occurring. Changes in self activities resulting from combination with activities originating outside the organism are termed *unit responses*.

After the environmental activity has been compelled to combine with the self activities in the sensory centres, however, it never appears again in pure or separate form. From that point on it is more logical and significant to think of the changes in activity as being parts of the *unit response*, which combines self and environmental part-reactions and possesses new characteristics not previously present in either reaction series.

Actions of the Hidden Machinery Constitute the Self

We divided this chapter, at the beginning, into actions of the hidden machinery and reactions of the hidden machinery. So far we have dealt with the actions of the hidden machinery in some detail and we have termed these actions, for convenience, the self. It seems worth while, in conclusion, to assume the bird's-eye point of view once more, before proceeding to a similarly detailed consideration of the reactions of the hidden machinery or unit responses.

The human organism is born already equipped with a set of reflex or intercommunicating mechanisms capable of setting the body in motion in different ways when adequately stimulated. The human organism also is natively equipped with a set of spontaneously operating stimuli, mechanical, physical, chemical, glandular, and genetic in nature which are adequate to stimulate the reflex mechanisms, and which actually do stimulate a large part of the reflex mechanisms constantly from before birth until after death. The human organism, therefore, by means of its reflex nervous machinery and its self activating stimuli driving this machinery, keeps itself in constant motion and activity throughout life. The human organism, in short, by the means thus described, *acts* constantly of its own initiative, regardless of all environmental stimuli whatsoever. These actions constitute the real human self.

In the next section we must consider how the self activities are modified by environmental influence.

B. Reactions of the Hidden Machinery

If we define *actions* of the hidden machinery as activity initiated by the organism's own stimulus mechanisms as explained in the last section of this chapter, we may define *reactions* of this same machinery as activity initiated by all stimuli having their origin in the environment. Since the actions of the human machinery are relatively constant, reactions of the same machinery must consist essentially of modifications in the machinery's actions. In other words, when environmental stimuli impose their influence upon the human machinery which is already in motion, the machinery reacts by modifying its movements in ways adequate to allow for the environmental influence and still continue functioning in the same general way as before.

According to the integrative basis of psychology proposed in the present book, the already moving machinery of the human organism has four elementary or primary methods of combining its actions with the new influences to activity imposed upon it by environment. We assume that new activities are set up by a passing environmental stimulus in the same integrative machinery consisting of nerves and connecting psychons which is already being kept active by the organism's own stimulus mechanisms.

Elementary Unit Responses

This new activity, in the first place, may prove antagonistic to the self activities already going on, and the new activity may be superior in volume or intensity to its opponent. In such case those self activities which conflict with the new environmentally imposed activities must *comply* or give way to the new activities. The compliance reaction combines old and new activities in a reaction which weakens the self activities and permits the new activations to control whatever reflex paths may best suit their direction tendencies.

The dominance response combines old and new activities in a reaction where self activities assert themselves by increasing their intensity or volume and thus compelling new activities to comply with self activities. In this form of reaction the self activities are actually increased and remain in unaltered control of the integrative channels of the organism.

The unit response of inducement occurs in the situation

where the self activities are stronger than the new activities as in dominance.   But the two sets of activities are in alliance with one another instead of being in conflict.   The inducement reaction combines new and old activities in such a way that the new activities are induced or attracted into the same reflex channels as those already activated by the actions of the organism.

The response of submission occurs when old and new activities are in alliance with new activities in command of the integrative situation.   Self actions are weakened to permit new activities to induce or attract self activations into new channels of reflex activity.

The Role of Part Reactions in Unit Responses

In a previous volume one of the present authors has attempted to show in some detail the integrative mechanisms of the four primary unit responses as far as these occur in the motor centres of the organism and without reference to sensory and connector centres.[1]   These motor centre integrations must be regarded from the view point of the present volume as motational part reactions in the total unit response. While it seems unnecessary in the present volume to repeat the detailed consideration of primary motor integrations just mentioned, it is still essential for our present purposes to consider briefly the roles which sensory and connector part reactions play in the total unit response.

According to our present view of the data at hand, any or all of the three principal part reactions in any unit response may be compliant, dominant, inducive, or submissive in type ; and there seems to be no factual reason why part reactions of different primary types may not be combined in a single unit response.

Let us consider for a moment the biological functions which the three types of integrative part reactions serve to perform. In primitive animals below the evolutionary level of the coelenterates the sensory-muscular response apparatus is not selectively differentiated.   The animals' reactions to environment are correspondingly crude.   The sensory apparatus is incapable of establishing clearly or definitely the animal's relationship to a given stimulus.   In the same

[1] W. M. Marston, *Emotions of Normal People*, p. 94 ff.

way the neuro-muscular apparatus is incapable of moving the animal in such a way as to bring about definitely a new and effective relationship to environment. This primitive type of organism, in short, is influenced by environmental stimuli of many different varieties in much the same way. And it reacts to these different influences with the same vague, random types of bodily movement.

The integrative nervous system of human beings, however, is designed to register definite types of relationship between stimulus and organism and to bring about equally definite types of relationship between the organism and its environment by means of selective bodily movements. The integrative machinery in the human organism may be thought of first as sorting environmental stimuli into appropriately labelled pigeon holes. This is done in the sensory centres and synapses. Secondly, the integrative machinery recombines and evaluates the sensory stimuli which have been previously sorted out. This is done in the connector centres. Thirdly, the integrative machinery determines what movements of the organism are best adapted to establish efficient relationships with the sensory stimuli which have already been assorted and evaluated. And it forthwith initiates the selected bodily movements. This is done in the motor centres and synapses.

A bird's-eye view of any unit response, therefore, would show that it was controlled by three integrative part reactions. The sensory part reaction determines the relationship between the new activity set up in the organism by a sensory stimulus and the old activity already taking place in the same sensory centres under the influence of the organism's own self activated stimuli. In other words, the sensory part reaction determines the relationship between the environmental stimulus and the sensory self. The connector part reaction which occurs next determines the relationship between the combined relationships of all new activities caused by the total pattern of environmental stimuli influencing the organism and the combined relationship of all the old activities initiated by the organism's own stimuli. In other words, the connector part reaction in any unit response determines the relationship between the mental self and the thoughts engendered by environmental stimuli. The motor part reaction determines the relationship between the new bodily movements which would tend to be initiated by the new stimuli and old bodily movements which are brought about by the organism's own self-stimulating mechanisms. The motor part reaction determines, in short, the relationship between new tendencies to movement emanating from environmental stimuli and the already acting motor self.

As noted above, the three integrative part reactions in any unit response may be predominantly of any one of the four primary types of integrative combination previously discussed : or they may more likely consist of combinations of the four primary integration types. The sensory part reaction might be predominantly of one integrative type, the connector part reaction of another type, and the motor part reaction of still another integrative type. For example, a motorist driving along the boulevard at night perceives a red signal light set against him. He reacts to this light by removing his foot from the accelerator pedal and jamming on the brakes which stop the car. This is a typical, every-day unit response with its three integrative part reactions fairly well defined. The sensory part reaction consists of the subject's " seeing " the colour red. The visual part reaction, red, according to the integrative theory of vision suggested in a later chapter, actually consists of a response of submission on the part of the sensory self to the sensory activities caused by the red stimulus. The sensory part reaction, then, is predominantly submissive in type. But the connector, or mental, part reaction which immediately follows is of the sort described in a later chapter as " mental grasping " of the stimulus situation. The integration which comprises an act of mental grasping in the connector centres contains both compliance and dominance with dominance in the ascendancy. The mental part reaction, then, may be described as prevailingly dominant. Finally, the motor part reaction which alters the existing motor activity of the organism to suit an antagonistic stimulus situation is clearly compliant. The red " stop " signal produces a motational effect of compelling the driver to concede the superior strength of his antagonist, the Law. This motational attitude is predominantly one of compliance.

Analysis of the every-day unit response just discussed reveals three, more or less separate, part reactions of distinctly different primary types. The sensory part reaction was submissive ; the mental part reaction was dominant ; and the motor part reaction was compliant. Looking at the entire unit response as a whole, which type shall we call it ?   Shall we say it is submissive, dominant, or compliant ?   Or should we call it a submissive—dominant—compliant response ? Selection of terms cannot be too rigidly logical but must conform as closely as possible to every-day usage.   A casual observer of the motorist's behaviour would judge the type of his response, perforce, by the sort of bodily reaction which eventually resulted from the intricate and diverse reactions of the hidden integrative machinery.   The externally observable behaviour of the motorist would probably be classed as predominantly compliant in type.   In short, the bodily movements expressive of a given unit response seem to conform most closely in type with the motor part reaction just preceding.   The motor part reaction of the automobile driver in the response to the red light stimulus was prevailingly compliant, and this compliance was revealed immediately thereafter in his bodily behaviour.   Common usage, therefore, would seem to classify a given unit response according to the primary type of its constituent motor part reaction.   For convenience, therefore, and not for any other reason we propose to conform to existing habits of thought in this regard. Instead of terming the above analyzed unit response a submissive-dominant-compliant response we propose to refer to it merely as *compliant*.

Is there a Law of Natural Sequence between Integrative Part Reactions ?

The answer to this question must be highly speculative. Since the suggested designation of primary integrative reaction type is itself theoretical, the hypothecation of any law which might be supposed to determine their inter-relationship within the same unit response can only rest upon a doubly contingent basis.   In the illustrative unit response which we attempted to analyze above there appeared no indication of any logical sequence of part reaction types.   It is hard to imagine any a priori reason why mental dominance should have followed sensory submission or why motor compliance should have followed mental dominance.

The writers have actually classified in class and clinic many thousands of unit responses with their constituent part reactions.   Naturally, however, there is no assurance whatever that such classification is correct since it depends solely upon

M

the judgment of the observers without objective measurement or verification. Discussion of the possible existence of a law of natural sequence between part reactions in the same unit response must be based upon an entirely different class of data.

The only data at present available, with reference to the question under discussion, are the facts derived from neurological researches on the structure and organization of the central nervous system. The entire nervous system might be thought of as a funnel. The wide mouth of the funnel represents the receptor organ end of the reflex machinery and the small outlet end of the funnel represents the comparatively small number of final motor outlets. A tremendous number of sensory receptor organs are found scattered throughout the organism. The number of receptor organs for cutaneous sensations alone is estimated at more than five million and there exists, very possibly, a total of ten million visual receptor mechanisms. In all, we might estimate that some twenty-five millions of separate receptor organs exist, each organ capable of generating its own individual nervous impulse of origin. But this huge volume of separate impulses must be greatly reduced in numbers while passing through the integrative machinery of the central nervous system, because a comparatively small number of final motor paths exist. The original number of separate sensory impulses must be gradually reduced in the various integrative centres of the central nervous system in order to permit a smooth and unified outflow of motor energy to the muscles and glands which eventually are moved.[1] In summary, then, we find a very large number of sensory nervous impulses originated by the receptor organs of the body ; and we find the number of these impulses gradually reduced as the spread of nervous excitement passes through the integrative centres toward the final common motor path.

These general facts are doubtless familiar to every student of neurology, but their bearing upon our present problem requires further explanation. It is simply this. The gradual combination of sensory impulses of origin into large, inclusive units must inevitably change the relative superiority or inferiority of any sensory impulse with respect to the previously existing excitations of the nervous system in proportion as the

[1] C. S. Sherrington, *op. cit.*, p. 333.

integration concerned approaches the motor side of the central nervous system. A single sensory impulse evoked for instance, by a blue light falling upon the retina, might easily prove superior to the visual self excitations existing in the visual sensory centres ; but the reverse relationship might be expected to obtain when the same excitation of environmental origin reached the motor centres of the organism. The blue impulse would meet in the sensory centres a comparatively small number of visual self impulses which chanced to originate in neighbouring receptors and to be received therefore in the same outlying sensory psychons. But as the wave of blue excitation travelled toward the motor side of the nervous system it must encounter increasingly massive combinations of self impulses representing combined units of constant excitation derived from many different systems of nerves and psychons. Eventually in the motor centres the blue impulse reaction unit must meet a vastly greater mass of self excitation thus combined than that which it was forced to encounter in the outlying sensory centres.

In light of the above situation the logical suggestion presents itself that quantitative relationships of superiority and inferiority between incoming impulses and self impulses may very well become reversed as between the sensory centres and the motor centres of the integrating machinery of the central nervous system. This quantitative reversal could not be expected to change the antagonistic or allied character of the stimulus excitation. If a blue impulse, for example, were antagonistic to the sensory self in the visual centres it might be expected to remain still antagonistic to the self excitations in the motor centres. But although the blue impulse might prove superior in volume or intensity to the visual self the strength of its ultimate influence would be expected to diminish relative to the strength of the self during its final integration with self activity in the motor centres.

Assuming, for a second example, that a yellow visual impulse may be allied to the visual self it might be expected also to remain allied to the motor self. But if the yellow impulse in the sensory centres were inferior to the visual self the resulting integration might be expected to send a relatively stronger battery of impulses toward the motor side of the system since the sensory self which proved to be the prevailing influence already commanded open channels of discharge through the entire integrative machinery of the central nervous system. Therefore, when this excitation, originally initiated by the yellow impulse, reached the motor centres it would seem likely to prove superior in strength to the motor self already existing there. The yellow impulse, therefore, would have remained allied to the self throughout its integrative course, but would have changed its relationship of inferiority to one of superiority by the time it reached the motor centres.

On the basis of such a possible relationship between sensory and motor types of integration we might expect to find a general tendency toward the following sequences in types of sensory and motor part reaction.

Sensory Part Reaction	Motor Part Reaction
Dominance	Compliance
Compliance	Dominance
Submission	Inducement
Inducement	Submission

Even if such a law of sequence as above suggested actually exists we should only expect it to take the form of a general integrative tendency subject to frequent modification and reversal by reason of unpredictable integrative influences exercised upon motor centre integrations by previously existing excitation of the correlation centres. It seems of little value to consider the possible influences which correlation centres might be expected to exercise over the total sequence of integrative part reactions in any unit response since these correlation influences must be extremely diverse in type and must depend largely upon the previous intellectual experiences and training of the individual organism. The entire question of natural sequence of part reactions resolves itself into an ultimate issue of experimentation rather than speculation. If the law of natural sequence suggested above were used as an hypothesis for experimentation along this line, it should be tested only in stimulus situations where motor part reactions seemed likely to follow sensory part reactions as closely as possible with a negligible amount of connector or intellectual activity in the total unit response.

CHAPTER VII

DRIVES : PART I

HUNGER DRIVE AND THE COMPOUND UNIT RESPONSES OF DESIRE AND SATISFACTION

Drives of the Self

So far, then, we have discovered a single spontaneous, dynamic " elementary activity " of the organism ; and that is the *general movements* comprising the " self ". In addition, we have discovered four types of elementary unit responses, Dominance, Compliance, Inducement, and Submission, which really represent four different types of change in the general self movements as a result of environmental influences of different sorts. The self does not move spontaneously into these four types of unit response. It is driven into them by the action of environmental stimuli upon the organism.

Suppose, then, that it becomes necessary or biologically useful for the organism to evolve new and more complicated types of unit response toward various types of object in its environment. And suppose also that it becomes efficient for the organism to be *driven from within* to effect certain definite types of relationship with certain environmental objects and with other organisms of the same species. How are such results to be accomplished ? Must the organism depend upon chance stimuli, outside itself, to build up new unit responses by compounding the four elementary types of unit response already discussed ? Has the organism any other " driving " mechanism, within itself, besides the stimuli to general movement already considered ? Is there any inherent, self-activating, stimulus mechanism within the organism capable of " driving " it towards specific types of objects in the environment, and capable of building up new and compound unit responses toward these objects ?

It is quite mystical and improbable to suppose, as did the

165

early instinctivists, that an organism could inherit some occult sort of ability to seek out food, for instance, or another organism of opposite sex, and then act in an elaborate and predetermined way toward the selected object, all on its own initiative. It is easier and more probable to suppose, as do the modern instinctivists like Woodworth, that the organism inherits some sort of "action tendency" which is set off immediately upon contact with the appropriate object. But this idea still leaves a great deal unexplained. Just what is an "action tendency"? Where does its "drive", or spontaneous activity, come from?

Let us go back to first principles, again, and see if we can discover a method whereby the organism may be expected to drive itself toward specific types of object, and to build up new unit responses toward them. We have already found the organism determining its four most elementary types of unit response to environment by determining its own *self activity*. This, then, seems to be the basic principle of its self-determinative behaviour. If new types of unit response are to be built up, they must be built up on the same sort of principle. The self, in its most usual condition, causes the environmental activities to combine with it in the unit responses of Dominance, Compliance, Inducement, and Submission self changes.

If, then, other and more complicated unit responses are to be created toward special objects for special purposes the self must change its own activities in such a way that the special unit responses to be created will occur in response to stimulation by the special stimuli designated. In short, if the organism possesses special stimulus mechanisms to change the self periodically, then the changed self will respond with new and special unit responses as long as it remains in its changed condition.

Suppose, then, that the organism periodically generates stimuli of its own capable of changing the self while these stimuli are in operation. Suppose that the self in its changed condition reacts selectively to certain special types of environmental stimuli. Suppose, further, that the spontaneously changed pattern of self-activity is such as to keep the organism constantly moving in ways likely to bring it into contact with the specially selected stimuli. And suppose, finally, that when the changed self comes in contact with the special stimuli which it is driven to seek, its changed pattern of self activity causes it to react with new and special unit responses to the selected stimuli.

Then you have a real " drive ", an inner, self-determinative propulsion of the organism toward a selected type of environmental stimulus, and a new, self-originated ability to react to the selected type of stimulus in new ways, with new types of unit response.

A drive, then, according to unit response psychology, must be described as follows. The organism furnishes some new and specially designed type of stimulus. The receptors to which this special stimulus is applied, activate the reflex conduction mechanism in a new way. The self pattern of activity is changed in such a way that several results follow : first, the organism becomes incapable of reacting measurably to any type of environmental stimulus save the type selected as object of the drive ; second, the organism's spontaneous activities are greatly increased ; third, when the object of the drive is encountered, the organism reacts to it with newly evolved unit responses, compounded by combining appropriate elementary unit responses, these new compound responses being determined by the changed pattern of self activity.

It is abundantly clear that two basic drives exist, each with its own peculiar stimulus mechanism, furnished periodically by the organism. These two are *hunger drive* and *erotic drive*. Hunger pangs furnish the special stimulus to hunger drive ; while menstruation, apparently, furnishes the stimulus to erotic drive (which seems to originate with the female, in man and the higher vertebrates, at least). In addition to these two basic drives, it seems fairly certain that we should include a third, the *procreation drive*, in both males and females. The initial stimulus mechanism for procreation drive seems to be the union of a pair of organisms, male and female. Yet the germ cells that begin to multiply rapidly after impregnation, are wholly spontaneous in their activities, and also completely determinative as to the nature of the stimulus that they apply within the body of the female. It seems necessary, therefore, to include procreation as a separate and unique drive, although it really represents a combination of hunger and erotic drives. Procreation, like the erotic drive, is one that originates with the female and affects the male secondarily, as a result of its initial modification of female activities and reactions.

We may now consider these three drives in turn, their stimulus mechanisms, and the compound unit responses that appear for the first time in the individual's behaviour during their occurrence.

Hunger Drive

The usual pattern of self activity calls for a preponderance of activity in the skeletal muscles, and a corresponding preponderance of action energy sent over the sympathetic branch of the autonomic nervous system to the blood vessels and glands that support and facilitate the actions of the skeletal muscles. The stomach and digestive tract, during this more usual condition of the self, receive some action energy, and a certain modicum, also, of blood supply and glandular secretions. But the balance of reflex activity is very clearly established in favour of the outside of the body, its heavy, striped muscles used in moving the limbs, and its supplementary effector apparatus contributing reserve strength in moments of great muscular exertion.

Now comes a sudden spasm of hunger pangs. These consist of stomach contractions, following one upon another, and usually becoming more severe and intense with each successive contraction. These hunger contractions, or pangs, are caused partly by a periodic, mechanical mechanism in certain outlying nervous system units called a " local automatism ", and partly by a chemical, or hormone, that appears in the blood when the tissues are in need of replenishing with fresh food materials. Later the subject of hunger pangs will be taken up further ; just now we are concerned with their effect upon the usual pattern of self activity. The first important point to emphasize, in connection with hunger contractions, is the fact that they are initiated by two influences emanating from the physiological processes of the body itself. In other words, the organism is furnishing its own stimulus to activity.

As soon as the hunger contractions are well under way, a measurable change occurs in the self pattern of reflex activity. The motor energy sent to the brain, and thence to the skeletal muscles, *increases*. The knee-jerk, measured by Carlson during hunger pangs, is found significantly increased. Blood pressure and blood volume in the limbs rise, *pari passu* with each individual hunger pang. The heart beat becomes stronger and more rapid. All these changes could be summarized by stating that the usual pattern of self activity has *increased* in intensity and volume.

When the stomach contractions of hunger become very severe, a new set of changes in the self activity appear. The blood volume in the limbs recedes and the systolic blood pressure drops somewhat. The attention of the person suffering hunger pangs can no longer be kept upon whatever he has been doing, no matter whether it be business or amusement. *The subject loses his ability to react to environmental objects other than food.* He becomes restless, and cannot think clearly. At the very height of each individual hunger pang, a small jet of salivary secretion is exuded through the salivary ducts. The blood supply to the stomach and intestines, also, and the various gastric secretions, are suddenly increased. This set of changes marks a radical alteration in the usual pattern of self activity. The ordinary balance is upset, and activity of the skeletal muscles is replaced by activity of the digestive viscera and the glands and blood vessels associated with the digestive tract. The ordinarily predominating part of self activity is increased, but so also is the ordinarily subordinate part of self action. And the usually subordinate portion of the self, that is, the digestive-visceral activities, is increased in proportion to the usually predominant portion, that is, skeletal muscular activity. All the self activity has *increased*, and the balance and pattern of self action has *changed*, so as to produce more activity, proportionately, in the stomach.

The result of this increase and change in the self soon becomes evident, either in adults or in new-born infants. The normal baby may have its first post-natal hunger pangs within two hours after birth. It immediately begins to cry. When the infant is a little older, it screams loudly when the hunger contractions grip its stomach, and it cannot be distracted from its howling by any of the toys that claim its interest and attention under other conditions. The normal adult, at the onset of hunger pangs, becomes inattentive to conversation with his friends, or to his reading or business. He becomes restless and irritable. He pushes his papers about, or paces about the room, or rushes off somewhere with an irrational excess of energy. He may not recognize the source of his restlessness and increased bodily activity for some tim⁚, but he cannot concentrate on anything until he does. Both infant and adult, when in the grip of hunger pangs, manifest *marked increase* of random movement and inability to continue responding to environmental stimuli that had previously held their attention.

We describe this compound unit response, in everyday life, by naming its emotional accompaniment. We call this compound response toward food, during hunger pangs, " desire ". Let us analyze out the two elementary unit responses of which desire seems to be composed.

The food, we observed, " gets a grip " upon the subject organism. This control of the organism by food can be made clearer by contrasting the reactions toward food during hunger pangs with the behaviour toward the same food when no hunger pangs are present. An old epigram states the matter quite clearly : " Hunger is the best sauce ". Many sorts of food are consistently rejected, by civilized people, merely because they never get really hungry enough for these foods to grip and control their responses. " Oh, I despise shell-fish ", or " I never eat raw vegetables ", are not uncommon remarks among city people. There is no special agreement, that we have ever discovered, as to the foods " despised " or " never eaten ". We have observed cases where various individuals consistently refused meats of all sorts, apples, bananas, grape fruit, any fruit with seeds or stones left in the fruit, oysters, clams, crabs, all fish as such, potatoes, carrots, butter, milk, coffee, tea, chocolate in all forms, all sweet candies with soft centres, etc., etc. These peculiarities of taste may have originated in some inherited peculiarity of the self, or, more likely, in some childhood experience or association. But in nearly all instances the individual will eat the food he " despises " with great eagerness if he is sufficiently hungry. We have obtained this result, in fact, in every case where proper experimental conditions could be maintained. Ordinarily, for some reason, the rejected food fails to get a grip upon the subject's organism, sufficient to make him respond to it. But the change in the self that occurs during hunger pangs, enables this same food to control the subject, and to force a response. Arctic explorers and persons lost in a wilderness eagerly chew bark, roots, unknown berries, and even their own leather boot straps, under the compulsion of cumulatively severe hunger pangs. Ordinarily, of course, they could not be persuaded to place any of these objects in their mouths.

Is this effect of hunger pangs limited to adults ? Is it, by chance, a " learned " type of response ? Undoubtedly the adult's distaste for various foods is very largely learned, and not native. But we see many evidences in the behaviour of young children, indicating that hunger pangs are frequently necessary to make them respond to food that they otherwise tend to reject. Once a child's sharpest hunger pangs are appeased, he frequently refuses to " finish " his food, much to the mother's displeasure. Children at play, who are not hungry, frequently refuse to come to meals when called ; although, if they suddenly become " hunger struck ", they leave their companions without ceremony and run home to demand food from mother or cook. In the behaviour of very young infants no proper contrast can be drawn between response to food during hunger pangs and at other times, since the baby sleeps most of the time, except when being fed, and shows little or no connected or organized response patterns except toward the bottle or breast. However, the converse effect of hunger pangs can easily be tested. A three-months old baby can be induced to respond to a rattle, or to a bright, moving toy, under ordinary conditions, but he is wholly unable to respond to these distracting stimuli when suffering from hunger pangs. Immediately upon presentation of food, however, the baby stops crying and moves mouth and lips in sucking movements. The food, certainly, has much more of an influence upon the young infant during hunger pangs than has any other stimulus ; and probably we may say that the food grips his organism more quickly and completely during stomach contractions of hunger than at any other time. It seems clear, on the whole, that learning is not an essential element in the control that food appears to exert over the behaviour of human beings and animals whose selves are being maintained in a modified " hunger " pattern by severe stomach contractions. Any sort of object with the slightest " food " characteristics gains instantaneous and undisputed control of the organism's major responses as long as severe hunger pangs continue.

The infant's howling brings him almost immediately to the

attention of any adults who may happen to be within hearing distance. The baby's crying can scarcely be termed *inducement*, for it constitutes about as disagreeable a stimulus to the ears of adults as any sound could. The infant's loud and unpleasant howling, however, *dominates* the nearby adults, who comply by bringing the baby his bottle. Or, if the infant's mother is feeding him from the breast, the howling interrupts whatever she may be doing and reminds her inescapably that it is feeding time. At all events, the baby's howling is a type of behaviour that tends to bring him into contact with the one thing he is then capable of reacting to—food. The adult's restlessness, similarly, takes him away from whatever he is doing and makes him move himself and his attention about, in a roving sort of way, which greatly increases the likelihood of his perceiving a restaurant or other place where food is dispensed. Food is the one object that he, also, is capable of reacting to while in the grip of hunger pangs.

This change in self activity, then, caused by the spontaneous stomach contractions of hunger, has three important aspects : first, it renders the subject incapable of responding to any environmental stimulus except food ; second, it greatly increases the random, spontaneous movements of the organism ; third, it produces a type of behaviour that tends to bring the organism into contact with food.

Now when food is actually contacted, so that it stimulates effectively the receptor organs of the organism, a new type of compound unit response immediately appears. We may describe this response roughly by saying that the food as a stimulus grips and controls the organism increasingly, while the organism, with all its increased energy, strives to grip and control the stimulus food. Carlson states that "in the new-born (baby) everything within reach goes into the mouth to be rejected or swallowed according to its chemical character or physical consistency ".[1]

Desire, a Compound Unit Response Combining Passive Compliance and Active Dominance

Can we describe this initial aspect of the compound unit response to food as one of those elementary unit responses

[1] A. J. Carlson, *The Control of Hunger in Health and Disease*, Chicago, 1916, p. 10.

already outlined in Chapter III ?   It would seem that control
of the organism's responses by a stimulus *opposed* to the self
in its given condition, so that the organism is compelled to
give up part or all of its reactions to other stimuli, constitutes
Compliance in its purest form.   We have already noted that
food controls the hungry organism and compels it to give up
all organised forms of response to other stimuli.   We have
not, as yet, determined whether the trains of reflex reactions
set up by food stimulation in the subject organism, are allied
with or antagonistic toward the self activities.

They are antagonistic.   Sight, smell. and handling of food,
as well as taste, chewing, and swallowing have been proved
to *inhibit* the hunger pangs, and also to *reduce* measureably
the increased self energy sent to the skeletal muscles and
adjacent viscera, by antagonistic *inhibition* of self energy
(that is, by overcoming and cutting off reflex conduction of
self energy at the psychonic connections in the nerve centres).

Says Cannon, " The sensation (of hunger pangs) can be
momentarily abolished a few seconds after swallowing a small
accumulation of saliva or a teaspoonful of water " ; also,
" repeated swallowing results in continued inhibition ".[1]   And
Carlson also reports that during hunger experiments the sight
and smell of food placed close to the subject just after he had
been awakened, caused the hunger contractions to become
weaker and the intervals between them greater, within a few
minutes.[2]

Food, therefore, as a stimulus during the hunger condition
of the self, evokes reflex conduction energy within the organism
that is *antagonistic and superior in strength* to the self activity.
The self decreases and readjusts its pattern under the compulsion of its superior opponent.   This is a clear case of
Compliance response.   While the organism remains in a
condition of wholly unsatisfied *Desire response*, that is, before
any food has actually been brought into the subject's possession, the major portion of the Compliance behaviour, compelled
by food, consists of giving up other responses to other stimuli
and in *passively* permitting the food to retain its grip over
the organism.   No active effort is made to *increase* the antagonistic control that food is exercising over the subject's activities.
We may regard this type of Compliance response as relatively

[1] W. B. Cannon, *op. cit.*, p. 254.
[2] A. J. Carlson, *op. cit.*, p. 152.

passive. One element of the compound unit response of Desire, then, is the elementary unit response of *passive Compliance*.

Curiously enough, the other element in Desire response seems to consist of behaviour precisely opposite to that just considered. In proportion as food stimulation grips the hungry organism, the organism attempts, frequently with aggressive fierceness, to grip the food. If you try to take his bone away from a hungry dog, the animal is apt to attack you despite his customary docility. Have you ever sat down at table in the " cook shack " of a harvesting outfit ? If so, you have seen the hungry harvest hands attack both their food and each other in a manner very close to that of the hungry dog just cited. Most men, in fact, when in the grip of severe hunger pangs, " wolf " their food like animals and fiercely resent the slightest interference or delay in the placing of edibles within their reach. Women also, during the first few moments of eating, sometimes show somewhat similar behaviour.

Going back once more to the native, unlearned behaviour of young infants, especially boys, we find a very similar attack upon food. Take the bottle away from a ten weeks old baby for a few moments, before he has eaten more than an ounce of milk, and he immediately moves his hands and arms about, in a " frantic " sort of manner, makes fretful noises with his vocal cords, and frequently bobs his head back and forth with exaggerated sucking movements of mouth and lips. If you still withhold the bottle, he begins to cry with short, apparently purposeful howls. In another moment he begins to screech, and passes rapidly into " rage " behaviour, as described by Watson.[1] When the bottle is put back, close to his mouth, his random movements increase in intensity, while his screams give way to more purposeful movements of attack, vaguely directed toward the nipple. The baby's general fierceness during these responses, is in every way comparable to the fierceness of the hungry dog, the hungry harvest hands, or the hungry working girls. (Girls who are idle or who are not kept away from food for several hours by classes or office duties, tend to nibble sweets and fruit constantly, and therefore never appear in a condition of severe hunger).

What type of elementary response is this fierce attack upon

[1] John B. Watson, *op. cit.*, *Behaviourism*, 1924, p. 122.

food, or upon whatever obstacle separates the hungry person from food ? Clearly it is *Dominance response*. The food, as we have seen, evokes antagonistic activity within the organism. Only part of this antagonistic activity is of *superior* force to the self activity. The hunger pangs, it will be remembered, were able to alter the balance of motor energy as between the skeletal muscles and the viscera, only at the very height of the severest stomach contractions.[1] In the same way the activity aroused by food within the reflex conduction mechanisms of the body is, for the most part, *inferior* in strength to the self impulses ; only the peaks of food excitation excel the self energy in strength. Therefore, during moderate hunger condition of the self, with food not yet in possession of the organism, there exists a larger increment of food activity weaker than the self, than the increment of food activity stronger than the self. This large increment of food energy which is both *opposed to* and *weaker than* the self activity, furnishes a perfectly adequate stimulus to *Dominance response*. The self *increases* its energy, *antagonistically to the food*. This is a clear case of Dominance response.

Since the hungry subject does not stop with maintaining his control over the food not yet in his possession, but responds with an *active* effort to increase his dominance over the weaker food stimulus by actually possessing it, we may regard this type of Dominance as relatively active. The secondary elementary response element, therefore, composing Desire, may be termed *active Dominance*.

Desire may be defined, then, as a compound unit response, composed simultaneously of passive Compliance and active Dominance responses, both adequately evoked by the same stimulus. Hunger pangs, initiated by the organism's own, inherited stimulus mechanisms, change the self in such a way that :

(1) they prevent the subject from responding to any environmental stimulus except food ;
(2) they increase the self activities of the organism, and change their pattern so that the probability of encountering food is greatly enhanced ;
(3) they change the inner balance of reflex conduction activities of the self in such a way that food, acting as an environ-

---

[1] W. M. Marston, *op.cit.*, pp. 212 ff.

mental stimulus, evokes a new, compound unit response, consisting of

a. passive Compliance, and

b. active Dominance.

Thus does the auto-stimulated hunger " drive ", leaving little to chance or to control by the environment, first change the self activities in such a fashion that the organism is brought into contact with food, and then alter the reactions of the organism so that it must respond to food with Desire, a compound unit response moving the organism to possess food, and to eat it. The element left to chance or to environment is the existence of food near enough to the subject and in sufficiently available form to be contacted and possessed.

Satisfaction, a Compound Unit Response Combining Active Compliance and Passive Dominance.

But Desire is not the only compound response built up under the influence of hunger drive. Desire moves the organism to gain possession of food, to chew it, and to swallow it. All these operations of Desire, in turn, modify the self activities evoked by hunger pangs, and eventually remove the hunger pangs themselves. The self activity then returns, gradually, to its more usual balance and quantity. During this gradual re-alteration of the self activity, under the influence of the ingestion of food, brought about by Desire activity, a corresponding change creeps into the compound unit responses toward food. The Compliance with food gradually becomes more active. The Dominance over food gradually becomes more passive. When these changes in both the Compliance and Dominance elements of the compound unit response toward food, have reached the opposite extremes from those obtaining at the beginning, a distinctively new compound response may be recognized. This is termed, in everyday parlance, " satisfaction ", a name that is intended to describe the emotion experienced during this type of compound unit response. Satisfaction, once it appears, may continue until the hunger self has been wholly abolished and the organism's reaction to food virtually ceases because of satiety. Satisfaction may continue further, however, without any observable outward stimulus, until the process of digestion is well advanced. This continuance of Satisfaction response

actually constitutes a reaction of the pressure of the eaten
food against the stomach walls and to the continuance of
various salivary and other reactions to the taste and smell of
the food just eaten ; all this may go on for as long as twenty
minutes or half an hour after the meal.[1]

Even the harvest hand, or the hungry animal, after eating
a certain amount of food, begins to show less ferocity of attack
upon the meal. He begins to look about him, to converse a
little or show friendliness vocally, and to pick and choose
between the various foods at his disposal. After he has
continued to eat a little while longer, he may begin to dally
with his food, and to seek sweets or special delicacies. He
would still protest rather effectively, if anyone tried to take
his food away before he had entirely finished with it ; but he
is content with the possession already established, and his
eyes do not rove ravenously in search for more. In short,
he still reacts with Dominance toward his food, but no longer
seeks to establish greater Dominance than he already has
achieved. This new, and less agressive, type of Dominance
may be termed *passive* Dominance.

On the other hand the food itself gains more and more
complete control of the subject's responses. The food masters
the eater in precise proportion as it stimulates effectively his
taste and his smell receptors. The dog or man who " bolts "
his food may eat a vast quantity of meat or other resistive
material, and still show little or no diminution in the fury
of his dominant attack. But the more æsthetic person, the
gourmet, who savours each dish delicately and stimulates his
sensations to the utmost with the sight, flavour, and chemical
emanations (odours) of food while he is eating it, thus deliberately gives the food stimulus more and more complete control
of the organism's responses. The salivary flow is greatly
increased, the gastric juices are more freely released, and the
rythmic relaxations and contractions of the jaw muscles are
increased in number. The food is chewed more thoroughly
and is more completely mingled with digestive secretions.
All these activities represent progressive control by the food
over the organism's behaviour. The self energy, flowing
toward the skeletal muscles and the allied viscera, increased
by hunger pangs, is now progressively inhibited by the reflex
conduction activity evoked by food stimuli ; and the hunger

[1] *Op. cit.*, p. 5   *Op. cit.*, pp. 235 ff., especially p. 246.

pangs themselves are gradually inhibited. The self energy that the stomach contractions had caused to be reflexly conducted back to the stomach and digestive tract, thus shifting the self balance in favour of this digestive organ outlet, is progressively replaced by a still greater volume of activity sent in the same direction by food stimulations. More and more blood is directed toward the alimentary canal and away from the brain and skeletal muscles, thus altering the usual balance of self activity even more radically than the hunger drive originally altered this balance, and in the same direction.

All these effects of food stimulation show a cumulatively increasing grip or control of food over the responses of the organism. When a person has " stuffed himself ", he can do little more than sit in a chair and digest the food that he has put into his stomach. This situation represents the acme of control of food stimulus over the bodily reactions. Each separate unit response toward food, during this portion of the eating process, tends to increase the control of food over the subject organism. The subject does not rest content with the Compliance already manifested toward food, but reacts more and more compliantly until food has gained complete control. This, then, is no longer passive Compliance response, but *active* Compliance.

The compound unit response of Satisfaction, then, may be defined as simultaneous *active Compliance* and *passive Dominance*, evoked by the same stimulus. We may now add a fourth result, accomplished by hunger drive :

(4) as a result of the Desire response, built up by hunger drive, the inner reflex conduction activities of the self are again changed in such a way that the stimulus, food, evokes a second compound unit response, Satisfaction, consisting of
    a. active Compliance, and
    b. passive Dominance.

Appetite Response.

Desire and Satisfaction responses are composed of identical elementary response units. Yet because of the difference of the background of self activity with which the stimulus activities must be combined to form unit responses, the responses actually formed are quite different. The man activated by Desire presents a picture of eager, active aggressive seeking of a desired object. The man activated by Satisfaction presents a picture of complacent, passive, pleased self-sufficiency. Yet it is comparatively seldom that we find, in everyday life, any individual expressing either pure Desire or pure Satisfaction. There is a very short interval, usually, in civilized life, between the occurence of hunger pangs and the obtaining of food. It may involve a walk of a few blocks to a restaurant, or a few steps to the family ice-box may suffice. Of course, desires for automobiles, fur coats, and new houses may persist much longer in an unsatisfied state. But, as we shall have occasion to note in detail in the chapter on Learning that follows, there exist a great many memories, or psycho-neural *retention* of past experiences of Satisfaction responses, and these retained satisfactions mingle with the present desire reactions in such a way as to mitigate and modify the present Desire response considerably.

On the other hand, satisfactions are apt not to be final or complete. There is nearly always something left to be desired, the present satisfaction mingles with a portion, at least, of the original desire that is not yet satisfied. Even if this is not the case, people tend to recall the original desire deliberately and to stimulate themselves by talking about it in order to make the attained satisfaction more pleasant. Satisfaction, therefore, like Desire, is seldom found in human behaviour without some mingling of the converse appetitive element.

Whenever there exists such a simultaneous mingling of Desire and Satisfaction responses, it is convenient to refer to the total, complex unit response as Appetite response. As we have already seen, there is a characteristic shifting, or transition, from Desire to Satisfaction throughout the major part of the duration of Appetite response. This transition from Desire to Satisfaction constitutes a reaction characteristic not inherent in either Desire or Satisfaction alone. Only when the two mingle in the definitely determined sequence fixed by the hunger pang mechanism, do we find this transitional element in the mingling relationship just described. We may say, therefore, that Appetite response possesses a characteristic not present in either of its elements ; the characteristic of *transition* from Desire to Satisfaction.

This transition includes several elements. Dominance response, as we have seen, gradually becomes less active and more passive, in proportion to its success in seizing and possessing food. Compliance response undergoes a transition, *pari passu* with increased stimulation by the food possessed, but in an opposite direction, passing from the passive to the active phase of Compliance. These are the two chief transitional elements that characterize Appetite response and form a graded interconnection between Desire and the Satisfaction that gradually replaces it. The other transitional elements concern changes in the self activity under the influences of hunger pangs and food respectively. But these transitions concern the *drive itself*, rather than the compound unit responses that the drive originates and builds up.

We shall have occasion to note, in a later chapter, how learning builds up the responses of Desire, Satisfaction, and Appetite still further by causing the subject organism to respond to many and diverse objects with Appetite responses, even though there is no hunger drive present. We learn to desire automobiles, clothes, money, objects of art, and material possessions of all kinds. But this does not signify, by any means, that an inner hunger drive, caused by hunger pangs or some equivalent mechanism, is operating in each instance. Desire and Satisfaction responses, once built up under the influence of hunger pangs and hunger drive, may thereafter be evoked by any material object whatsoever that we have learned to regard as an effective stimulus. It may be, of course, that the inner hunger drive is also evoked by the object desired; or more likely, by some stimulus situation of hardship, unpleasantness, or need, which we have learned to respond to with hunger drive. But the drive and the appetitive responses are two wholly distinct behaviour elements, and either may occur without the other.

Learned Hunger Drive.

It seems to be a fact that we learn to respond with a real hunger drive, or increase of self energy and change of self pattern, to many environmental situations, once this hunger drive has been sufficiently built up in the organism as a result of the body's hunger pang mechanism. Huge business organizations, political intrigue, giant construction projects, and lifelong ambitions to be a great physician or scientist seem to require an element of sustained, inner hunger drive that cannot be found in a mere succession of Desires and

Satisfactions evoked by passing environmental objects. The hunger pang stimulus, of course, builds up this hunger drive, as we have seen ; but hunger pangs build it up toward a specific type of environmental stimulus, namely food. Hunger pangs, while they endure, would not permit the hunger drive to be directed toward building a bridge across the Amazon, or toward studying brain surgery. Yet the hunger drive certainly builds up, in the retentive nerve connections of the reflex conduction system, a new self pattern with increased energy capacity. This is a capacity for selective concentration upon a single stimulus object and with sustained compulsion to respond to that object with the compound unit responses, first of Desire and then of Satisfaction, after the Desire responses are successfully executed. If this retained hunger drive pattern of self activity can be evoked by other needs and other stimuli than those of hunger, then the hunger drive pattern of self activity may be evoked and maintained, selectively, toward the type of object determined by the stimulus that evoked it. Apparently such is the case.

Any sort of *danger* situation that does not completely overwhelm the self activities, seems naturally capable of evoking the hunger drive condition throughout the reflex conduction system. A baby dropped on a pillow, clutches the air and moves his legs and arms about wildly while left without support in the air. Later, infants spontaneously retreat from a stimulus that has partially overwhelmed their own self actions, such as a loud noise close to the head, an animal that has bitten or scratched, or another child who has taken their toys away on the preceding day. The child shows a certain amount of *sustained drive* to seek safety or some remedy for the unpleasant stimulation that is oppressing him. In short, this type of stimulation seems capable, from a very early age, of putting his self activities into the typical *hunger drive pattern*, which causes him to respond with Desire and Satisfaction to whatever object *protects him from the danger or removes the unpleasant stimulus.* This seems in every way comparable to the hunger drive initiated by hunger pangs.

Still later in life, any stimulus situation that impresses upon the child a *need*, or a *lack*, reinstates hunger drive in the same way. He may see other children riding velocipedes, or bicycles, or ponies. The pony or bicycle may not, in themselves, arouse any true Desire response in the child, because he has had no experience of them and does not understand their nature. But the fact that his playmates are going off together, doing something that he cannot do, sets up a hunger drive that may be said to have a need situation as a stimulus. The hunger drive to be able to play again with his companions, makes him respond with Desire toward the pony or bicycle.

Of course, in adult life, hunger drive may be evoked by needs, dangers, and also by the more intangible stimulus condition known as "ambition". A man or woman with ambition, is a man or woman who has developed a very strong and persistent hunger drive, which is evoked, apparently, by almost any situation where there appears to be something useful or sought after by others and which is not yet possessed by the ambitious person himself or herself. It is possible, of course, that a man like Julius Cæsar, who was said by Plutarch to have an insatiable "passion for honour", i.e. ambition for power over others, had had built up within him a hunger pang mechanism perhaps more powerful and unpleasant than the average. A hunger drive condition of self activity would result, which seldom abated, and so he would become focussed upon whatever environmental stimulus presented itself. Certain it is that the extent of the hunger drive depends, not so much upon environmental stimulation as upon the condition of the self activity pattern; a pattern that might be permanently held in a hunger drive condition by hunger pangs themselves, or by a variety of other stimulus mechanisms operating spontaneously within the organism.

This is evidently the phenomenon upon which Alfred Adler bases his conception of "inferiority complex", with which he supposes everyone to start and which they then gradually compensate for and conquer by combative activity. Adler also has a concept of "organic inferiority", which, he supposes, is the original cause of the inherent inferiority feeling. Adler's concepts seem to be remarkably penetrating when we consider that they are reached from a purely subjective point of view. But to call hunger pangs, or threat of danger, or some endocrine or organic over-activity an "organic inferiority" seems altogether inaccurate. The stimulus mechanisms responsible for hunger drive, whether hunger pangs or something else, seem rather to consist of *over*-active, or *superior*, stimulus mechanisms of one sort or another. The hunger driven individual is not trying to *compensate*, he is trying to compel his environment to supply his needs. Even in fleeing from danger to the protection of a tree or house, there is most certainly no reaction based upon weakness, but rather a response directed toward securing some weapon or assistance that can be compelled to serve the subject's need against a threatening danger.

It is easy, however, to see the origin of the inferiority and compensation ideas in connection with hunger drive. The stimulus, whether hunger pangs, danger, or bodily need, is both stronger and weaker than the subject. He complies with it insofar as it is stronger than he ; that is, he does not seek to combat it without assistance. He ultimately seeks to dominate it, but in a roundabout way, by dominating food, or weapons, or other objects, by means of which he can destroy the stimulus to hunger drive and get rid of the drive itself. If a drive to enlarge one's powers and possessions or to overcome an opponent is a " compensation " response, then the hunger drive may be so regarded. Such a description seems to us, however, to be in the main inaccurate.

Not only may the hunger drive be evoked by truly adequate stimuli other than hunger pangs, once it has been sufficiently built up, but also it may be evoked in adults by inadequate stimuli to which the subject has *learned* to respond with hunger drive. Thus a business or professional man learns to respond with a sustained hunger drive toward certain objects or people, and toward situations in his profession or occupation, simply as a matter of custom or habit.

CHAPTER VIII

DRIVES: PART II

EROTIC DRIVE AND THE COMPOUND UNIT RESPONSES OF PASSION AND CAPTIVATION

Introductory: the Genital Systems

BOTH sexes possess two types of genital organs, the external and the internal. The internal genitals are, in each case, differently innervated than the external genitals. The internal organs are connected with the ganglia of the sympathetic branch of the autonomic nervous system; while the external genitals are connected with the sacral division of the same system. The internal genitals, therefore, through their sympathetic nervous connections, belong to that part of the self pattern of activities that receives a preponderance of motor discharge during the usual condition of the self. The external genitals, on the other hand, though a normal tonus activity is maintained in them, bear the same relationship in the self pattern to the internal genitals, as do the digestive organs to the skeletal muscles. More energy, in short, flows through sympathetic channels to the internal genitals than flows through sacral channels to the external genitals. When love (" sex ") activities involve a great deal of activity in the internal genital organs, there is likely to be an accompanying increase of activity in the skeletal muscles and adjacent viscera. When the external genitals are unduly excited, on the other hand, there is likely to be marked decrease of energy in skeletal muscles (" sexual lassitude "), sometimes with a sharp decline in the strength of the heart beat, as evidenced by a drop in systolic blood pressure.

Periods of " heat " occur in female animals, and a distinct cycle of erotic excitement in women, closely connected with the menstrual cycle. Our studies show[1] that women experi-

[1] W. M. Marston, *op. cit.*, p. 322.

ence marked increase of activity in both internal and external genital organs, during and just following menstruation. External genital excitement, moreover, seems clearly to predominate. The menstrual flow apparently furnishes a certain amount of mechanical, and possibly also chemical, stimulation to the clitoris, the female external genital organ, with its associated viscera sacrally innervated. Erection of the clitoris, like erection of the male external organ, the penis, is readily subject to observation, and both depend upon increase of vaso-dilator impulses to the blood vessels of the organ, with consequent engorgement and erection.

This excitement of the external genitals, following menstruation, does not appear to interfere substantially with the activity of the brain or skeletal muscles.[1] Nor does it depress the systolic blood pressure, although this drops somewhat during menstruation itself.[2] The phenomena involved in menstruation appear to concern primarily the balance of motor discharge as between internal and external genital organs, the other parts of the body being affected incidentally rather than primarily. As we have already noted, there seems to be very little inhibitory action of the genital organ excitement upon the usual functions and activities of the body. Reflex excitations connected with erotic drive show a high degree of alliance, one with the other, the change in self pattern being rather a question of change in balance, with all usual activities retained.

It is possible that there exists in the human male, also, an erotic drive mechanism, or mechanisms, capable of shifting the balance of activity in favour of the external genital organ. Various writers have suggested such erotic stimulus mechanisms in connection with urination and other functions.[3] But we have seen no evidence for such theories, nor do our own studies confirm them in any way. Physiologists have sought in vain, in many researches, to discover a male erotic cycle corresponding to that of the female. Despite all these failures to obtain positive results, however, the possibility still remains that there exists an erotic stimulus mechanism in the average male organism. If so, the most probable source of such an

---

[1] *Ibid.*, p. 322.   [2] *Ibid.*, p. 322.
[3] J. B. Watson. *op. cit., Behaviorism.* F. H. Allport, *Social Psychology.*

erotic stimulus is to be found in a gonadal hormone of some as yet undetermined sort.

Changes in the self activities, following menstruation and constituting the erotic drive, may be summarized thus. Increased activity is present in both the internal and external genital organs. The balance of activity as between these two poles of the genital apparatus is changed markedly in favour of the external genitals. Other activities of the body are not substantially interfered with; but the presence of preponderant motor discharge to the external genitals apparently renders the woman extremely susceptible to adequate love stimuli, and less susceptible than usual to the influence of other types of stimuli. The change of pattern in self activities, as between internal and external genital organs, also has the effect, as we shall note, of *decreasing* the relative power of the self with respect to the strength of an appropriate love stimulus.

Causes Underlying Love Behaviour

" Sex ", or more properly love behaviour, appears in definite form in both sexes at adolescence. It is at this period that the interstitial cells of the ovaries begin to mature and to act as true endocrine glands, called by Steinach and others the " glands of puberty ". It is the endocrine products of these glands, apparently, that determine secondary sexual characteristics. Also, the addition of this hormone, with the other endocrine changes it brings about, creates a permanent change in the self activities of both sexes.

In the male there appears a condition of almost constant susceptibility to erotic response, on sight of or contact with the female body, as already said. There seems little doubt, from a consensus of observation and opinion concerning men's behaviour, that the male organism, from adolescenece on, shows much more constant erotic excitability than does the female organism. The continuous condition of excitability, however, appears to lack one of the essential characteristics, at least, of a drive, as we have defined the term. It does not (except perhaps during part of adolescence and under exceptional conditions later in life) turn the male from other pursuits of an appetitive nature and spontaneously drive him hither and yon until the object of the drive is attained. The male excitability, also, does not seem to be periodic, or to follow any fixed cycle, at least none that has as yet been discovered. This male gonadal hormone, therefore, in its stimulus effect upon men's behaviour, assumes more the character of a constant element in the male self activity, rather than of a specialized, erotic drive. It shows one element of the typical drive, nevertheless, and that is its apparent power to compel men to respond to attractive females with a certain, definite type of compound love response, customarily termed " passion ".

The behaviour of adolescent girls, during and following menstruation periods, shows certain characteristics apparently attributable to changes in self activity brought about by the menstrual phenomena. This typical effect of menstruation is frequently obscured by pain and other physiological abnormalities connected with the menstrual function. But in cases free from these complicating factors, the behaviour changes may readily be observed.

First, the girl frequently shows marked inattention to school work, household tasks, or any physical or mental work requiring sustained concentration. She becomes much absorbed in day-dreaming and frequently shows both physical and emotional lassitude. She may also grow " moody " and sometimes depressed, and shows petulance when kept in the house or away from her girl, and especially her boy, friends. Some girls, of more robust and healthy constitution, may become especially dutiful and affectionate at home, during and after menstrual periods. Such girls are able to perform routine duties effectively under the direction of their mothers or of other girls whom they like. But they still show a marked loss of spontaneity and interest in the work itself. About the first or second day of the menstrual period there usually occurs a noticeable drop in systolic blood pressure, indicating a certain decrease in strength of heart beat. It seems probable that other muscular and sympathetically innervated activities share in this cardiac depression.

Second, there is quite likely to appear, also, in the typical adolescent girl's behaviour, at this time each 24–28 days, a tendency to wander about aimlessly and to seek constantly to be with other people, preferably with girls and boys of her own age. The girl may become quite restless or show a certain hectic activity, mainly devoted to pleasure-seeking of one sort or another. Nothing seems to satisfy this type of girl for more than a few moments at a time ; she is constantly rushing off to find something new, of the nature of which she has no idea. Although this restless over-activity is quite inconsistent with the usual lassitude and decrease of outwardly directed energy mentioned in the last paragraph above, both phenomena frequently may be observed at the same time in a girl's general behaviour. This restless, unsatisfied seeking element, when present, seemingly furnishes the essential drive characteristic of changing the individual's behaviour in such a way that there is increased probability of encountering a special type of stimulus object toward which the drive is really directed.

Third, there is a marked increase in the susceptibility of girls to masculine attraction. Some " problem " cases studied by the writers[1] show extreme instances of this trait, wherein girls of good home training accost nearly every male whom they may happen to meet on the street. Another case of a seemingly average adolescent girl, showed repeated hallucinations of men staring at her, attacking her, looking in at her window, and so on. Thus even when no man is physically present, the same tendency to respond to memories and ideas of men persists. There seems also to be an undeniable tendency to yield to men's advances, together with a frequently increased suggestibility, and general " weakness " of resistance toward the influence of persons of both sexes, but especially males. This general characteristic of girls' post-menstrual behaviour represents the third essential chacteristic of drive, i.e. a new type of self activity which, when coupled with the first two, tends to bring the subject organism into appropriate contact with the special type of stimulus object.

Passion ; a Compound Unit Response Combining Passive Inducement and Active Submission

When the love-seeking female comes into contact with the male, the erotic drive compels a new type of compound unit response, commonly called passion. As we have already noted, a predisposition toward this same response is created in the

---

[1] W. M. Marston, op. cit., p. 295.

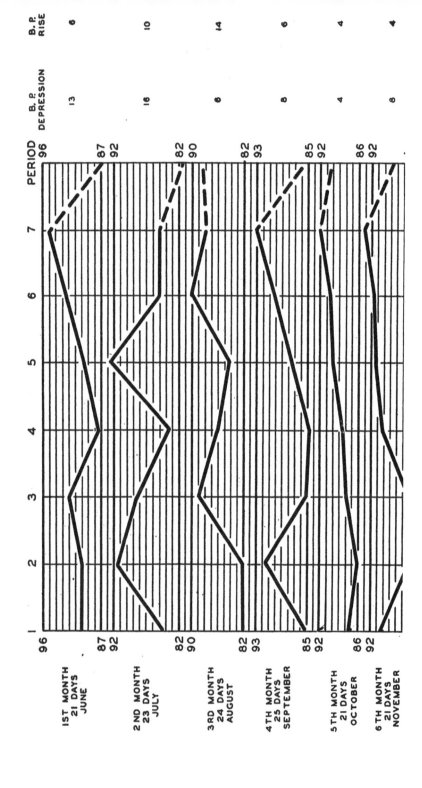

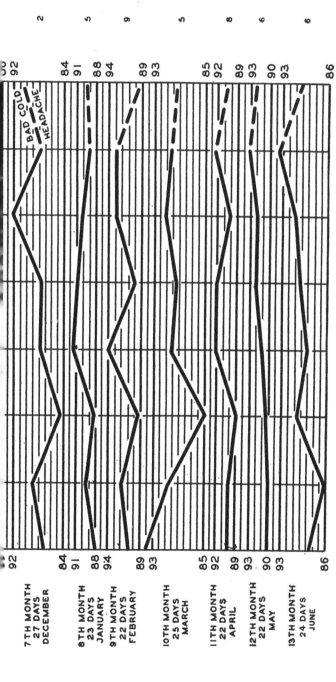

Fig. 37

STUDY OF BLOOD PRESSURE DURING THE MENSTRUAL CYCLE

The above graphs summarize a study of female blood pressure made by E. H. Marston for the purpose of determining the influence of menstrual function upon female blood pressure. The subject was twenty-seven years old, married, and in normal health. During a period of one year, seven readings were taken each morning immediately upon the subject's awakening. This was done to minimize the effect of mental and emotional disturbances during waking hours.

Since the menstrual months were of unequal length they were fractionated for the purpose of the above summary and the averages for each of the seven parts, together with the average blood pressure during the menstrual period, plotted as above.

The table at the right of the graph indicates the actual blood pressure depression during each menstrual period, measured from the blood pressure level at the beginning of the period and is expressed in millimetres of mercury as taken from the original complete records. The table also shows the total blood pressure rise from the beginning of the lunar month to the blood pressure level at the beginning of the period.

At the left of the graph the number of days in each lunar month is indicated, as well as the calendar month during which the greater part of the lunar month occurred.

male organism, evidently by an appropriate hormone stimulus mechanism, so that the male reacts in kind upon sight or contact with the female.

Now a word of caution may perhaps be required before attempting to describe the inter-sex love responses. For various reasons, principal among which is the fact that our social laws, customs, and taboos are man-made and not woman-made, love has long been considered an impolite, and even an illegal, subject to discuss ; especially with regard to the bodily expression of sexual relationships. Whether this strange taboo upon the most pleasant and constructive aspect of human behaviour makes for the uplift of humanity, or for its downfall, seems a question peculiarly within the province of psychology to decide. Most certainly we claim the right, as psychologists, to investigate this question to the fullest possible extent, without fear or favour toward moralists, however vociferous. On the other hand, we have no further concern with the subsequent use by moralists of psychological discoveries, once they have been made, since this does not fall within our province. At the very least, when the *facts* are finally ascertained, there will be something more solid to build upon than the prejudices and superstitions that only too obviously form the insecure supports of much modern " morality ". The present writers sincerely believe that sex and love relationships should be studied and taught by competent authorities in precisely the same manner that all other aspects of human behaviour are studied and described. Certainly modern scientific opinion, and the opinion of enlightened child students and other progressive social workers is in accord with us in this matter. It is no longer illegal to offer competent scientific instruction in matters of love and sex, with the exception, in some states, of birth control information, a subject in any event outside the scope of a psychological book.

While under the influence of erotic drive, i.e. in " heat ", the female of the higher animal species permits the male to approach her, establish sexual contact, and complete the act of copulation. The female, in most cases, will drive the male away or prevent him from establishing sexual connection at times when she is not herself erotically excited. Human behaviour follows closely the behaviour of other vertebrate species in this particular. Although the male animal, as well as the male human being, seems as a rule to be aroused at all times to erotic behaviour by sight of or contact with the female, the average woman or female animal apparently fails to respond by yielding to male advances except at the times already mentioned. Just as a person of either sex who is busy with other matters of interest, does not respond readily to food stimulation, although desiring that same food intensely when hungry, so the female animal or human may reject the very sexual contacts to which she readily yields when under the influence of erotic drive. The rule would appear to be that the choice, in all species, is made by the female, who in turn is largely influenced by the cycle of her erotic stimulus mechanisms, as previously described.

On this point we may quote from Howell, as follows : " The phenomenon known as heat (or oestrus) in lower mammals resembles, in many essential respects, menstruation in human beings, and they may be regarded as homologous functions. Heat is a period of sexual excitement which occurs one or more times during the year and during which the female will take the male. The condition lasts, as a rule, for several days, and in the female is accompanied by changes which resemble those of menstruation. . . . The changes during heat must be considered as physiologically homologous to those of menstruation. The sexual excitement that attends the condition in the lower animals is not distinctly represented in man, although it is commonly said that in the period following menstruation the sexual desire is stronger than at other times, but in the changes undergone by the uterus and the fact that these changes are connected, as a rule, with the liberation of an egg from the ovary (ovulation), the two phenomena are physiologically similar."[1]

To proceed with the description of erotic drive, we have already referred to the female's initial role as one of yielding or surrendering herself to the male. She also captures the male's attention and strives to hold his interest. In other words, the female initially responds to the male by surrendering herself to him and by attempting to secure his surrender to her to the extent, at least, of giving up other interests and responding to her exclusively. This initial unit response, resulting from erotic drive, has been wrongly referred to as " desire ", in popular speech and literature, apparently ever since

[1] W. H. Howell, *A Text Book of Physiology*, 1913, pp. 948 ff.

literature began to record popular ideas and misconceptions.
But a moment's thought will show that the woman's initial
love response is precisely the opposite of desire. Erotic drive
makes the woman respond as if she were the food, rather than
as if she were the seeker for food. Her initial effort is to feed
the male with herself, as it were, rather than to feed herself
with the object of passion.

Another totally perverted idea of woman's love response
is that she is stimulated to passion by the male, and that he
is the aggressor and initiator of her reactions in yielding
herself to him. We have noted that the female, even in
animal species, does not respond to the male except when
she is driven to respond from within. And the male is so
constituted that he reacts almost continually to the female
with Passion response, no matter how the female may be
behaving toward himself. The true interpretation of this
relationship, therefore, seems to be, not that the male seeks
to capture the female and that she finally yields herself to
him, but rather that the male continually tries to give himself
to the female so that she may excite him still further, and
that the female only experiences a corresponding response of
giving herself to the male when the inner, self-stimulated
condition of her organism compels her to do so. It is only
under the latter circumstances that natural sex relationships
are consummated. The mistaken popular (and obviously
masculine) notion that woman yields herself under the influence
of male love attractions, apparently refers to a circumstance
peculiar to the love responses and precisely opposite to the
organization of the appetitive responses, which are much
better understood. This peculiarity of the love responses
lies in the fact that the *passive*, yielding, self-surrendering part
of love (true Passion response), comes *first* in the time sequence
determined by erotic drive, and the *active*, capturing, making-
the-lover-surrender part of the love response, comes afterward.
In love behaviour the woman first gives herself up, a love
captive ; then she quickly utilizes her position as love captive
to capture her apparent conqueror. This second phase is
Captivation response, and it is a wise man who understands
this female sequence of love behaviour.

Let us put the matter in everyday terms, using non-psycho-
logical words such as " want ", and so on. In appetite, the
food does not want to get itself captured and eaten. Its

interests are antagonistic to those of the hungry animal or person. If the food were able, so to speak, it would immediately turn on its captor and destroy him, the moment his vigilance relaxed. Therefore the hungry food-seeker *desires* to capture and utterly subdue his food, first. Only when the dangerous and independent attributes of the food are wholly within his control, does he dare to yield or to comply with the food to any great extent. He must first master it ; then he may safely permit it to control him.

In love each lover is a prospective slave of the other, so to speak. Both slaves want to be captured and subdued to the uttermost. Why? Because capture and enslavement does not mean being eaten or destroyed. Quite the opposite ; it means great increase of pleasure for the captive. The interests of the prospective captive and prospective conqueror are not antagonistic, as with food and its captor ; they are *completely allied*.

The erotic drive, therefore, compels each participant to surrender *first;* then, having completely surrendered to her lover, the woman is able *safely* to capture and control him. Her interests are identical with his by virtue of her initial surrender ; in capturing and controlling him she does not risk making him do anything destructive or unpleasant to himself, and so run the immediate risk of losing her love captive.

Love control of one person by another depends wholly upon the extent to which the captor is able to give the captive greater pleasure than the captive is able to give himself. A simple, scientific fact that is seemingly very difficult for many people, especially men, to understand, is that self-surrender must come first, and conquest of the lover afterward. The more complete the initial self-surrender is, the more powerful the subsequent erotic (love) control of the captive may be.

If one compares appetite and love responses, one must think of them as opposites in all respects. Active Appetite, or Desire, comes first ; active Love, or Captivation, comes last (if it be a complete Love response, and not merely Captivation used for amusement or profit, as in seduction and " gold-digging " behaviour). Passive Appetite, Satisfaction, comes last ; passive Love, Passion, comes first, enforcing immediate surrender of oneself to the lover at the very beginning of the true love behaviour. The almost total lack of scientific understanding of Love response undoubtedly springs from the attempt to warp it into the pattern of Appetite, whereas the two are actually totally distinct and opposite types of response, to two wholly different types of stimuli. Desire seeks to destroy its object in order to utilize it for self purposes. Captivation seeks to stimulate its object to greater erotic pleasure, in order to control it for its own happiness. Satisfaction permits the self to be controlled by food for the benefit of the self and the final destruction of the food. Passion voluntarily seeks to get the control of the self into the hands of another person, for the benefit of the loved one and the increased pleasure of both parties. Appetitive power depends upon belittling one's opponent and magnifying oneself. Love power depends upon increasing the pleasure of one's lover and adapting oneself to the lover's response mechanisms.

With the bugaboo of confusion between Appetite and Love responses temporarily disposed of, let us consider in greater detail the compound unit response of Passion, to which the female organism seems to be impelled by periodic erotic drive, as is the male organism by continual hormone balance.

When a woman, under the influence of erotic drive, surrenders herself to a male, she yields utterly and eagerly. Of course this active type of surrender is frowned upon by occidental social conventions and customs, so that only those types of women who are freest from conventional restraints and inhibitions permit themselves the luxury of natural love behaviour under the influence of erotic drive. The essence of this yielding element in Passion response consists, apparently, of Submission response in its purest and most active form. The subject seeks to be controlled and caressed by the lover increasingly and to the fullest possible extent. Other responses of the subject fall, for the time being, completely under the control of the Submission response, and the woman is willing and anxious to perform any task or take any pains or trouble to please her lover and carry out his wishes. This is *active Submission* response. By means of it *the subject is controlled by the object person.*

Simultaneously with Submission, however, the woman responds with Inducement. She exhibits herself in such a way that she may control the attention and love responses of the man. She dresses to please him (Submission) but she also pays especial attention to her clothes and physical appearance in order to attract and hold him (Inducement). She uses the technique of flirtation with other men, " come and catch me " behaviour, and she limits her Submission to the extent of denying the caresses her Submission tends to bestow, in order to "keep him interested ". All this represents a response of passive Inducement.

It is Inducement, clearly enough. And it may be regarded as passive because the woman is only striving to keep her lover's attention away from other objects of response, to hold his present interest in her until it culminates, naturally and spontaneously, in a proposal of marriage or of some appropriate form of love relationship. She does not seek to make him do this or that under her direction, at first, but only acts in a way calculated to fix his already aroused love response upon herself. By means of this passive Inducement response, *the subject controls the object person.*

Passion response, then, consists simultaneously of an attempt to gain passive control of the lover and an attempt actively to surrender to the lover's control. Passion is a compound unit response, simultaneously consisting of passive Inducement and active Submission, adequately evoked by the same stimulus person, under the influence, in the first instances at least, of erotic drive. Passion response, with the corresponding response that it elicits from the male, turns both organisms from other activities and brings the two together in a relationship that makes each available for a consummated Love response toward the other.

Captivation; a Compound Unit Response Combining Active Inducement and Passive Submission

Just as the decisive shift from Desire to Satisfaction occurs at the moment the food is fully possessed and taken into the mouth, so we may also discover a natural line of demarcation between Passion and Captivation responses at the moment when the woman is completely possessed by her lover and the external male genital organ is taken into the female vagina. Prior to this moment, contacts and caresses from her lover have only stimulated the woman's lips and the outside sensory organs of her body, including to a certain extent the female external genital organ and adjacent tissues. But the moment the bodily relationship is completed, a different set of receptors, and a different set of afferent and

motor nerves, are brought into play.   The vagina is regarded
by physiologists as an *internal* organ, since it is innervated by
sympathetic nerves.   Direct stimulation of the internal
genitals, of course, tends to counteract the original menstrual
stimulus, with its resulting change of balance of self activities
as between the two sets of genital organs.   That is to say,
direct stimulation of the internal genital organs tends to excite
these same organs to greater activity than before ; and *pari
passu*, to restore the usual self pattern of activity in favour
of the internal genitals.   Thus the change from erotic drive
back toward the previous self balance and pattern, begins with
the first direct stimulation of the vaginal receptors, just as
the change from hunger drive back to the previous self pattern
began with the direct food stimulation of taste and digestive-
visceral receptor organs.

We have already remarked that the internal genital organs
belong to the same group of tissues as the brain and skeletal
muscles, in so far as the organism's general activity pattern
goes.   We may expect, therefore, to find increased muscular
activity and brain activity along with the increase in motor
energy flowing to the internal genitals.   Such increase in
outward-flowing bodily energy does, in fact, occur, as indicated
by increased strength of special movements of the thighs and
legs, and so on.   All this increased energy in the self pattern
results in a cumulative change in the woman's Inducement
response, from passive toward *active Inducement.*   That is,
she gradually, by positive and active stimulation, induces
new movements in the behaviour of the male.   These skeletal
muscular movements of the male are no longer wholly the
result of his own Passion response, given an opportunity to
direct itself toward the female, but represent also Passion
responses directly enforced and controlled by the female's
active stimulation of his body.

Correspondingly, during this phase of love behaviour the
balance of energy flowing into the female external genital
organs, naturally subsides.   The degree to which she is
controlled by her lover diminishes, *pari passu*, becoming more
passive in type.   The Submission element in the woman's
behaviour, while it persists throughout intercourse, eventually
consists merely of permitting herself voluntarily to remain in
her lover's control so far as concerns the exclusion of other
reactions, and in suffering passively the external stimulation

of the male's body. The Submission of the total response, in short, changes gradually from active Submission to *passive Submission*.

These two love stimulus effects may be contrasted, for greater clarity, with the two stimulus effects of food in the appetitive shift from Desire to Satisfaction response. Food stimulates directly the receptors most intimately concerned with the anti-self balance and pattern of the reaction. The external genital organ of the male, on the contrary, stimulates directly those receptors most intimately connected with the woman's own self balance and pattern of action. Food stimulation, therefore, tends more and more to control the organism's total responses, the more of it is eaten. Male organ stimulation, on the contrary, tends more and more toward control of the male by the female, the longer it is maintained. Food stimulation results in more and more passive control of the food by the organism, while male organ stimulation brings about increasingly passive yielding of the female to the male.

It must be noted, in passing, that there is no possible means by which the internal male genitals may be directly stimulated during the entire course of the love response. Instead of a gradual increase in activity of Inducement and passivity of Submission, therefore, in male behaviour we find an apparent piling-up of Passion response until a certain threshold is reached within the central nervous system, and then a sudden, explosive shift from Passion to momentary Captivation response, expressed in the male sexual orgasm.[1] The whole mechanism is central, rather than being attributable to any change in external stimulation. This difference between male and female bodily love mechanisms has the effect of initiating an immediate change in female behaviour from Passion to Captivation, as soon as bodily union is begun ; whereas in male behaviour, Passion response is seemingly prolonged and retained throughout the entire act, with only a momentary flash of Captivation response at the ultimate climax. Contrary to popular, male-made ideas of love relationships between the sexes, therefore (with the notable exception of Bernard Shaw's *Man and Superman*), man is so constituted that he must play the role of love captive from the very beginning until, literally, the last moment.

[1] W. M. Marston, *op. cit.*, p. 325.

Woman's body, on the other hand, begins with a similar erotic surrender to the male, but very quickly changes the response to a type of Captivation behaviour naturally designed to assume and exercise love leadership throughout the major portion of the inter-sex relationship. Man is evidently the appetitive leader, by virtue of an apparently superior hunger drive ; while woman is similarly equipped, by virtue of her menstrual stimulus mechanism, her resulting erotic drive, and double genital mechanisms capable of direct love stimulation, to act as love leader.

How may we reconcile the above account of woman's natural control of inter-sex relationships with the current popular notions of " man's place " and " woman's place ", in courtship and the home ? This task is not so difficult to-day as it would have been during the last century. In Victorian days, " woman's place was the home " ; a masculine dictum which meant something very different from its purported intention. This rule for women actually meant, " Man is leader, appetitive leader and love leader as well. Woman's place is to remain at home awaiting her husband whenever he may choose to come home, and bearing children." Woman was merely one of man's pleasures, and one of his servants. Under this regime, it is quite true that all the love captivation that was done must officially be done by the male. The woman was indulgently permitted to do a little " flirting " before her marriage and it was greatly to her credit if she could lead as many men as possible into thinking that she loved them, so that they would propose marriage to her. Still she must not do this in the way provided by nature, i.e. exhibiting her body and bestowing her caresses upon prospective customers. She must remain inaccessible, prim, and very haughty, repelling all lovers' ardour with a scornful (dominant) glance. Once safely married, however, with her property rights and those of her prospective children secured, the whole picture of woman's supposed conduct changed. She should then become an " obedient and submissive wife ". Which meant, apparently, that she must give up what little Captivation she had been able to work up during her courtship days, and shift permanently into the passive love role, turning on her Passion, as it were, like a tap whenever her husband demanded, and never seeking to control his behaviour except in so far as an adequate amount of food and clothing was concerned. This male delusion concerning woman's natural love role still persists, to a considerable degree. But, of course, it is utterly impossible for woman really to behave that way. She never did. She never will. Since the Great War, when woman found she could conduct business, drive ambulances, and even fight precisely as well as man, the more loving sex has ceased to pretend that they are playing out the part assigned them by Victorian playwrights.

Recent studies in the four elementary emotions corresponding to the four elementary unit responses of C, D, I, and S indicate that woman's Inducement response is very much stronger and more frequent than her Submission response.[1] This finding merely verifies the clinical observation apparent in our studies some years ago,[2] that woman's love behaviour is falsely interpreted as predominately Submissive, and passive. In reality, it is principally active and Captivating. As a matter of fact, as noted elsewhere,[3] woman's Passion behaviour is actually at a minimum because of the lack of any type of male individual capable of being predominately captivating. Men are dominant, and forcefully appetitive, in their responses, but never capable, for physical reasons, of sustained Captivation response. The male Passion response, which naturally forms by far the largest part of masculine love behaviour, tends to be disorganized and promiscuous because men's Dominance does not permit them to seek love training at woman's hands. Women, internally driven to love attitude, as we have seen, accept the male disinclination to be love controlled and trained in coitus at its face value ; and they try, therefore, to please men as the men represent themselves to be rather than trying to build up male pleasure and happiness by openly assuming an active love control of male lovers, and building up and organizing the naturally predominating male Passion response.

Also, of course, women who depend upon men for financial support, or even for love companionship which they fear to have taken from them and transferred to some other woman, are in the position of an excess commodity in a buyer's market ; they are glad to get the semblance of love (with easy financial

---

[1] " Bodily Symptoms of Elementary Emotions," *Psyche*, October, 1929, p. 20.
[2] W. M. Marston, *op. cit.*, p. 299.
[3] *Ibid.*, p. 324.

support) in exchange for themselves, without risking the loss of a sale by demanding too great a price. The only natural and normal price is female Captivation control of the male, with power to organize and develop his love responses.

All these conditions have led to an exceedingly unnatural, perverted, and appetitively suppressed condition of the love behaviour of both sexes. It is this great underlying, but meticulously concealed flaw in the present love life of civilized people that has recently been discovered by Sigmund Freud and his pupils. Although Freud has perverted the idea of love response fully as appetitively as have the people whom he is attempting to analyze and readjust, his keen insight, nevertheless, has penetrated the mask of Victorian hypocrisy behind which the fundamental love longings of humanity have long been buried. Freud is quite correct in his assertion that the " sexual libido " or, love drive, is wholly out of tune with the present social environment and occidental laws and conventions ; and that this disharmony is responsible for a major portion of the existing psychological abnormalities of human kind. It seems likely, however, that normal and enlightened love development represents a portion of the organism's behaviour which has merely lagged behind the appetitive portion in its evolution and outward expression. Appetitive responses, because they are most primitive, might naturally be expected to evolve first, and to delay, somewhat, by their own evolution, the proper evolution of love behaviour. Clear psychological understanding of the natural, normal love responses, and wide-spread dissemination of this knowledge can do more than any other single factor to push human evolution onward, in this aspect, to its next necessary attainment. Appetitive suppression and perversion of love should not be looked at as something humans have " fallen " to, from some high and goddess-like estate, but rather as a crude, primitive, animal-like condition of behaviour consisting of control and inhibition of erotic drive by hunger drive, a condition that humans have not yet evolved out of.

If the bodily love mechanisms, as we find them, may be taken as the standard of nature and normality, then we may interpret the most successful type of inter-sex relationships as closely approximating the normal compound unit responses of Captivation on the woman's part, and persisting Passion response on the part of the man. Many cases studied show such behaviour.

In summary, Captivation may be defined as a compound-unit response, built up and conditioned by the female, erotic love drive, and *consisting of simultaneous active Inducement and passive Submission responses to the same stimulus person.*

Love Response and Erotic Drive

Love response represents the combination of Passion and Captivation responses, with the latter gradually outweighing the former; precisely as Appetite response represents a

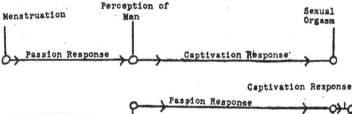

WOMAN'S RESPONSES

FIGURE 38

Normal Relationship Between Erotic Responses of Women and Men

The diagram indicates the normal relationship between woman's erotic drive, with its resulting compound responses and the compound erotic responses of a man as affected by a woman's behaviour. It is necessary to emphasize the fact that the normal time relationship between the responses, as described in the text and indicated in the above diagram, seldom, if ever, occurs in untrained subjects. The reason for this lack of normalcy in sexual relations seems to be the inability of the male to sustain passion and delay captivation behaviour until after the female orgasm or simultaneously therewith. The result of premature initiation of male captivation response is to bring about the sexual orgasm in the man before the woman's captivation response has run its natural course, leaving her still in a state of uncompleted erotic excitement which is both physiologically and psychologically unhealthy.

similar combination of Desire and Satisfaction. Because of the interference between the Appetitive and Love responses which we have already referred to at some length, we find one or the other elements of Love response without its companion part, more frequently than we find either Desire or Satisfaction alone in human behaviour. Men are frequently passionate, with little or no Captivation in their behaviour, as when some immature youngster, of wealthy family and inadequate emotional development, becomes helplessly captivated by a chorus girl or night-club hostess. Cases of this sort, which have come to our attention, indicate almost sheer Passion on the boy's part, and frequently, also, extremely well-developed Captivation on the part of the girl, her Captivation being controlled, in turn, by Appetite reaction (Desire for money and gifts). On the other hand, certain cases of girls who are uncontrollably promiscuous in their sex relationships, which have been brought to our attention in consultation practice, show an opposite condition, with Passion apparently controlling the girl's behaviour exclusively. Some men, of the " sheik " type, seem quite cold so far as passionate surrender to women is concerned, and report themselves as enjoying erotic excitement only in the process of captivating a woman who resists their masculine charms. We have been unable to verify these male self-observations. But it does seem clear that Passion response may appear without any appreciable mixture of Captivation in the behaviour of both sexes ; and that Captivation response frequently appears by itself in female behaviour.

The characteristic of completed Love response, which does not appear in either of its components taken alone, seems to be a progressive change from Passion to Captivation. The Inducement elementary response, passive in nature in Passion, changes gradually to a more active type of Inducement in Captivation responses, as the normal love response proceeds toward its completion. The elementary unit response of Submission, however, changes in the opposite direction, beginning at its most active extreme, and shifting gradually toward greater passivity. *Love response*, in the large as it were, *is characterized by control of the lover's behaviour by the interests of the beloved ;* whereas either Passion or Captivation responses, by themselves, may show an ultimate control of the unit love response by self-interest, or Appetite responses.

Review of our foregoing discussion of the Love responses shows that erotic drive, in the female organism, directly produces the following results in female behaviour.

1. It interferes with the subject's responses to environmental stimuli other than persons, especially of opposite sex, and breaks up any organized response to other stimuli.
2. It decreases some self activities and increases others, so that the probability of encountering possible lovers is increased.
3. It changes the inner balance of reflex conduction activities of the self in such a way that attractive persons, especially of the opposite sex, acting as environmental stimuli, evoke a new compound unit response, *Passion ;* consisting of
   a. passive Inducement, and
   b. active Submission.
4. As a result of the Passion response, the inner reflex conduction activities of the self are again changed in such a way that the stimulus, a loved person, evokes a second, compound unit response, *Captivation,* consisting of
   a. active Inducement, and
   b. passive Submission.

Thus erotic drive, like hunger drive, changes the total self activity in such a way that a dynamic, inner cause is set up in the organism by means of a spontaneously acting stimulus mechanism, resulting, first, in behaviour tending to bring the organism into contact with a specially selected type of stimulus ; and, secondly, resulting in special compound unit responses capable of fulfilling the object of the drive by bringing the subject organism into the appropriate relationship with that stimulus.

The erotic drive, like the hunger drive, seems to be something more than the aggregate of compound unit responses which result from it. A woman may learn the unit responses of Passion and Captivation so completely that they become perfectly definite behaviour patterns. She may learn to respond to a certain person or persons with either or both of these responses. Yet it is quite possible that even such habitual stimulus persons may not possess the power to evoke within her the erotic drive condition of self activities. If the drive itself is not evoked, then it is a case of " out of sight out of mind " as far as concerns responding with Passion, Captivation, or completed Love response to the stimulus person in question. When actually in the presence of this individual, the woman may respond lovingly. But when away from him (or her) there will exist no continued, dynamic behaviour element, within the woman's organism, to compel seeking behaviour tending to re-establish contact with the lover.

On the other hand, certain persons (husband or male lover, children, or occasionally, greatly loved persons of the same sex) may acquire the power, through psychoneural retention (see chapter to come), to evoke not only isolated love responses, but also the love drive itself within the female organism ; and also, it would seem, within the male organism, to a somewhat lesser degree.   The absence of the loved person, in such a case, results in continued drive behaviour, tending to reunite the subject with the absent loved one.   In many women, there seems to exist a love drive of much more generalized type.   This appears in her behaviour in a form not unlike the so-called " gregarious instinct " of earlier psychological writings.   The woman thus driven seeks companionship and the company of other persons continually. Many women who have no important love relationships of an organized or fixed character, manifest this vague, general, love restlessness, which seldom accomplishes any fully consummated love responses, and therefore continues, seemingly, throughout mature life.

The love drive of men, in so far as we have been able to find evidences of the existence of such a drive, appears to be of much more limited scope and partial character.   It consists seemingly and for the most part, of vague and unreciprocated Passion, either for one woman, for several selected women, or for women in general, as such.   In the latter case of course, it results in destructive promiscuity.   This male drive, as we have already noted, is really less a " drive " in the definite sense in which we have defined the term, than it is a self pattern of activity with a strong erotic element more or less continually active.   This erotic self characteristic may be enhanced by the presence or memory of women once loved, or simply by the accumulation of physiological conditions (hormones ?) creating it.   When thus enhanced, it assumes something of the apparent characteristics of true erotic drive which is, nevertheless, as a totality, present only in the female organism following menstruation or by processes of retention and recall.

CHAPTER IX

DRIVES

PART III: PROCREATIVE DRIVE AND THE COMPLEX UNIT RESPONSES OF ORIGINATION AND TRANSFORMATION

Procreative Drive

THE creative behaviour of human beings seems to be little better understood, on the whole, than is human love behaviour. Perhaps the reason for this mystery about creative responses is that love responses play a controlling part in creation of all sorts. Before discussing the question of creative drive, therefore, it becomes necessary to outline and analyze the creative behaviour to be accounted for.

Not all human beings, by any means, are spontaneously creative, except as some fragmentary creations become essential in the course of satisfying the desires of everyday life. Women, of course, need not be, and frequently are not creative in their love relationships, nor as a result of love relationships (child bearing). Nevertheless, creative behaviour is extremely important to any fundamental understanding of human psychology. It seems to constitute, naturally, the complete pattern which combines in the only normal way *all* the compound responses of Appetite and Love. Creative behaviour represents, apparently, the normal synthesis of all simpler responses. It may be considered, therefore, the final desideratum of human behaviour, with all possible types of unit response present and normally combined.

Creative behaviour has two fundamentally different aspects. One aspect is concerned principally with human reactions to inanimate *things;* the other is concerned principally with reactions to living *people* (and animals). The first type of creation endows inanimate materials with human emotional meanings, as in the case of artistically created statues, paintings, etc.; and, in the case of procreation, endows food materials with actual human life, in the form of a newly-born infant. In this form of creation, the creator *endows inanimate substances* with human stimulus values, or with human life *drawn from within himself or herself*. This aspect of creative behaviour is concerned with originating a creation.

The second type of creation response endows living organisms with new types of response, new abilities, and new bodily forms and parts, through the process of natural growth directed by the creator. In this type of creation, the creator endows other human beings with new human values drawn out of inanimate things, with which he stimulates other people.

The creator, for example, gives an apple to a hungry child. The child takes the apple, eats it, and his hunger pangs cease. Moreover, the child digests the apple in such a way that nutritive values are extracted from it and added to the bodily tissues of the child. The child's body actually changes and grows as a result of being stimulated with the apple. No bodily tissues are really originated by the mother's creative act of feeding the child with an apple. But the child's body is substantially *transformed* by the mother's creative behaviour. This second type of creation response therefore, may aptly be called " transformation " response. It really consists of stimulating other human beings in such a way that they will be transformed by the effect of the stimulus upon them, the transformation being of a relatively permanent nature and the part transformed being a portion of the true self activities.

Origination and Transformation responses naturally occur as successive parts of the same creative behaviour pattern, just as Desire and Satisfaction naturally form successive parts of the same complex Appetite response.

A creator endows materials less animate than himself with a part of his own animation, of his own individuality. A creative writer, for example, expresses his ideas and emotions in the form of a book—that is Origination response. Then the same creator, through the agency of his publishers, stimulates the minds of thousands of individuals with the book which he first originated. The readers of this book, or many of them, develop new ideas, attitudes and emotions of their own as a result of the stimulation administered to them. These readers, in other words, are transformed to a certain extent by the book. This is Transformation response.

The creation is now complete. An original object, the book is created, endowed from the personality of the creator with characteristic values as a stimulus to other human beings. Other human beings are then transformed by applying this stimulus effectively to their organisms. The book, which is a thing, was endowed with human values by its originator. The readers of the book, who are human beings, are endowed with new consciousness values by the inanimate stimulus object, the book. Such appears to be the invariable method of creation by human beings.

A mother creates, within her own body, special tissues and nutritive blood supply which are built out of the very substance of her body itself. She has endowed less animate materials with the individual forms and chemical characteristics of her own organism. She then surrounds the impregnated ovum (which is a separate germ plasm entity previously kept isolated within the ovaries and testes) with the nutritive stimulus materials and protective tissues which she has created. As a result of this stimulation, the germ cells multiply rapidly. The impregnated ovum is transformed into the embryo and foetus. This process of successive Origination and Transformation continues for nine months within the mother's body. At the end of that time her completed creation, a human infant, is born. This process seems to be nature's own physiological creation pattern.

Nature compels both animal and human mothers to continue the same creation process toward the child after birth, which had been carried on physiologically within the mother's body prior to birth. Within two or three days after birth the mother's mammary glands originate a new food substance, milk, especially adapted to nourish the organism which she has just created. The baby's mouth and digestive tract are stimulated with this newly originated substance. As a result the infant's body is gradually transformed by the natural processes of nutrition and growth. Here we see identically the same type of Origination and Transformation responses on the mother's part and the same results in creating a new human being, as those previously noted.

But the creative behaviour imposed upon the mother by nature forms only a small part of her total pattern of creation responses toward her child. She acquires fruits, vegetables, and other food substances, and prepares them according to her own ideas or those prescribed for her by a doctor, for the nourishment of her child as he grows older. Cooking, in short, and artificial preparation of food is the simplest of Origination responses. The mother then teaches her child to eat the food which she has prepared for him, this process frequently involving great patience and skill. Stimulation of the child's organism with the materials originated for that purpose is no longer an easy or simple task. When it is accomplished, however, the child's organism is transformed by processes of growth and development in just the same way as before. Origination in cooking food and Transformation in administering it to the child form a completed act of Creation.

Thus we might follow Creation responses on the mother's part throughout the entire period during which her offspring remains under her immediate charge. She " brings up " her child physically, emotionally, and mentally. That is to say, the mother originates food and clothing for her child's body and transforms his body by applying these stimuli to it. She originates games, work, activities, and innumerable expressions of her own love in words, gestures, and caresses, and she transforms the child's emotional responses by applying these stimuli to his organism in appropriate ways. She also originates, at least during the early years of her child's life, many intellectual stimuli in the form of words, and variously exercises guidance of the child's ideas and activities ; and transforms the child's rapidly maturing mind by applying these stimulations to it. Thus we may note that a conscientious mother's creative responses toward her child are by no means limited to simple bodily creation. They also extend into the fields of physical, emotional, and intellectual training and education.

In precisely the same way, though perhaps in lesser degree, adult human beings are continually influenced by the creative responses of some of their fellows. Scientists originate scientific theories and these theories, applied in many forms to the daily lives of millions of people, transform the organisms and activities of the individuals to the individuals thus influenced. Creative artists write books, mould statues, paint pictures, write music and design houses, buildings, and structures of various types. These original creations are usually applied to the organisms of the great masses of people throughout the world by an entirely different set of people.

Some of these people are artists, though they are usually not designated as creative artists. Actors on the legitimate stage and in the motion picture studios enact the stories and plays which have been originated by writers. Stage directors, and motion picture directors, and many other types of artists assist in these tasks. Musicians and singers play and sing the music originated by the composers. Editors and illustrators arrange books and articles in attractive form for the public. Art exhibitors arrange statues and paintings with favourable lightings and backgrounds for the enjoyment of those who come to see them. Thus we find a second group of non-originating artists whose chief occupation is the reproduction of original creations in a form most effective for stimulating the organisms of the people who are ultimately to be transformed by these creations.

Along with the reproducing artists a second group of artistically inclined, but commercially motivated, individuals assist in applying these artistic stimuli to the public. We refer, of course, to stage producers, musical promoters, motion picture producers, publishers, booksellers, and the like. These people make appetitive use of artistic creations for their own financial advantage, but nevertheless, in the present organization of society, form an essential link in the total chain of creative behaviour under discussion. The responses of this group of individuals, however, cannot be regarded as Creation responses from the point of view of these individuals themselves. Only from the point of view of social psychology could we regard the entire group activities concerned with placing original artistic creations before the public, as typical Transformation behaviour. At all events, though a complex social group of creators be required to complete the creation, we nevertheless discover the same succession of Origination and Transformation activities underlying artistic creation and its transformation effects upon public morals, emotions, and social customs. This is a sort of wholesale or mass creation, in fact.

Creative influences are exercised in the same way over large numbers of people by teachers, ministers, philosophers, statesmen, newspaper writers, popular athletes, and many other types of social leaders and mentors. In each of these creations even a casual analysis will reveal a succession of Origination and Transformation activities similar to those above considered. From the standpoint of the individual creator in every case Origination response represents a basically different pattern of simple and compound unit responses than does Transformation response.

In order to discover the nature and arrangement of these complex response patterns, we must consider, briefly, the mechanism of the creative drive, and how the organism behaves under its influence. Although creative behaviour, apparently initiated by a true creative drive, occurs in a great many cases not connected in any obvious way with pro-creation and care of offspring, the female mechanisms of child-bearing nevertheless offer the best example of what we can surely identify as spontaneous, creative behaviour. Let us, therefore, briefly review maternal creation, regarded as a natural creative drive.

Maternal Procreative Drive

The first two requisites of a drive are easy to discover in the mother's child-bearing activities. Nine months' pregnancy, labour, and delivery of the child, accompanied by pain and followed by depletion of the bodily tissues (hemorrhage), engorgement of the breasts two or three days later and persisting six to eight months or more, and an extensive set of physiological changes throughout the body accompanying these phenomena, suffice to direct the mother's activities away from ordinary pursuits, and also to direct her attention towards the child. Maternal drive, unlike hunger and erotic drives, not only enforces a greater likelihood of the organism's giving up previous pursuits and seeking adequate stimuli for special responses to follow, but also actually produces the adequate stimulus itself, a new-born child. Human or even animal mothers cannot escape some response to the child as a direct result of maternal creative drive ; and the creative responses to the child thus enforced, will be prolonged for an extended period unless the mother destroys or abandons her offspring, which is the exception rather than the rule, even in animal behaviour.

Two types of complex unit responses toward the child seem to be brought about by the procreative drive mechanisms just described. These two creative responses brought about by maternal drive appear to offer natural standards for Origination and Transformation behaviour patterns. The precise details

P

of the innervations of these complex creative responses are not as yet clearly known, but the maternal behaviour resulting seems definite and remarkably uniform.

Mother's Origination Response

Of the two, the mother's Origination response seems less well understood, as far as the exact physiological functions involved are concerned. But the Origination behaviour of both animal and human mothers has long been known and described, usually under the term " maternal instinct ". It begins, of course, with the impregnation of the ovum by spermatozoon, and consists, essentially, of increased desire for food substances which may be eaten and assimilated into the mother's blood stream, thence carried into the embryo, and finally utilized in building up the rapidly multiplying body cells of the new organism being created. " Pregnant desires " in human mothers are frequently observed. They sometimes seem wholly irrational, as desires for chalk or coffee grounds ; sometimes more ordinary, as desires for strawberries, cantaloupe, or rice and tomatoes mixed together. Medical examination frequently shows, also, an engorgement and hyper-excitation of the external genital organs. Several cases studied by one of the writers revealed greatly exaggerated Passion responses, apparently brought about by this external genital excitement. (These responses were especially marked during the early months of pregnancy, before the cumulative strain of carrying and nourishing the heavier foetus began to produce bodily symptoms which obscured the passion responses). Thus during the early part of pregnancy period, there appear both Desire and Passion responses, seemingly produced simultaneously by the procreative drive in the same way that Desire and Passion responses have been shown to occur separately as results of hunger and erotic drives, respectively. The joint effects of these pregnant Desire and Passion responses is, of course, to increase the mother's appetite, and also to increase the flow of nerve energy and blood supply to her internal genitals where the embryo is being nourished. In short, she is made to ingest more food materials into her own organism, and then to offer her own bodily tissues, thus enriched, to the embryonic offspring. The ultimate results of these responses occur, of course, on a physiological level, and remain largely unconscious.

After the offspring has actually emerged from the female body, the Desire and Passion responses both tend to become fixed upon the newly created organism as adequate stimulus. A curious effect of this sudden fixing of Desire upon the newly born offspring appears in the behaviour of some animals below man, notably the rabbit, a naturally herbiverous animal. The mother rabbit frequently eats the bodies of her young, just after birth, leaving the head alone uneaten. At other times the female rabbit may only bite the young, or devour a small portion of the bodies of one or two out of a litter. Seldom does she eat all the offspring, her Desire apparently becoming satiated, or perhaps normally controlled again by Passion response toward the young, after she has eaten a small amount of flesh. A piece of meat, put into the cage from which the young have been temporarily removed, sometimes serves as an effective substitute in satisfying her exaggerated Desire response until it becomes normally controlled.

Carnivorous animals, including human mothers, give evidence of somewhat better control of the Desire element in the complex Origination response toward their young. The mother frequently attacks her mate, driving the male away, and often slashing him fiercly with her teeth. She fights with complete self-abandon any intruder who approaches her young, and if her nest or hiding place has been discovered, she frequently carries the young animals away to a new and secret place, as in the behaviour of cats. Before the birth of the young, the mother usually prepares some sort of nest, or home, apparently beginning to respond with the Desire-Passion combination to *her own body* before the appearance of the young. The female rabbit at this time, tears out mouthfuls of fur from her own breast and belly, and lines the nest with this soft, warm material. It is rather improbable to suppose that the animal mother has any premonitory or instinctive reaction to offspring not yet born. Rather she seems activated by the maternal drive mechanisms of pregnancy which change her self-pattern of reflex nervous conduction in such a way that she is compelled to seek some adequate stimulus for the complex unit response pattern of Desire-Passion, and which permit this response only toward herself or her offspring. The details of this complex change in the self pattern of activity, and the precise reasons why it causes Origination response selectively toward appropriate stimuli are not yet known.

As the Origination response becomes built up and maturely organized in the behaviour of the mother, she hunts special food for the young, leads enemies away from their nest (quail, foxes), warms them with her own body, and sometimes finds for them sources of drinking water and other necessary supplies (salt-licks in case of sheep, etc.) In all the activities the mother reacts toward her offspring with passionate self-surrender and service, (as evidenced by her frequent self denial, and by her self-abandon in fighting off enemies) ; and she reacts toward food, shelter, other supplies, etc., with special desires intimately combined with and apparently springing from her Passion responses to her offspring. In brief, the mother animal desires various materials *for* her creation, her offspring.

The average human mother reacts in precisely the same fashion, but with greatly enlarged scope in her Origination behaviour. She desires for her baby minute care and attention; gifts of all sorts from her friends and relatives ; pretty clothes and playthings which are of no practical value to the child ; and her passionate adoration of the child is frequently so extreme as to become ludicrous in the eyes of other people not under the influence of maternal creative drive. Like the animal mother. the human creatress is constantly on the alert to detect and eliminate dangers to her offspring, whether imagined physical dangers at the hands of the baby's father, or nurse, or possible dangers of sickness or insufficient nutrition. The whole picture presented by the Origination responses of human mothers follows in a striking manner the same pattern of responses in animal behaviour, but with exaggerated and enlarged scope. The mother, in short, goes on building her baby up, and trimming it with every imaginable embellishment just as she did in a simpler physiological way during the preceding nine months of pregnancy. She gathers physical materials of every sort and shapes them according to her own ideas and emotions for eventual application as stimulation to the infant organism. This is true Origination response.

It should be noted, in these maternal Origination responses, that the baby is treated, to all intents and purposes, like an inanimate object. The mother seeks building materials and a favourable environment under which to add these benefits to her creation. She eliminates dangerous and undesirable objects and environmental influences in the same way, with the infant in the role of passive beneficiary. The mother *does not seek to make the infant do anything*, nor does she expect any guidance or appreciation from him with respect to her Origination activities. The infant's food, clothing, and other appurtenances are moulded according to the mother's combined Desires, plus Passion on the infant's behalf. She endows these materials with her own characteristics, just as she endowed the bodily tissues and nutritional supplies made for the infant within her body before birth, and just as she endowed the milk secreted by her mammary glands for the baby after birth. The mother, in short, *originates* many different types of physical objects for her infant by endowing various materials with her own characteristics. And her complex unit Origination response, under analysis, reveals a simultaneous combination of Desire and Passion responses evoked within her organism by maternal procreative drive.

Mother's Transformation Response

Origination response which we have just considered, is only one aspect of the mother's creative behaviour which begins as soon as the ovum is impregnated. At that moment a new and separate biological entity begins to function. The embryo has living structures of its own, capable of using the materials presented to it for its own growth and development. It is impossible to regard the embryo as a true part of the mother's own body even in its very early stages of growth. The two sex cells, ovum and spermatazoon, had been isolated from the body cells of the mother and father respectively throughout the lives of these parent organisms. The germ plasm, thus set apart, is really as old in its separate existence as the family tree of the organism within which it resides. We may, therefore, legitimately regard the united sperm and egg cells as a distinct and separate individual for whom a mother originates nutritive and protective materials and who is capable of creative transformation when stimulated with these substances.

The mother's body then originates a protective covering with which a growing embryo is surrounded. The mother's own blood stream becomes connected with that of the embryo, thus the chemical food materials originated in the mother's body are brought into contact with the embryo. When thus stimulated the embryo absorbs into its own tissues the materials originated by the mother and is transformed by the nutriment which it receives from these supplies. The mother, therefore, physiologically originates and transforms throughout the entire period of pregnancy.

Within a few days after birth the mother's breasts become engorged with milk. As we have already noted this milk is originated from the mother's own organism for the nourishment of her child. With this milk the mother satisfies her baby's Desire for food, just as she satisfies her own Desires by stimulating the mouth and digestive tract with food. The first component of the mother's Transformation response towards her child would appear, therefore, to be a Satisfaction response. Instead of being directed toward herself, however, this Satisfaction response is clearly focussed upon the child. While nursing, the little one's lips stimulate the mother's breasts ; this stimulation, if not too painful, is ordinarily reported as giving the mother erotic experience of the active or captivating type. From our knowledge of the nervous system, we may feel reasonably sure that the reflex motor discharge resulting from nipple stimulation reaches the internal genital organs[1], thus giving evidence that the unit response is of typical Captivation pattern.

We find, therefore, that the mother is responding simultaneously with Satisfaction and Captivation responses. The unit response patterns of both responses are fairly clear and amply evidence the mother's supplementary behaviour. By word and action she expresses profound Satisfaction in the supplying of her child's needs. By hugging and patting and caressing the child, as she holds him in her arms, she clearly manifests Captivation response. This Captivation behaviour, in fact, on the mother's part frequently interferes with keeping the child in the most efficient position for nursing.

The mother's complex Transformation response to her child after birth appears from the above analysis to consist of simultaneous Satisfaction and Captivation responses evoked by the child as a stimulus. The specific adequate stimulus is no doubt the baby's need. She satisfies his hunger in order that she may captivate him and bring him closer under the love control which she longs to exercise over him. Thus she serves his needs and not her own. She stimulates the infant

[1] Marston, *op. cit.*, p. 346.

with materials which she, herself, originated in order to transform him through the natural processes of growth and development, of which his organism is capable. This behaviour of the mother's would appear to constitute nature's own pattern of a characteristic Transformation response.

Transformation responses on the mother's part form an increasing proportion of her creative behaviour toward her offspring as the child grows older. The mother is able to originate an ever smaller proportion of the materials necessary to supply her child's needs. But on the other hand, she finds it increasingly necessary to satisfy his desires with many kinds of stimulus objects in order to win the child's love and control his behaviour by maternal Captivation. This entire Transformation response has for its object, of course, the training and development of the child's body, emotions, and mind.

Animal mothers show Transformation responses of precisely the same type. It is necessary for animal mothers to teach their young the adult technique of food hunting. Mother cats bring live mice to their kittens, thus teaching the kittens to pounce upon and kill the prey, which they fail to do in some cases unless they have received this training.[1]

Human mothers, of course, have a tremendous amount of teaching and training to do. The child's condition and his developmental needs must be constantly studied, and training, or Transformation responses, must be undertaken to teach the child to form habits of behaviour which will enable him to care for these needs by himself later in life. If a human infant be left to form his own habits by trial and error methods, the result is almost invariably unfortunate for his adult life. He must be taught to dress himself, to eat, to control his excretory reactions, to observe social customs, " manners " of doing things, etc. In every case the mother follows precisely the same response formula in her child training. She satisfies the child's Desires by stimulating him with appropriate objects or environmental surroundings. And she captivates him, thus, into learning new and more mature methods of behaviour.

The doting and over-indulgent mother is one whose Transformation response contains too great a proportion of Satisfaction of the child's needs and too small a proportion

[1] C. S. Berry, " An Experimental Study of Imitation in Cats," *Journal of Comparative Psychology and Neurology*, 1 8(1908), pp. 1–26.

of Captivation. This is the type of mother whom psychologists justly inveigh against. Unless Captivation controls Transformation behaviour towards children, the child's reactions to the mother become controlled by Desire rather than by Submission. The child, as a consequence, demands an increasing number of Satisfactions while himself yielding a decreasing quota of submission to parental authority. The wise and intelligent mother must make sure that every Desire of her child which she satisfies, is used to increase her love control of the little one. In this way the child's Submission is made to control his dominant Desires and he accepts his mother's judgments with regard to the quantity of Satisfactions which he shall receive. Thus a proper Captivation-controlled Transformation response on the mother's part paves the way for increasingly effective Transformation of her child's behaviour as he grows to maturity.

The maternal Creation behaviour, then, directly resulting from procreative drive, includes both Origination and Transformation responses, evoked by the child, and controlled ultimately, in each case, by constituent love responses tending to enlarge and benefit him and not the mother. At the beginning, a preponderance of Origination response appears in the mother's creative behaviour pattern ; then gradually more and more Transformation creeps in, until the proportions are reversed, somewhere near adolescence, with Transformation responses greatly predominating. The gradual replacement of Origination by Transformation responses in creative behaviour may be compared with the similar transition from Desire to Satisfaction in Appetite, and from Passion to Captivation in Love.

We may summarize the results of the procreative mechanisms, or procreative drive, in the mother's behaviour, as follows :

1. It interferes with the mother's responses to environmental stimuli other than her child, or other than objects connected with her child's uses or needs.

2. It practically eliminates many of her usual self-activities, and substitutes the child-bearing activity which actually produces the procreative stimulus and forces it upon her attention.

3. It changes the inner balance of reflex conduction activities of the self in such a way that the child, acting as adequate

environmental stimulus, evokes a new, complex, unit response
Origination ; consisting of
> Desire and
>
> Passion, combining to form passionate Desires to originate necessary materials for the child's needs.

4. It also changes the inner balance of reflex conduction activities of her self in such a way that the needs of the child similarly evoke a second, a new complex unit response, *Transformation,* consisting of
> Satisfaction and
>
> Captivation, combining to captivate the child by satisfying his desires.

Other Types of Procreative Drive.

While we have as yet no specific knowledge of physical procreative drive mechanisms other than those of the mother, just discussed, observations of the life behaviour of many creative individuals of both sexes justify the conclusion that some sort of procreative drive mechanisms are active within their organisms. We have observed creative writers, for example, who seem utterly unable to work consistently at anything but creative writing. In this type of individual, the drive appears to result preponderantly in Origination responses. We have also observed sculptors, painters, inventors, and creative scientists who seem to be driven constantly to devote themselves to creative work at the expense of all other activities. Many of these individuals have not shown marked talent in their chosen line of creative work. Thus it would seem that special talent and physical or mental adaptability to creative work have no essential connection with the procreative drive which compels such work to be undertaken.

We have also observed several types of individuals who seem driven to undertake creative work of a preponderantly transforming nature. We have observed at least one young man who seemed irresistibly driven from within to religious preaching and attempted moral leadership of the people around him. This man did not seem to experience any sudden " call " to the ministry, and, in fact, never completed his theological training or sought to be ordained as a minister. He preached and taught religion, however, in school, college, and also in a factory where he earned college expenses for a time. He taught classes in Sunday School, Y.M.C.A., and social settlement houses. He became janitor of a church, and at one time led the Salvation Army meetings. Insofar as we could determine, this man seemed irresistibly driven from within to transform other people religiously. And his Transformation behaviour could not be traced to training or environmental influence insofar as we could discover. Other types of individual whose behaviour indicates the presence of a creative Transformation drive mechanism controlling their actions in greater or lesser degree throughout life, are reformers, social theorists, some radical leaders, many teachers, and several different types of social and religious leaders.

It may be, of course, that the marked Origination and Transformation behaviour just discussed, does not result from the presence of any specific procreative drive mechanism. It may be that such behaviour is brought about merely by a peculiar or characteristic balance and connection between the hunger and erotic drive mechanisms. Creative behaviour of the types mentioned, in fact, might result merely from the union of well developed unit response patterns of Appetite and Love, and these constituent responses might have been built up by special training rather than by organic drives of unusual strength. Whether or not, therefore, there exists a true procreative drive mechanism other than the maternal drive mechanisms analyzed above, must remain for the present an open question. Further psychological and physiological observation and research directed to the solution of this problem, may be expected to produce results of great practical value.

CHAPTER X

MOTIVATION

PART I: ANIMAL AND HUMAN MOTIVATION

Introductory

MOTIVATION of behaviour means *internal* determination of behaviour, according to presently accepted psychological usage. A boy steals an apple from the neighbourhood fruit stand. What was his *motive*, we ask? Or, in more exact, psychological language, how was his act of stealing *motivated*? This motivation does not include the external causes which contributed to the boy's act, such as the brightness of the sun's rays shining upon the red cheeks of the apple, or the fact that the fruit vendor had gone to the back of his store. Those physical factors constitute the stimuli, of course, or part of the stimuli, which helped determine the boy's act. But they are stimuli which happen *outside* the boy's organism, and independently of his organism, and hence are not regarded as part of his " motivation ".

If, on the other hand, certain hormones were working inside the boy's body, resulting in stomach contractions called hunger pangs, these hunger pangs would be considered part of the boy's motive in stealing the apple. The hunger pangs are part of the total stimuli determining the act of stealing, but they are stimuli which occur *inside* the subject's organism, and which are themselves a part of the organism's total functioning. Hence they are part of his motivation.

Two types of motives.

If, then, we consider as motives merely the causes, or factors⸴ inside the subject's organism which predetermine his reactions to external objects, we find two different varieties of such internal causes, or motives. First, we have the drives, considered at length in the last chapter. Second, we have the native integration mechanisms which determine what

219

variety of unit response to the external stimulus situation shall occur. Sometimes these two types of internal causes are working together, reinforcing one another to produce the reaction which appears. Sometimes the two types of internal causes are in conflict, with the final response representing a partial victory for one or the other internal cause, or motive.

For example, the boy stealing an apple is a case of this later type, where the drive motive and the unit response motive are in conflict. The boy, let us suppose, is undergoing hunger pangs. The pangs immediately initiate a hunger drive, causing the boy to seek food and to cease responding to other objects. At the same time, we will suppose, the boy has been punished for stealing, and so reacts to the threat of authority with the unit response of compliance. His total motivation, therefore, contains two conflicting elements. Hunger drive influences him toward taking the apple ; compliance with punishment influences him toward letting the apple alone. Both internal influences are parts of his total motivation. At last the hunger drive wins out, and he grabs the fruit. But the fact that the punishment motive is still influencing his behaviour is attested by the quick and furtive way in which he snatches the apple and his subsequent running away down the street.

On the other hand, we may easily find examples of behaviour where the drive motive and the unit response motive are in perfect harmony, and hence tend to reinforce each other in the total reaction. For example, let us suppose that the same boy is whittling a stick in his back yard when the hunger pang occurs. At that moment his mother appears at the door, saying, " Come to dinner at once, Johnny, or I'll take your allowance away for a week." Johnny has been deprived of his allowance before, and realizes it is no idle threat. His natural unit response, therefore, we will suppose, is compliance with his mother's command. This punishment motive, therefore, coincides precisely with the hunger drive initiated by hunger pangs with respect to the final reaction which both tend to produce. With all motives in harmony, no furtiveness or other inefficiency is evident in the boy's conduct. He rushes into the house at top speed, and is seated at the table demanding his food before his mother has time to place the meal on the table before him. In this behaviour there are two motives of different types, a drive motive and a unit response motive.   But both motives tend to produce identical final action, so both may be said to be in harmony with one another, and mutually reinforce one another's influence on the subject's behaviour.

Formerly the word " motivation " was used only in connection with human beings and their behaviour.   Now its use is extended in many text books to the behaviour of animals less complex than man.   This use of the word " motivation " as applied to the internal, or predisposing causes of animal reactions is surely warranted from the wholly objective viewpoint of the present volume.   Any organism whose behaviour is properly within the range of psychological description possesses *motives* to action of the same two types possessed by humans, namely drives and unit responses. The unit response motives are imposed upon the behaviour of the animal by the integrative mechanisms, their innate laws of functioning, and the existing conditions of tonic nervous excitation natural to that particular organism.   The drive motives are imposed upon the animal's behaviour by the hormones and other spontaneous bodily stimuli causing changes in the natural or usual state of tonic nervous excitation, as described in the last chapter.   Both the tonic nervous excitement regulating unit response, and the changes in tonic excitation comprising drives, are forces generated within the animal's own body, as a part of its natural, spontaneous functioning.   Therefore, both types of internal cause are true, dynamic motives for resulting reactions.

What Motives Cause Animals to Learn ?

Several questions concerning animal motivation immediately come to mind.   These questions should properly be answered by experiment, as in any physical science.   First, what are the actual motives that drive animals to perform their everyday actions ?   In trying to find an experimental answer to this question, we may set certain problems before the animal, and try to discover what motives will most effectively influence him to solve them.   Many experiments on animal motivation have been performed by use of an apparatus called the maze.

The maze consists of a series of complicated passages,

leading one into another. Some of the passages are blind alleys, and some lead in the ultimate direction of the animal's reward, which may be an escape from punishment (electric shocks), food, or an animal of opposite sex. The animal must learn to run through the passages, making the correct turns from one passage to another, until he reaches his reward.

When a white rat, for example, is placed in a maze, or problem box of any kind, he first begins to move about very actively, but at random. Some experimenters call these spontaneous movements exploratory movements, others call them random movements. In the present book we have already explained that random, spontaneous movements result from the constant, tonic reflex activity within the animal's brain and nervous system, initiated mostly by intra-organic stimuli. Exploratory spontaneous movements are really unit responses of the types already studied, combining the random, tonic movements, and the reflex activities initiated by outside environment through the sense receptors of eyes, ears, nose, etc. If the box or compartment into which the rat is first placed contains no other animal, nor odour of other animals, then we may be fairly sure that the initial unit responses will all be of compliant or dominant varieties. In other words, the rat's preliminary behaviour in the maze is motivated by unit responses of compliance and dominance types. He is compelled to comply with the superior, antagonistic strength of the walls that shut him in. He tries unceasingly to dominate these walls by finding some way through them, under them, or around them. We may say, therefore, that the rat is acting from compliance and dominance motives of unit response type.

In some classical learning experiments with the maze this trial (dominance) and error (compliance) type of behaviour, motivated only by the animal's tonic energy and its unit responses, has proven sufficient to drive the animal into solving the problem, i.e. learning the path through the maze to a food compartment. But other motives, primarily of the drive variety, are frequently added. Even if the rat reaches the food box the first time merely as a result of Dominance-Compliance unit responses, his subsequent trials are influenced by a new motive, since he has found food, and his hunger drive or appetitive response is thereby aroused. Let us not confuse, however, the compound appetitive responses of desire, satisfaction, and appetite, with the real hunger drive. The animal, if pretty well fed, will still respond to food in the destination compartment with *desire* responses. But these are only compound unit response motives, precisely similar in type to the simple unit response motives of Dominance and Compliance which brought exploratory movements. The rat, on smelling or tasting food, responds by *desiring* it, which is to say that he responds by simultaneously complying with it and trying to dominate it. Were this the whole story, the food-seeking must still be regarded as motivated only by the unit response type of motive.

But we know from the researches of Cannon[1], Carlson[2], and others that very frequently the sight, smell, and taste of food will itself initiate hunger pangs. And whenever hunger pangs begin, the hunger drive begins simultaneously. Thus it follows that the rat's motivation changes and becomes more complex immediately following his first taste of food in the food compartment. Whereas, just before tasting food, the animal was motivated by unit responses of desire only, just after tasting food he becomes motivated by hunger drive as well.

In the same way, if an animal of opposite sex is placed in the destination compartment, we find our animal subject, at first, threading the passageways of the maze at random, motivated by exploratory dominance and compliance responses. Then he finds the other animal, and is permitted some brief contact with her before starting the problem again. The first smell or bodily contact with the female doubtless adds some Passion reaction to the Compliance and Dominance motives. Passion reaction, however, although composed of the simple unit responses of Inducement and Submission, instead of the exploratory Compliance and Dominance, is nevertheless the same general type of motive, just as Desire is a compound unit response motive. But still no real drive motive has been added to the rat's total motivation. When, however, a persisting condition of erotic (sexual) excitement has been induced, with appropriate glandular activity and release of increased quantities of the sexual hormones, we find the organism yielding to a real erotic drive. This erotic drive is added, therefore, to the compound unit response

[1] W. B. Cannon, *op. cit,* pp. 6, 8.
[2] A. J. Carlson, *op. cit.,* p. 162.

motive of Passion, and to the simple unit response motives of Compliance and Dominance, making the rat's total motivation a complex one, composed of both types of motives, unit responses and drives.

This is only one way in which the drive motives may be added to unit response motives in the animal's behaviour. A still surer way of accomplishing this same result is to starve animal subjects for several hours or even days before the tests, thus ensuring strong hunger drive motivation in the natural way. Or, if erotic drive motivation is desired, a female animal in heat may be selected for the tests. When this procedure is followed, we have the hunger or erotic drive as the principal motive controlling the animal's behaviour, with unit response motives of Desire or Captivation added to the initial drive motive as soon as the food or the sex object is perceived.

There is still another manner in which experimental animals may be motivated. This is the punishment method. A rat, for example, may be placed in a compartment of a maze the floor of which is made of electric grids, charged with alternating current. As long as the rat stays in this compartment, he will suffer a series of harmless but painful electric shocks. He rushes about with great energy, seeking to escape this punishment until he finds an opening into another compartment. The method can be carried further by arranging the maze in such a way that the rat will receive electric shocks in all the passageways and compartments that do not lead in the right ultimate direction. Thus the animal experiences pain every time he makes a mistake, and continues to experience it until he gets into the right path again.

Yerkes[1], in his early work with animals in a maze, frequently combined punishment and reward, placing food or another animal in the destination compartment, and administering a shock to the animal every time he entered a wrong passage. Yerkes found the punishment method, in fact, more effective in motivating the animal than reward methods.

Now insofar as punishment results in simple withdrawal or escape reactions, the motivation appears to consist of a simple unit response of *Compliance*. The stimulus, an electric shock, is antagonistic to the organism, and also is decidedly stronger.

[1] Yerkes, *Introduction to Comparative Psychology.*

Therefore, the organism complies by giving up, or by decreasing whichever of its spontaneous, tonic movements are incompatible with the stimulus. In other words, the animal retreats or withdraws from its antagonist, without attempting to give battle or assert itself. That is the essence of the simple unit response of Compliance.

Where punishment is the only motivation used, therefore, in compelling animals to learn the maze, our analysis shows only the unit response variety of motive behind the animal's behaviour, and that unit response a simple one, Compliance. Where punishment and reward are both used, then the animal is motivated more complexly.

If food is the reward combined with punishment, then we find unit response motives of spontaneous Dominance and Compliance, simple Compliance (with punishment), Desire (Compliance and Dominance compounded), and finally, after sampling the food, perhaps hunger drive also is present. All these motives are comparatively harmonious, and certainly tend to reinforce one another to a considerable extent as experimental results show.

If sex reward is combined with punishment, we also have complex motivation, but the interrelation of the motives seems quite different. Appetitive responses of Desire and Satisfaction are composed of Compliance and Dominance, compounded. Additional compulsory Compliance response from punishment, therefore, would seem to have a very good chance of combining harmoniously with a motive of Desire for food, at least when the Compliance with punishment is actually showing the way to food. The Captivation and Passion responses are composed of Submission and Inducement, two unit responses of alliance with the stimulus, another animal of opposite sex waiting in the destination compartment of the maze. It would seem, therefore, theoretically at least, that punishment shocks administered whenever the animal enters a wrong passageway, must tend to inhibit rather than to enhance the Passion or Captivation motives. The electric shock is an antagonistic stimulus, and, being much more immediately powerful than the sex stimulus, throws the entire organism into a condition of antagonistic motor set, thus inhibiting all love response. It has been shown, in fact, that any intrusion of antagonistic stimuli during sexual excitement tends to inhibit and supplant the sex with escape or attacking reactions[1]. This punishment does not effect a combination of its resulting Compliance response with pre-existing Passion or Captivation responses. It rather inhibits the love motives altogether, replacing them with simple Compliance motivation.

Comparative Effectiveness of Different Animal Motives

So far we have been concerned in discovering what motives cause animals to solve problems, and to learn to follow a specified path through the maze. Now the question naturally rises in our minds, which of these motives is most effective? Which type of motive causes the animal to solve his problem or to learn the maze, most quickly and effectively?

The early experiments with animals bear only indirectly upon this issue, because the experiments were designed primarily to investigate the psychology of learning, and not the motivation behind the learning process. Nevertheless a great many sidelights were thrown, by these investigations, upon the relative effectiveness of different types of motives in animal behaviour. For example, as we have already said, Yerkes found that punishment (meaning the simple unit response of Compliance) was a more effective motive than others and that it always increased the effectiveness of the total motivation when added to other motives. Others, however, obtained somewhat different results, and on the whole these earlier experiments were inconclusive as regards motivation.

When we come to the later experiments, we find that some of these were designed expressly to test the relative effectiveness of different motives in animal behaviour.

Among these we may mention first the experiments of Moss. He chose a very ingenious way of evaluating different motives by setting up simultaneously an antagonistic motive and then testing the animal to see which motives were best able to overcome the antagonistic one.

Moss placed an electrified grid across the animal's path to the destination compartment. Then he tried giving the animal different motives to see which would most readily cause it to cross the grid that the animal had already learned would give him a painful electric shock. He found that hunger pangs constituted the most effective motivation, that sex was next in effectiveness, while still weaker was the maternal

[1] W. B. Cannon, *op. cit.*

instinct. In our own terms these three motives would be described as hunger drive motivation, the motivation of the compound unit response of Captivation, and the motivation of the procreative drive. Moss also found that food and sex were superior to punishment under the conditions of the experiment and thus that both hunger drive and Captivation exceed in effectiveness the simple unit response of Compliance.[1]

Moss' findings are not altogether substantiated by later investigators. Specifically, Warden at Columbia has recently carried out experiments in animal motivation. His results, at the time of writing, are not yet available, but we are informed that the preliminary conclusions are not entirely in harmony with the work of Moss.

It is possible to say, however, that some of these methods of measuring the relative effectiveness of different motives, are open to one fundamental criticism. The Compliance response evoked by punishment shocks on the electric grid, has a much more powerful inhibitory effect upon erotic drive and Captivation response motives (usually known as " sex " motives) than it exercises upon hunger drive and Desire response motives. This more powerful inhibitory effect upon love behaviour is due to the integrative laws of the animal's central nervous system and to the contrasting nature of Compliance and Love, rather than to any relative weakness in the effect of love motives upon the animal's behaviour, while the love motives are permitted to act. In other words, the readiness with which the erotic motives are inhibited by antagonistic motives is by no means a significant test of the strength of the erotic motive itself, while the latter remains uninhibited. We might as well argue that fire is less powerful in consuming paper than is nitric acid, because fire can be very easily extinguished by water, whereas nitric acid does not yield so readily to the antagonistic effects of water. The only adequate way in which to compare the relative effectiveness of fire and nitric acid as destructive agents, would be to equate the amounts of these applied agents, and then to measure the respective quantities of paper or other material destroyed. Just so with Love and Appetite response motives and with hunger and erotic drive motives. To compare their relative effectiveness in animal behaviour, we must measure their

[1] F. A. Moss, " Study of Animal Drives," *Journal of Experimental Psychology*, 7, 1924, pp. 165-85.

respective effects in causing the animal to act, when both the contrasted motives are at their height, or otherwise equated, with no selectively antagonistic, inhibitory motive simultaneously acting.

The work of Moss and others does show, however, that the effectiveness of hunger drive increases, up to a certain limit, in direct proportion to the time the animal is deprived of food. That is to say, the effectiveness of hunger drive in motivating animal behaviour is in direct proportion to the intensity of the drive itself.

Another investigator, Simmonds, performed a series of experiments[1] upon white rats to investigate the relative effectiveness of various " incentives " when applied to the learning process. For this purpose two mazes were used, one of simple construction and the other of more difficult design. This enabled the experimenter to ascertain whether the results obtained in both simple and difficult learning problems were comparable with respect to the incentives used. These incentives consisted of bread and milk, sunflower seed, escape from punishment, return " home " (to the accustomed cages), sex attraction, and maternal appeal. The standard of comparison was the incentive offered by the bread and milk. The most effective incentive proved to be the bread and milk, and this was also proved to be relatively more effective in the cases of both the mazes. This work supports many of the previous findings that the most effective motivation of all is furnished by the hunger drive mechanisms.

It would appear from the foregoing results of experiments upon animal motivation that the hunger drive is the most effective motive. This is followed by the compound unit response of Captivation ; and the simple unit response of Compliance would seem to be the least effective of all.

Human Motives

Human motives present, of course, a much more complex picture than do animal motives, and are consequently much more difficult to analyze experimentally. While some experiments, as we shall see, have proved profitable, especially in the field of social motives, by far the most extensive and penetrating studies of human motivation have been made by

[1] R. Simmons, " The Relative Effectiveness of Certain Incentives in Animal Learning," *Comparative Psychology Monograph*, 7, 1924.

the psychoanalysts who use a strictly clinical method of analysis and build their studies frankly on a basis of mystical theory. For the " libido ", the ultimate source of all motives according to the psychoanalysts, cannot be described in physical or physiological terms.

The libido, according to Freud, is entirely " sexual ". It is dynamic, sexual energy, constantly striving for expression. It therefore acts upon the brain and body, in some manner undetermined, to drive man and woman toward " sexual " ends. There are six types of sexual behaviour, all abnormal, toward which this hidden libido tends to drive human beings according to Freud. They are : autosexual craving, (that is, erotic excitement over ones' self) ; homosexual craving, (erotic excitement over persons of the same sex) ; incestuous craving, (erotic excitement evoked by persons of opposite sex in the same family) ; sadistic craving, (erotic wish to inflict painful subjection upon other persons of opposite sex) ; masochistic craving, (erotic longing to be painfully subjected by other people of opposite sex) ; and exhibitionistic craving, (erotic wish to display one's own body or genital organs to persons of opposite sex). The fact that Freud regards all the natural, or innate expression tendencies of the libido as abnormal, is extremely significant. It makes the Freudian doctrine very similar to the older type of religious theory which maintained that all human beings are " born in sin ", and can only be redeemed by changing their nature through aceepting the religious precepts offered.

The Freudian doctrine of motivation may be reduced to this. There is a fundamental erotic drive, which motivates all human behaviour, no matter how incongruous may seem the act and the hidden erotic motive. This hidden erotic drive (which is constantly disguised in consciousness by a sort of mental protective mechanism called the " endo-psychic censor ") results not in a single type of conduct, but rather in six specific types of behaviour. These six, named above, are all abnormal. They are all specific, and actually con- stitute six separate drives with one common characteristic, i.e. an erotic element.

There is no other type of motive, according to psycho- analytical theory, except the drive type of motive, taking its origin from the hypothetical libido, nature unknown.

Freud has examined an immense number of dreams, which

he regards as symbolic expressions of one or more of the six erotic drive motives. Everyday behaviour, also, represents an expression either of the erotic drive itself, or of the censoring mechanisms functioning to disguise the true erotic motive striving for self-expression.

Freudian and psychoanalytical theories have been ridiculed and discounted by many critics[1] on the ground that the " libido ", " endopsychic censor ", etc. are all imaginary, mystical creatures of theory and not of fact. But the truth remains that study of thousands of cases of mental abnormalities has yielded much clinical data indicating that the erotic (" sex ") motive, and its suppression are among the most important motivations of human behaviour even if they are not the sole motivations.

Further proof of the ultimate importance of the love, or erotic, motive in human conduct is furnished by the psychoanalytical method of controlling the mind and behaviour of the patient for the purpose of effecting a cure. The ultimate result of the treatment may be questionable, but there seems little doubt of the effectiveness of the emotional control established by the successful analyst over his patients. This control is admittedly a love, or " sex " control. It is called the " transfer ", which means a transfer of the patient's love attachment to the practitioner. Every psychoanalysis which is said to be " successful ", is so regarded because the transfer is complete, and the psychoanalyst has succeeded in establishing a complete erotic, or love control over the patient's personality. The writers of this book have studied many cases where psychoanalysis has been attempted, and we have found that love control, or transfer, has never once been complete (in the cases studied) where both practitioner and patient are of the male sex, even though erotic bodily relationships may have been established.[2] On the other hand, we have found, almost invariably with expert practitioners, that complete transfer has been effected when practitioner and patient are of opposite sexes. We have also found a considerable number of cases where complete transfer has been obtained by a woman psychoanalyst treating girl and woman

[1] F. H. Allport, *Social Psychology*, 1924, p. 355. F. A. C. Perrin and D. B. Klein, *Psychology, Its Methods and Principles*, 1926, p. 180. L. T. Troland, *op. cit.*, 1926, p. 156. J. Jastrow, *The Place of Emotion in Modern Psychology*, Wittenberg Symposium, 1928, p. 24.

[2] W. M. Marston, *op. cit.*, pp. 315, 316.

patients[1]. In at least one case of the latter type, the female analyst was unable to re-transfer to anyone else the love control which she had established over the emotions of a girl patient. All these facts simply go to indicate that the strongest and most effective motivation of human behaviour which can be used by the psychoanalyst to compel human beings to alter and reorganize their entire personalities, is the erotic drive, and the unit response of passion, evoked in persons who submit to psychoanalytical treatment.

Freud, although properly regarded as the founder of psychoanalysis as a clinical method of diagnosis and cure, is by no means unanimously followed by other psychoanalysts in his exclusive emphasis upon the " sex " (erotic) nature of the libido. Alfred Adler of Vienna, a former pupil of Freud, has gone quite to the opposite extreme in his theories of human motivation emanating from the libido. Adler maintains that the libido is primarily a unit of self-assertive, aggressive drive. We spend our lives, according to Adler, trying to compensate for whatever inferiorities of brain or body may be especially impressed upon our organisms. The sole motive of human life is to attain superiority over our environment, and especially over other humans who compose our social environment. (It never seems to occur to Adler that the fundamental nature of a drive to control other people is quite different from the fundamental nature of the drive to control inanimate objects.) Adler's theory, in substance, maintains that the libido supplies to the organism a constant dominant drive motive, which is behind all human behaviour. That Adler thinks of this drive as a simple dominant drive is proved in his unvarying method of treatment, which is to stop fighting or opposing a patient and agree with whatever he says. In short, he *complies* with them and so removes their dominant drive by permitting them to consummate their dominance without opposition.

In contrasting the theories of Freud and Adler as to the nature of the libido, it is interesting to note that Freud bases himself exclusively upon " sex " or love drive, maintaining that our actions toward inanimate objects are merely disguised love acts, while Adler bases human motivation exclusively upon dominant drive, and maintains that all our actions toward other human beings and animals are merely disguised

[1] *Ibid.*, pp. 315, 316.

dominance responses. This failure to differentiate between human motives toward *things*, and human motives toward *people* prevents either the theory of Adler or that of Freud from attaining adequacy, in the opinion of the writers. Each theory presents half the picture, and the value of each is attested by a large number of case analyses of human behaviour which chanced to be motivated, predominantly, by love or dominance, whichever the particular psychoanalyst was looking for in the first place. Of the two, Freud's doctrine contains the more fundamental discovery, i.e. that the erotic drive gives human beings their greatest pleasure, and consequently should constitute the ultimately controlling motive in all average human behaviour where love motives enter at all. That erotic drive motivates all human reactions is certainly open to question.

Moreover, even where erotic drive is attempting to express itself, Freud's own theory points out that the mechanisms for suppression of the " sexual libido " frequently prove stronger than the drive itself, and so distort and repress the erotic motive. The " endopsychic censor ", in fact, is an imaginary creature, or symbolic concept, invented to explain human conduct wherein the ego drive, or dominance reactions overcome erotic drive in one way or another, by repression, inhibition, or perversion. It does not occur to Freud that there must be another part of the " libido ", or nucleus of driving energy, which drives human beings toward dominant self-assertive behaviour, at the expense of love motivation. In all those instances where environment defeats the erotic motives, Freud seems to think of the repressive influence rather as something mechanically imposed by environment. This is very like a unit response of Compliance, which is stronger in most instances, according to Freud, than the erotic drive from within. We must not forget, too, that Freud actually describes the six native forms of erotic drive as abnormal ; so that only the Compliance response remains normal, according to this theory, though it is responsible, directly or indirectly, for all mental conflict, suffering, and abnormality.

In brief, you have an erotically driven organism, compelled to comply with an anti-erotic environment stronger than itself. The environment, since it is stronger, *must* be the more normal of the two, according to this line of reasoning. The organism, then, can only become normal by becoming unnatural under the influence of environment. This is the ultimate upshot of the Freudian doctrine of " sublimation ", or expression of natural erotic drive in unnatural ways like physical exercise, art, or business. There is also, perhaps, a suggestion of compromise, or combination in the doctrine of " sublimation " ; the natural erotic drive combining with the Compliance response to environment in such a manner that the Compliance response dictates the manner in which the erotic drive shall express itself.

It is quite incompatible with the writers' observations of human behaviour that a simple unit response of Compliance should ultimately control human conduct in the absence of a dominant, or hunger drive from within stronger, even, than the erotic drive in most cases. It seems to the writers that Adler's dominant drive does exist, and that it is responsible for training the organism to respond predominantly with Compliance or Dominance when there is a conflict between these responses and the erotic drive or unit responses of love. There undoubtedly exist a great number of human acts which spontaneously seek self-enlargement, and which are not attributable by any stretch of the imagination to the influence of environment outside the organism itself. These actions are motivated by hunger drive from within. Most desires fall into this class, especially those vague, undefined desires which are not, at first, fixed upon any specified object in the environment. Adler's concept of a drive for dominance, or superiority seems to be a somewhat incomplete attempt to describe this hunger drive, which surely constitutes the motive responsible for a tremendous amount of human behaviour.

Carl G. Jung, a mystic psychoanalyst of Berne, Switzerland, adds another concept of motivation to those proposed by Adler and Freud. Jung is more eclectic than either of his confreres in that he accepts both erotic and dominant departments of the libido. In addition to these two drive motives, for which the libido is held responsible, Jung also introduces a concept of " archetypes ", or controlling ideas which the world soul is supposed to have derived from its previous experiences of incarnation in various races of human beings. It is not altogether clear whether the archetypes are supposed to possess dynamic force in themselves, and so constitute drive motives ; or whether they are thought of as being determinative patterns of thought, which determine the forms of actions set off originally by the libido, and which also determine the form of reactions to outer environment. Perhaps the archetypes can best be thought of as potentially dynamic causes of action, since Jung himself refers to them as " dispositions to modes of thinking ". In short, archetypes seem very close to unit responses ; they are potentially dynamic tendencies, ready to be set off by appropriate influence from within and without.

Of course, the archetype concept is vague, undefined, and very mystical, whereas the unit response concept is specific and based upon neurological fact. Also, unit responses contain a constantly dynamic element, i.e. the self-activity which changes in some way during the response as a reaction to an outer or inner stimulus ; while we cannot be certain that archetypal patterns are conceived of as animated or energized prior to the animation from some other source which occurs during the response that the archetype determines. These are the differences between the archetype concept of Jung, and the unit response concept of the present writers.

Despite these differences, however, there is a fundamental similarity in the two concepts. Both the unit response and the archetype concepts are based upon the recognized fact that the organism itself dynamically predominates the manner in which it shall respond to environmental stimuli. Both concepts, in taking account of the total motivation of higher animals and human beings, emphasize the importance of these self-impulsions to certain types of actions not attributable to drives. Both describe mechanisms within the organism by which these self impulsions are believed to occur ; the one (archetypes) a vague, undetermined mechanism ; the other (unit responses) a particular psychoneurological mechanism. In brief, Jung's concept of archetypes really shows a recognition of the fact that there is another type of motive to be considered, besides the drive type of motive. This second type of motive is precisely the same as that insisted upon in our earlier discussion, and designated as the unit-response type of motive. It is a spontaneous, dynamic impulsion of the organism from within, which nevertheless only occurs under the influence of appropriate environment.

If, then, we combine all the motivations described by the leaders of psychoanalytical theory, we find a fairly close approximation to the motivations described by the writers at the beginning of this chapter. Freud and Adler describe the two fundamental drive motives, love (Freud) and hunger (Adler), while Jung adds the unit response type of motive, (archetypes). No attempt has been made by the psychoanalysts, however, to discover the physical nature or basis of these various mechanisms of motivation.

Let us turn now to what might be called the psycho-analysts' practical experiments in motivation ; that is, their methods of influencing their patients' behaviour for the purpose of effecting a reorganization of personality, and a readjustment of reaction to environment. There are different types of motivation methods used by the psychoanalysts to influence patients.

First there is what has come to be known as the " cathartic " method. This consists of encouraging the patient in every way possible, to unburden himself of his troubles, his repressions, his hidden fears and complexes, by confession to the analyst. The belief is that this unburdening process, in itself, without any attempt at advice or persuasion to change the self in any way will actually remove certain types of mental abnormalities. While we are not concerned, at this point, with theories of therapy, and therefore need not consider the efficacy of this mode of treatment from a medical point of view, we are at present concerned with the methods by which the analyst causes his patient to confess and unburden himself.

The principal device whereby hidden information about himself is sought from the patient is the method of " free association ". The patient is asked to relate his dreams to the analyst. Then the central object or word in a dream is selected by the analyst, and the patient is told to give all the words and ideas which occur to him in connection with this object or word ; i.e. all his " free " associations with the stimulus word. In this way the patient is dominated by the analyst, in that he is compelled to reveal certain otherwise concealed brain connections, or associations between various objects, ideas, and thoughts, without in the least realizing that he is doing so. Thus the " unconscious " or " subconscious " resistance of the patient is overcome, and his mind and emotions are forced open, as it were, to the analyst's inspection and analysis. By superior skill and knowledge, the analyst attempts gradually to dominate the patient completely, insofar as the patient resists revealing his innermost feelings and secret strivings.

Put in its simplest terms, the situation is just this. A patient, suffering from some hidden emotional conflict, comes to a physician. The doctor must motivate the patient, in some way, to reveal the hidden emotions from which he is suffering. The patient's most primitive and uncontrollable dominance reactions are evoked by each direct question which touches the secret and repressed complexes. But the physician to effect a cure, must compel the patient to reveal the very emotions he is trying to conceal. Which is to say that the analyst must first dominate the patient completely and evoke from him complete compliance in his most secret and personal emotions. By the free association method, already mentioned, and by analysis of dreams, where there is much less emotional inhibition than in waking life, the analyst cleverly spies upon the inner emotional workings of his patient, until he is satisfied that he knows all he needs to know. Then he tells his patient what he has learned, and compels him to acknowledge as true the hidden emotions discovered. It is just as if a detective concealed himself behind the curtains of a bedroom, and then suddenly stepped out face to face with the occupant at precisely the moment when the latter had removed all his clothes. The person spied upon is suddenly forced to realize that he is being compelled to reveal himself just as he is.

The shock produced upon the patient by this procedure was considered, by G. Stanley Hall, the most important result of psychoanalysis. It constitutes an extremely ingenious method of establishing a fundamentally compliant attitude in the patient toward the analyst. The doctor is regarded, unconsciously, as a superior antagonist from that time on, and all his commands or questions tend to become dominant stimuli capable of evoking compliant responses from the patient. The patient, in short, is thenceforth motivated in his reactions to the analyst, by unit response motives of compliance.

The doctor then takes the next step, which is to use the patient's compliant attitude to evoke Submission responses. To do this, the analyst changes his own attitude from Dominance to Inducement. He adds persuasion and personal charm to his treatments of the patient, talking kindly and intimately about the patient's life and innermost emotions.

Presently the patient begins to find these personal talks with the doctor increasingly pleasant. He (or more likely she) begins to look forward to the daily hour of psychoanalysis, and enjoys the feeling of being mastered and directed by the physician. At this point the patient has begun to submit. It is as though the bedroom occupant, once having been caught nude, finds that the intruder takes a friendly and intimate interest in improving his personal appearance, and so begins to enjoy revealing himself at command, without restraint. Once the nude person has been completely mastered, he feels he has no more to lose and begins to enjoy the new relationship to another human being of superior but kindly strength. Henceforth, the patient is motivated by unit response motives of Submission as well as Compliance.

At last comes a time (perhaps after many months or even years of psychoanalytical treatment) when the analyst's attitude towards his patient becomes still more personal and intimate. The physician is genuinely absorbed and personally interested in his patient. This submissive stimulus offered by the analyst evokes a wish on the patient's part to hold the doctor's attention and interest. The patient begins not only to submit to the physician's wishes, but also to offer himself spontaneously, and volunteer facts and submissive acts to the doctor, in the hope of intensifying the latter's personal interest in himself. This constitutes a unit response of passive Inducement on the patient's part, which combines naturally with the active Submission response already evoked to produce passive love, or Passion response, by the patient toward the analyst. When this final motivation has been established, the " transfer " is said to be complete. The physician has made himself a captivating stimulus to his patient, and thenceforth can evoke Passion responses from the patient at will. By means of these Passion responses, the patient can be made to reorganize and change his entire personality, and to adopt totally new types of behaviour at the psychoanalyst's dictation. This is the Freudian method of motivating patients to effect the personality readjustments considered necessary for a cure, and it has proved amazingly successful in a large number of cases. These cases, therefore, may properly be regarded as clinical experiments in human motivation.

Summarizing the patient's motivation, we may say he is

first made to acknowledge the physician as his master, and comply with him. Then he is made to regard the doctor as his friend, and to submit to him. Finally he is made to feel the captivation of the analyst's personality, and responds with Passion. When thus motivated, the patient can be made to do almost anything the psychoanalyst directs. The final state of motivation, with a completely compliant individual responding also with Passion, probably represents the strongest possible control which one human being can exercise over another. It is the control which a fascinating woman exercises over her lover or husband, and, when coupled with a wish to reform the man's character, constitutes the literarily well-known " influence of woman " in regenerating a man's character. One of the present writers also has shown elsewhere[1] that many mothers evoke Passion responses from their adolescent daughters, and are thus able to mould their personalities by establishing an emotional influence over them which frequently endures for many years after its purpose has been served.

Summary

We may summarize the Freudian type of clinical motivation experiments as follows : human beings respond with almost complete Compliance when their resistance to revealing their hidden ideas and emotions is dominated by the psychoanalytical experimenter. While in this compliant attitude, the subject appears extremely susceptible to the analyst's Inducement, and Submission reactions are readily evoked. Once a submissive attitude has been added to the compliant one, the subject's Submission may easily be changed into the unit response of Passion directed toward the analyst. Compliance-Passion response appears to furnish extremely effective motivation, resulting in partial or complete reorganization of personality, and change of deeply inwrought habits of behaviour.

Other Types of Motivation in Psychoanalytical Therapy

Adler's system of clinical treatment is quite different from that of Freud. Adler's results, therefore, furnish us with a second type of clinical motivation experiment. Adler starts with the assumption, as we have seen, that the patient is

[1] W. M. Marston, op. cit., p. 235.

aggressively seeking a fight, or contest for personal supremacy with everyone he meets, and especially with the psycho-analyst. His method of therapy is to remove the desire for conflict by agreeing completely with the patient. This consists, primarily, of the analyst's adopting a completely *compliant* attitude toward the person to be treated and thus permitting the subject to exercise his Dominance as freely as he chooses. (Contrast this with the Freudian methods just described, which seek to *dominate* the patient initially, compelling him to respond with *Compliance*.) Mixed with the patient's drive to dominate, however, we find a wish to *induce*, i.e. personally to master and control the other person. Adler does not differentiate between these two basically different motives, which are inextricably mixed up together whenever the opponent to be mastered is another human being. Because of this complication, Adler's compliant attitude leads naturally into Submission, and the patient responds to this submissive stimulus by becoming friendly (allied) and superior to the experimenter. In other words, the physician complies until the patient's Dominance is all expended (even to the point of beating the doctor with his fists, scratching his face, etc.). Then he submits to the patient's will (by agreeing entirely with the patient, or by binding up a hurt, etc.), and the patient responds by becoming inducive (a unit response expressing an alliance with the stimulus) instead of dominant (a reaction of antagonism to the stimulus).

It is not altogether clear how far the Adler method is able to influence the patient from this point on. Certainly the control exercised over the patient's personality must be largely an indirect one, the doctor, perhaps, refusing to submit to the patient unless the latter improves in one way or another. From Adler's own accounts of clinical treatments, one gathers that the patient benefits largely by the very fact that he is acting from inducive rather than from dominant motives. If this is so, then Adler's results must be regarded as establishing new motivation habits in the patient's personality, rather than as influencing and controlling the patient's behaviour directly by means of a motivation which brings the patient under the doctor's direct control.

Regardless of the degree to which the doctor controls his patient, however, Adler's results demonstrate clearly that human beings can be motivated by Dominance-Inducement responses to behave in a peacable, friendly manner toward the experimenter.

Contrasting the Freudian and Adlerian results in clinical motivation experiments, we may say that the Adler type of motivation is easier to establish in the patient (provided the experimenter himself is willing to risk being hurt physically by the unresisted dominance of his subject) ; while the motivation sought by Freud is much harder to establish in the patient. It is easier, in other words, to evoke Dominance-Inducement responses from human beings than to evoke unit responses of Compliance-Submission. On the other hand, the Freudian motivation, once established, appears to give the physician much more influence over the patient than the Adler motivation. To make the patient express friendly Inducement toward the doctor may be intrinsically good for the patient. But it does not give the doctor any very powerful control over the patient's behaviour. When the patient is made truly to submit, on the other hand, the doctor's control is great, and this control probably becomes maximally powerful when the compound unit response of Passion is evoked in the patient.

CHAPTER XI

MOTIVATION

PART II : UNIT RESPONSE MOTIVATION

Introductory

OUR own clinical observations and experiments lead us to conclude that nearly all the simple and compound unit response motives can be evoked in the minds of human beings, by use of appropriate stimuli. Likewise the three drive motives frequently make possible the establishment of associated unit response motives, and sometimes are themselves evoked by a previous establishment of an associated unit response motive, but on the whole cannot be dependably established experimentally in adult human beings, because of the complexity of human personality and mental organization. You can easily starve a white rat, and thus evoke hunger drive which will make him seek food. But human beings, if starved, may subordinate the physical hunger drive to other unit response motives of contrary nature, and consequently may even refuse food altogether. Similarly, female animals may be experimented with during heat, with predictable results of this drive motivation. But women may frequently develop mechanisms of suppression or inhibition, so that their sexual behaviour becomes actually more cold and inhibited during the periods following menstruation, when their physical condition furnishes the strongest erotic stimulus. It is our conclusion, therefore, that the drive motives in human conduct can best be studied and observed through their associations with component unit response motives.

Compliance

A great proportion of human conduct is controlled by this Compliance motive, even though it is apparently a wholly acquired motive[1]. We may think of Compliance motive as virtually identical with the " censor " mechanisms emphasized by Freudian types of psychoanalytical theories. The censor, or suppressive influence of environment, is the great anti-erotic, or anti-libido motive demanding disguise and distortion of natural " sexual " or erotic drives. It is absurd to try to think of this self-repressive behaviour as unmotivated, while its opposite, erotic behaviour, is motivated by the libido. Unless there were some motive intrinsic in the nature of the organism which causes the organism to repress and alter part of itself to suit its environment, we should have to regard the self-repressive reactions as purely mechanical, and not spontaneous or voluntary. Such would be contrary to fact. We shrink from fire spontaneously, " to avoid pain ", as we say. That action, then, has its *motive*, a spontaneous effort of the organism to protect itself. After the baby's hand has been burned in reaching for the candle, he positively inhibits or represses his dominant reaching and grasping movements at sight of the candle flame, just as adult human beings inhibit or repress both dominant and erotic actions when threatened by an antagonistic environment which they have learned has the power to hurt them. Their *motive* in thus inhibiting or repressing parts of their spontaneous activities is *Compliance*.

Any control of human slaves or prisoners by force represents the maximum use of the Compliance motive in controlling human behaviour. Confinement within physical barriers which are far too strong to be overthrown, constitutes one form of dominant stimulus which enforces continuous Compliance upon the persons confined. Most prisoners cease all active efforts to escape once they become convinced of the impregnability of their prison. In other words, they comply by giving up a great part of their natural, spontaneously sought freedom of movement. This is passive Compliance.

But modern prisoners, like the slaves of ancient times, are compelled to work for their keepers by threat of painful punishment if they fail to comply. Roman galley slaves were chained securely to their benches and to their oars. They were then whipped mercilessly by an overseer who walked up and down between the rows of slaves. As long as a slave pulled strongly and evenly at his oar, he received only occasional and perfunctory blows of the master's whip. But

[1] W. M. Marston, *op. cit.*, p. 191.

if he slackened even slightly in his efforts, then he was given a terrific lashing. To escape the pain, he *actively complied* with the dominating slave driver, an antagonist stronger than himself, by pulling the oar with all his might.

Prisoners in many states to-day are compelled to work in precisely the same way, with the whip. The number of blows which can be given in one whipping is usually limited by law, and the type of whip to be used is prescribed to safeguard against permanent injury to the prisoner. But the method of control by force, or Dominance, is precisely the same, and the prisoner's response of active Compliance is the same, also. Besides the whip, there are many other forms of physical torture which may be applied to compel active Compliance from prisoners, notably the " third degree " procedures when a confession is to be forced from a suspect, the straight jacket, the dark solitary cell, handcuffing the prisoner's arms above his head for long hours at a time, making the prisoner " ride the mule " (sit astride a wooden beam) until the pain is intense, and many other forms of physical torture which break the prisoner's Dominance and evoke active Compliance without marking the prisoner or leaving a permanent disability.

In milder degree, any form of threatened punishment to avoid which normal people comply actively or passively with the law, utilizes the same motivation. Compliance motives may also underlie various forms of social conformity such as styles of dress, living in a " fashionable " neighbourhood, speaking with a markedly " cultured " accent, and refraining from natural love behaviour of all kinds whenever other people are looking. There is also much geniune Submission motivation in all social behaviour, and it is often difficult to distinguish between Compliance and Submission motives. A test may always be applied, however, which will differentiate the two without fail. If the person who conforms to social rule would continue to do so even though he gained no appetitive advantage by conforming, then he is conforming because he enjoys being ruled by others, and his motive is Submission. If, on the other hand, he acts quite contrary to peoples' wishes in a situation where there is nothing to lose by it, then his former motive was Compliance. Compliance motives, though often inextricably interwoven with other types of motivation, are extremely important in normal adult life, and undoubtedly constitute the major motivation underlying all self-restraint, self-repression, and inhibition of natural impulses and behaviour, especially of love behaviour as emphasized by Freud.

No human being can be controlled completely by Compliance motivation, because there are always parts of the organism and its activities which do not come under the control of the dominating person or stimulus, and which cannot be observed in order to tell whether or not they are in conformity with command. These parts include implicit part-reactions such as sensations, thoughts, emotions, etc., which go on hidden within the organism.

Moreover, it is extremely difficult, if not impossible, to compel active Compliance continuously, because of the difficulties attendant upon exercising Dominance continuously upon the subject. Prisoners and slaves must always be closely guarded, and at best they do only a small fraction of the work, per person, that they are capable of doing if spurred on by other motives. In this respect active and passive Compliance, as human motives, are sharply contrasted. It is comparatively simple to enforce passive Compliance by means of permanently placed physical obstacles such as prison walls, chains, prohibitive laws, and social taboos. Thus it happens, as Freud repeatedly points out, that self-repressions and inhibitions occur, actually motivated by passive Compliance ; while no positive, active outlet can be found for the suppressed energy for the very reason that active Compliance cannot be measurably enforced. It is comparatively easy, in short, to evoke passive Compliance by making people give up some natural activity ; but it is always difficult to evoke active Compliance by making those same people, instead, perform a different set of acts prescribed by the dominating persons. Such are the limits, roughly, of Compliance motivation in everyday human behaviour.

Dominance

Actions motivated by dominance begin to occur, in all probability, before birth. Human infants a few days old grasp a rod which is pressed into their hands, and when the rod is pulled away, the child clings to it tighter and tighter, until his whole weight may be suspended by the grasp of one hand upon the rod. This spontaneous increase of strength to overcome an opposing force is an example of Dominance motive. Unlike Compliance, Dominance is apparently an unlearned unit response ; or perhaps it is learned prior to birth. During the first few months of life, Dominance motivates a large proportion of the infant's behaviour. Any antagonistic stimulus which tends to interrupt or hamper the child's spontaneous movements evokes a response of dominant type. All stimuli, it seems, impress the infant as weaker than himself and are, therefore, to be dominated. Only when a painful stimulus like the candle flame, or an over-intense stimulus like a sudden, loud noise close to the baby's head overwhelms the child's psychoneural resistance, and so interrupts his natural movements, does the response of Compliance replace that of Dominance. And several repetitions of a painful stimulus may be necessary before the baby learns that it is actually stronger than himself, and therefore not to be dominated but rather complied with.

The "naughty" or rebellious child is a child motivated by Dominance not controlled by Submission or defeated by compulsory Compliance. "Temper tantrums" seem to represent misdirected and unrestrained Dominance, of similar type to that described by Watson in the behaviour of young infants under the term "rage". "Determination", "stubbornness", and "aggressiveness" in child behaviour represent Dominance motives more purposefully directed.

Pure Dominance motives play a decreasingly important role in human behaviour as the individual grows older, while Compliance motives conversely increase in importance with age. When a child is very young, Dominance responses may be evoked by almost any sort of opposition to his natural movements. Just as no opposing force is recognized as superior in strength, so also no opposing force is regarded as too trifling to be dominated. As the individual grows older he learns that a great majority of antagonists are stronger than himself, and so must be complied with. He also learns that many antagonistic stimuli are so trifling and unimportant that Dominant responses to them are a waste of time. Thus an intelligent adult is comparatively hard to motivate, experimentally, by offering stimuli that provoke to Dominance. And women are much harder to evoke Dominance responses from than are men.

For instance, a test of intelligence, or of special skill, may frequently fail to arouse any more than a languid " interest ", with correspondingly lackadaisical efforts to pass it successfully. The test, in short, evokes very little Dominance response from the subject ; usually because it falls partly into the class of antagonists that are of too trivial importance to dominate, and partly into the class of opponents that are accepted as obviously too difficult to overcome. In either case, Compliance motive has replaced the Dominant motive.

We well know that youth is more ambitious than age ; more aggressive, more contentious, and more eager to overcome obstacles just because they are difficult and dangerous. Youth is more adventurous, more restless, quicker of temper and less tolerant of other people's annoying peculiarities. All these types of behaviour, characteristic of youth as contrasted with age, are clearly products of Dominance motives. In other words, the behaviour of youths is much more completely motivated by Dominance than the behaviour of persons of more mature age.

Also, there is a tendency with age to shift from motives of active dominance to motives of passive dominance. Older people become " set in their ways ". They are less eager, no doubt, to seek new fields to conquer, but they resist passively, with considerable tenacity, any attempt to budge them from a field already possessed. Their Dominance motives gradually shift, in short, from active to passive types of Dominance response.

One individual can use Dominance motives of another person to control that other person's behaviour by stimulating the other fellow to rash deeds of Dominance or by the method known as " giving him rope enough to hang himself with ". " Pride goeth before a fall ", and " him whom the gods destroy, they first make mad " are two proverbs intended to warn against being controlled or destroyed by permitting our Dominance motives to be too easily or too intensely evoked. The overdominant emotional set known as " pride " causes an adult person to fail to discriminate between antagonistic forces that are weaker than himself, and antagonistic forces stronger than himself. Like the untrained, naive child, he tries to dominate a stronger antagonist just as readily as a weaker one, and is himself injured or destroyed as a result. Now if " the gods ", or some shrewd human antagonist, can make any human being "mad" enough, (which is to say dominant enough), that person will surely destroy himself by attempting to dominate antagonists superior to himself. This method is frequently employed with great success in professional boxing contests. One man passes a slurring and insulting remark to the other. The other man loses control of himself ; he goes "mad" in a fury of attack, leaving himself wide open to the coolly directed blows of his self-controlled opponent, and, as a result, the "mad" man may exhaust himself, and yield, eventually, to an opponent who was originally weaker than himself in all but psychological knowledge of human motivation. When you "give him rope enough to hang himself", you permit the dominant individual to go on with his conquests unchecked, until his overdeveloped Dominance motive causes him to attempt the impossible, in which attempt he destroys ("hangs") himself.

But, on the whole, Dominance motives offer comparatively unimportant means whereby one person can control another's behaviour. Dominance responses mostly innure to the benefit of the dominant individual. Dominance is the prevalent motive of infancy and childhood, diminishing gradually in importance and singleness of quality as human beings grow older. In normal adults, Dominance motives occur less often than Compliance, and are more or less completely held in subservience to Submission and love motives. Dominance represents, nevertheless, the great primitive, self-preserving and self-enlarging motive underlying all others in the life-long behaviour of average human beings and animals.

Inducement.

During early infancy, there are very few evidences of real Inducement motives in child behaviour. When a baby compels its mother or attendants to serve his needs by bringing food, or by making him more comfortable in some way, he does so mostly by loud and prolonged crying. Infant crying behaviour seems motivated by Dominance rather than by Inducement. The child is increasing his tonic energy, or self energy, to overcome some antagonist—perhaps hunger pangs or a hard metal toy which has become wedged beneath him and is causing discomfort. There is no evidence that the baby differentiates between the antagonistic object which is hurting him, and the mother who relieves him of the hurt, as far as his crying and howling goes. He soon learns that the mother's coming brings relief. But his method of bringing her to him remains the same—a prolonged and unrestrained howling. Until she relieves him, the mother is reacted to, apparently, as the antagonist for the very reason that she has not yet helped him. And as long as the child is simply compelling an opponent to do something, his motive must be simple Dominance, and not Inducement.

When the baby is only a few months old, in most cases, he begins to experience a real enjoyment of being taken up, hugged and fondled. In several cases observed by the writers, the baby begins at the age of four to seven months, to hold out his arms spontaneously at sight of persons who have frequently petted him, including the mother. Watson[1] also, has noted this same type of spontaneous behaviour. The apparent purpose of holding out the arms in this fashion is to *invite or induce* the older person to pick the baby up and fondle him. The infant's motive in such actions would seem to be real Inducement. He has learned to regard a certain adult as friendly, or *allied* with himself. He *increases* his activity in stretching out his arms to make the other person lift him, but yet remains wholly allied to the stimulus person throughout the entire action. We may easily contrast this action with the behaviour of ill-trained babies in crying and howling every time the mother leaves them, or whenever an adult who has been amusing the child leaves him. Such actions are motivated by *Dominance*, the mother or adult being treated as antagonistic to the child until the adult returns to pet and amuse the little one. Cessation of petting, in short, makes the adult an *opponent*, whom the infant seeks to dominate. But in the case where the child holds out his arms, the adult in her capacity of prospective petter is an ally, whom the child seeks to control by Inducement.

The degree to which Inducement motives supplant Dominance motives as the child grows older, seems to depend very largely upon the training and experience of the child. The typical " spoiled " child is one who has never been taught that other human beings should be controlled by Inducement and not by Dominance. The spoiled child has always succeeded in getting what he wants merely by demanding it,

[1] J. B. Watson and Rosalie R. Watson, "Studies in Infant Psychology," *Scientific Monthly*, 1921, p. 494-515.

which is to say *dominating* the person who gives it to him. If members of his family do not yield immediately to his demands, this type of child cries, howls, and perhaps goes into a temper tantrum. He complains bitterly, and makes himself as disagreeable as possible. In short, he treats his relatives as *opponents* whenever they refuse him anything he wants, and attacks them until they yield. His motives are almost purely dominant.

The well trained child learns, during early infancy, that he must *dominate things*, and *induce human beings* and animals. Male children learn more quickly than girls to dominate *things* successfully and not to cry and give in (comply) when the task proves hard. But little girls learn to induce *people* rather than to dominate them, much more readily than do boys. Girls spontaneously flirt with grown ups of both sexes. They quickly learn to persuade their fathers and mothers to grant various concessions by making themselves attractive and agreeable to the parent. When a little girl climbs into her father's lap and begins to pet him, it is frequently a signal that she wants him to grant her some childish favour. Child behaviour of this sort is clearly motivated by *Inducement*. It is exactly opposite to the spoiled child's method of persuasion. The spoiled child tries to compel others to give him what he wants by making himself as disagreeable (*antagonistic*) as possible ; the little girl who climbs into her father's lap, tries to persuade him to grant her request by making herself as agreeable (*allied*) as possible. The spoiled child is motivated by Dominance, the flirtatious little girl is motivated by Inducement.

During adult life human beings must learn to control others by Inducement rather than by Dominance if they would maintain permanent social relationships with others. Organized society is controlled by the Inducement of its leaders. According to civilized law, Dominance control may be used only upon those individuals (" criminals ") who are incapable of being controlled by Inducement. Laws are passed and executive orders issued by political leaders, theoretically at least, for the benefit of the people who must submit to these laws and commands. And curiously enough, from a practical point of view, laws which are dominant rather than inducive cannot be enforced. Legislators and officials of the government must remain *allied* with the people they govern, or with a majority of them, in promulgating rules and regulations, if these rules are to become effective. Any law which is antagonistic to a substantial majority of the people, can never be completely enforced, and will always be overthrown, sooner or later, frequently entailing along with it the over-throw of those who made the law. It is an axiom of political science that any government which becomes too oppressive (i.e. antagonistic and *dominant* toward the people governed) will be overthrown sooner or later. The growth of civilization, like the social development of the individual, is really the growth of inducive methods of government and the decline of dominant methods.

For example, let us consider two laws now in existence in the United States, and let us compare the degree to which these laws are enforced. There is a law in every state which prohibits murder ; and there is also a national law prohibiting the manufacture, transportation, and sale of alcoholic beverages. Both the laws are integral parts of the Constitution of the United States. Now the threat directed toward compelling people to obey both laws, strangely enough, is approximately equal. Death in the electric chair, or life imprisonment (actually meaning about 20 years or frequently less, with time off for " good behaviour ") is the legal penalty for a wilful murder ; death at the hands of the " high-jackers ", rival bootleggers, gangsters, etc., or ten years in prison, is the risk encountered in transporting and selling liquor. The threatened legal penalty for murder is slightly more severe than the risks attached to bootlegging, but the likelihood of conviction for first degree murder is much more remote than the likelihood of being " taken for a ride " by rival gangsters in the liquor business, which just about evens the actual risks involved. Comparing the degree to which both laws are obeyed, we find that a very small percentage of the total population of this country commits murders, (even with the marked increase in this percentage due to illicit liquor traffic) ; while a comparatively high percentage either buy or sell liquor in violation of the constitutional prohibition law. Assuming that there is a different murderer for every person murdered (which is far from true, because most bootleg murders are committed by professional killers), we still find that only a fraction of one per cent. of the population violate the law against murder. With approximately 32,000 speakeasies in New York City alone, and with the annual importation of illicit liquor from Canada *only*, officially estimated by Canadian officials (1928) at 1,392,109 gallons of whiskey, 239,105 wine, 3,557,333 beer, etc.,[1] it is obvious that a pretty substantial percentage of our total population violate the law prohibiting liquor.

Comparisons of these two laws, then, gives us a very fair comparison between the relative effectiveness of Inducement and Dominance controls of society by legislative and executive leaders. Nearly every inhabitant of the United States abhors murder, and is consequently completely in alliance with a law which forbids it. A large percentage of American citizens, on the other hand, enjoy alcoholic beverages, and a still larger percentage believe that liberty to drink or not to drink should not be interfered with by law; consequently the prohibition law is antagonistic to a considerable percentage of citizens, and the law must prevent their drinking, if at all, by Dominance rather than by Inducement. The dominant control exercised on these persons is practically nil; whatever effectiveness the law has, is exercised over people who are in alliance with it either because they do not drink alcoholic liquor, or because they believe that it is best to prohibit its sale for the benefit of other people. On the other hand, when a law is truly inducive, like the law against murder, and people are allied with it in the first place, then not only is its Inducement effect very powerful, but its Dominance control is also enhanced. An average person who commits murder, violates the Inducement appeal of the law, which results in an experience of "guilty conscience"; and while the individual is in this condition, the dominant threat of arrest and punishment becomes trebly significant, resulting in an attitude of over-compliance and fear. Contrast this with religious fanatics, and crusaders for a "cause", who deliberately violate laws which they regard as antagonistic to themselves and others, and subsequently manifest not the slightest dread of punishment or Compliance to escape punishment. We may conclude that any law which lacks high Inducement appeal, has little chance of controlling people by means of its Dominance threat; while any law which possesses high Inducement value, increases, pari passu, the effectiveness of its Dominance control. The initial attitude of the people

[1] From Records of the Dominion Bureau of Statistics.

governed must be controlled by Inducement rather than by Dominance, if a stable social order is to be secured.

Control and guidance of children, at home and in school, depends upon the Inducive powers of parent or teacher. Modern methods of child training have abandoned whipping, frightening of children, and other dominant methods of child control almost entirely. The behaviour of most women toward children seems to be naturally motivated by Inducement, for the most part. But in the untrained mother or teacher there are frequent lapses into Dominance when children become unusually stubborn or irritating. Maintaining Inducement as a constant motive in child training requires much experience and training, even on the part of naturally well-balanced mothers.

Modern business salesmanship is motivated mainly by Inducement, when it is successful. The dominant, pushing, nagging salesman who attempts to force his goods upon the attention of the buyer, does not get very far. But the salesman who makes himself agreeable, charming, and allies himself with his customer in discussing business needs and available goods on the market, is the man who gets the trade and keeps it. Modern advertising, in a similar way, must be motivated largely by Inducement. The picture or headline of modern advertisements frequently has nothing whatever to do with the commodity advertised. For instance, a very interesting picture of a prizefight, with one fighter landing an uppercut on the other man's jaw, constitutes the Inducement stimulus for an advertisement of cast-iron pipe. The caption reads : " That baby has a cast-iron jaw ! " and the reader's mind is then gently led around to the idea that " cast-iron " has come to be used, in everyday language, as a term synonymous with strength and durability. Therefore, if one desires strong and durable pipe, one should buy cast-iron pipe. No attempt is made, in this style of advertising, to force the reader's attention upon the goods advertised. Rather the advertisement copy writer allies himself as completely as possible with the taste and interest of his readers, and gives them a picture and a caption dealing with a sport they are already interested in. That is the essence of Inducement.

In our modern American civilization advertising and publicity constitute the greatest sources of real power. A man can no longer be elected president of the United States, for example, by sheer force of money or military threat. In the days of Julius Cæsar a politician without military power, which, of course, was essentially dominant, was in a very precarious position. Usually he was destined to lose, first his office, and then his life. Julius, after completing his first consulship, organized an army and waited just outside the city of Rome until he had dictated the next Roman election of public officials. Cicero, by far the most inducive of the Roman politicians of that day, never became a permanent political power apparently because he never resorted to military or financial influence.

In recent years we see precisely the opposite type of event taking place. Foch and Joffre were both unable to control French political opinion and non-military politicians ruled France throughout the great war. Similarly in England, Lloyd George, that consummate inducer of public opinion, outweighed such military geniuses as Kitchener of Khartoum and Sir Douglas Haig. Thus we see a real change of motivation in the political leaders of civilization from Dominance, in the old days, to Inducement in modern times. Such men as Theodore Roosevelt and Woodrow Wilson, radically different in personality though they were, demonstrated repeatedly the power of publicity and oratory over the political destinies of the United States. In their policital manipulations of public opinion both men were motivated primarily by Inducement rather than by Dominance.

Submission.

Submission is the most baffling and difficult of human motives to study objectively. Submission is intricately mingled with Compliance in nearly all human behaviour. Compliance, moreover, operating as it does in the form of an inihibitory or repressive mechanism, tends to prevent Submission in itself from being consciously recognized as a human motive at all. Compliance with appetitive laws, customs, and leaders has led to a social stigma attaching itself to any action which is frankly submissive. Submissive behaviour is characterized as childish, impractical, simple minded, and by similar terms of opprobrium. Yet Submission, nevertheless, is the basic motive underlying all human companionship and organized society.

The earliest form of Submission appears in infant behaviour

during the first few weeks of life. The average child, as Watson[1] points out, responds readily to stroking of the skin, especially in the erotic zones. The infant also responds to cuddling, hugging and petting. If a child is crying he stops, his muscles relax, and he frequently smiles or makes cooing noises apparently indicative of pleasure. Before a child is one year old he begins to manifest more marked Submission activities. He watches friendly adults closely when in a responsive mood, and makes obvious efforts to act in accordance with their wishes. A child of nine or ten months may be taught, for example, to put his hand on his ear in response to the stimulus word " ear ". When the child is in a friendly mood he will always carry out this response when his mother calls for it. But when the baby is obviously irritated or dominantly intent on some reaching or crawling activity, he pays no attention whatever to the stimulus word " ear ". In short, infant responses of this type appear clearly to be motivated by Submission. We have observed instances where an infant's attention may be held for fifteen minutes or more by a mother who is patiently trying to teach the child the word " mamma ". In one instance observed, the baby was too young to control his vocal chords in the manner required. Yet he moved his lips in close imitation of the mother's and made throat movements in an apparent effort to repeat the sounds his mother was making. It seems safe to interpret this behaviour as motivated by simple Submission

It would seem to us that all spontaneous, naive imitation behaviour on the part of both animals and human beings is motivated by Submission. The older instinct theories usually included imitation as one of the primary instincts. Moreover it would seem that all imitative behaviour must contain an element of submissive motivation even though the behaviour as a whole may be controlled by dominant or compliant motives.

Young children between the ages of three and ten years old take obvious delight in Submission to their mothers or other beloved elders. Little boys, especially, frequently help their mothers in wiping dishes, picking up articles about the room, or following the mother about to carry something for her. It seems significant that these spontaneous services usually consist of actions which can be performed in the

[1] J. B. Watson, *op. cit.*, p. 123.

mother's presence and under her immediate direction. The child frequently rebels if asked to run errands which take him a considerable distance from the mother. It would seem probable that the mother's physical presence is the natural stimulus to Submission and that action at a distance from her becomes merely compliant in motive. Since Submission is always positively pleasant and Compliance only mildly pleasant or indifferent, Submission constitutes by far the stronger motive. When Submission motives cease to operate, the entire behaviour pattern is usually controlled by totally different motivation which results in unit responses of a totally different type.

Marked sex differences in Submission behaviour appear at adolescence. Prior to this period there is evidence that Submission motives have played a larger part in the behaviour of boys than of girls (the reverse being true of Inducement motives). But with the onset of sexual maturity boys' behaviour would seem to manifest greater Dominance and Inducement while girls' conduct evidences increase of Submission motivation. From this period on through adult life, however, Submission, whenever it appears, is likely to be found compounded with Inducement in the erotic compound response of Passion. Adolescent girls develop passionate attachments towards their mothers, teachers, and girl friends as well as toward males. Frequently an adolescent girl forms such strong habits of Submission to her mother during this period that she is utterly unable to break these habits of behaviour later in life. Through the girl's Submission, the mother is able to control her daughter's dress, her tastes, the major trends of her personality, and even her love affairs. The habit of Submission in these particulars makes for most inefficient behaviour on the girl's part after she has become a woman herself.

Hero worship which begins in adolescence and frequently lasts throughout adult life is a form of behaviour which seems motivated quite simply by Submission. Respect and admiration for prominent persons and those whose publicity personalities have been attractively built up play a great part in " mob psychology " and the control of public opinion.

In the last section we discussed the Inducement motivation of modern political leaders and of course Submission motives on the part of the public are the counterparts of the leader's

Inducement which make it possible for the public to be controlled in this manner. Nevertheless there seems to be no marked development in Submission motivation in modern times corresponding to that of the modern Inducement development. Submission motives are developed most naturally and effectively through free exercise of love passion and this is an emotion which has been especially repressed throughout the Christian era. It seems probable, in fact, that a good deal of the dominant control of the public in older times was partly ascribable to the natural Submission motives of human beings which prevented the great masses of the populace from becoming as dominant as their tyrannical rulers.

However this may be, it can easily be demonstrated that criminals, both ancient and modern, are primarily lacking in Submissive motivation. One of the writers, acting as psychologist in a penitentary survey of Texas, interviewed 3800 prisoners of both sexes in an attempt to analyze their personalities. Complete physical records, records of the crime, and records of the convict's behaviour during his imprisonment were available for this research. The outstanding result of this study insofar as criminal motivation was concerned, was the conclusion that every criminal act and attitude (except those concerned with sex offences, which formed less than two per cent. of the whole) showed a subnormal admixture of Submission motives.

The habitual criminal seems unable to believe that any human being truly enjoys Submission to other human beings for its own sake. Criminals of this type are convinced that persons who obey the law do so from motives of Compliance. They believe that the law-abiding person's apparent enjoyment of Submission to persons in authority is merely an hypocritical pose motivated by Inducement ultimately controlled by Dominance, (which is the general motivation of all types of deceptive conduct.) The criminal feels that only persons like himself who recognize the hypocrisy of Submission to authority are sufficiently allied with himself for him to submit to in the way of friendship or close association.

A study of the sexual histories of these same criminals showed that a large majority of them were motivated by strong Inducement in their sex relations with little evidence of well developed Passion. The startling conclusion suggests itself that many criminals might actually be made into law-abiding citizens if their love passion were deliberately stimulated and developed to the point where they *enjoyed* Submission to persons placed in authority over them.

While the world longs for peace and seeks to attain it largely by dominant methods, it would seem pertinent to remark that development of true Submission motives in human beings of all races and stations offers the only possible psychological hope for permanent peace between any two or more human beings living together. We are reminded of the Christian maxim that " unless ye become as little children ye cannot enter the kingdom of heaven ". It may be that the uninhibited Submission motives of the natural child were the characteristics referred to as making possible the " heaven " of peaceful human relationships.

Compound Unit Response Motives.

In adult behaviour motives are seldom simple, though compound unit responses motivating a given act may be analyzed into simple unit responses as we have attempted to do in the preceding paragraphs. In order to sketch a more comprehensive outline of human motivation, however, it seems advisable to mention briefly the principle compound unit response motives.

Desire.

Nearly all human behaviour of the acquisitive type is motivated by desire. Acquisitiveness, however, is to be distinguished from ambitious striving for power, fame or position. Motives of ambition may very probably contain some admixture of desire but this desire motive is clearly distinguishable from ambition motive. Desire motives result always in efforts to possess some concrete thing or object. Ambition motives underlie behaviour which seeks to attain high esteem or admiration of *other people*, or possibly power over other people. Political office-seeking is typically motivated by ambition while commercial trading and money making activities are typically motivated by desire. Of course the politician may hope to use his office for financial gain in which case desire forms a subsidiary part of his total motivation. Business men similarly may hope to use their money and commercial prestige to secure public appointments

S

or public favours of some kind. This indicates the presence of other motives joined with desire. Ambition would appear to be a complex motive containing the elements of Dominance and Captivation variously combined and directed toward dominating opposing forces in such a way that captivation of other people is thereby procured.

Desire is the human motive which makes possible all trade and commerce. A merchant controls the behaviour of his customers to the extent of obtaining from them the price of his goods by utilizing the customer's motives of Desire for the goods purchased. Primitive peoples seem to understand the Desire motive in people and animals with considerable accuracy. The Desire motives of animals are utilized to lead them into traps where food which arouses their desires is displayed. The Desire motives of fellow tribesmen are utilized by offering goods or services to bring about profitable trade.

Anglo-American law recognises as legitimate the control of one human being by another through arousing and utilizing Desire motives. If a merchant can arouse the Desire of his customers strongly enough he can make them pay a high price for his goods. The law sanctions this proceeding. But if the customer's Desire is evoked by his own organic drives the law tends to place a limit upon the degree to which the resulting Desire can be utilized by merchants. For example, the hunger drive compels all human beings to experience intense Desire for food. Nearly all governments from ancient Egypt and Rome down to modern times have forbidden profiteering in common food commodities. In psychological terms these governments have passed laws prohibiting merchants from taking extreme advantage of Desire motives resulting from bodily drives which people cannot possibly escape.

In modern times this same regulation of commercial utilization of other people's Desire has been carried still further. Governmental commissions such as the United States Trade Commission, and various state rent and food commissions have passed regulations prohibiting high prices of numerous commodities, the public Desire for which had been artificially built up by the merchants themselves. In short, modern law tends to recognize distinct limitations on the commercial utilization of human Desire motives, no matter how these motives may have been aroused in the first place.

Desire motivation within reasonable limits results in wholesome, constructive, and well organized acquisitive behaviour. When carried to extremes, however, Desire motives result in restless, insatiable cravings for inaccessible objects ; in wandering, aimless travelling about from place to place ; or in feverish, unbalanced seeking for excitement or pleasure which never satisfies the seeker.

Satisfaction.

Human conduct which is motivated by Satisfaction is for the most part peculiarly distasteful to other people who observe it. The miser, gloating over his gold is an extreme case of conduct expressive of Satisfaction motives. In more moderate degree the connoisseur, the art collector, the stamp collector, or the collector of antique furniture represent people whose behaviour in poring over the objects which they have collected is motivated by Satisfaction. Usually the antique furniture collector's collection is of far less interest to other people than it is to him. His friends may try to be polite (Submission motives) when they are called upon to admire a newly acquired piece but they actually find the collector's Satisfaction enthusiasm extremely boresome. People try to escape from observing other people's Satisfaction behaviour as quickly as possible and this escape behaviour itself would seem to result from the fact that Satisfaction is a motive which it is very difficult for another person to ulitize for his own benefit.

Very wealthy persons who acquire magnificent estates customarily surround these show places with high walls and fences to keep out the public at large. This conduct in itself is motivated by the passive Dominance element in Satisfaction. Thus, the poorer people whose desires to see and experience unusual luxury and beauty of environment might find agreeable Satisfaction in mere inspection of the millionaire's show place are prevented from seeing it by the owner's Satisfaction in its possession. The wealthy individual's friends, on the other hand, whose desires to view luxury have long ago been satisfied, are called in to admire the place and thus further enhance the Satisfaction of the owner. In both instances the owner's Satisfaction-motivated conduct fails to give any satisfaction whatever to persons other than himself. Thus we may describe most Satisfaction behaviour as " unsocial "

There is one important social application of Satisfaction

motives, however. There is a business maxim to the effect that " a satisfied customer is our best advertisement ". This maxim is essentially true. A person who has purchased an article which gave unexpectedly great satisfaction is likely to show off the article to his friends and to tell them what a wonderful purchase he has made. This behaviour on the customer's part is largely motivated by Satisfaction and such behaviour is, of course, extremely useful to the merchant who desires to sell more articles of the same sort. Thus we see that in commerce Satisfaction serves to direct the future Desires of satisfied customers and their friends toward the store where the satisfying goods were purchased. Moreover the customer's Satisfaction tends to produce in him a favourable psychological condition for the arousing of new Desires for the same and similar types of goods.

It would seem that Satisfaction in combination with various love motives plays an important role in marital faithfulness and constancy. A person may be capable of strong love for a short period yet wholly incapable of keeping this love fixed on one individual or on a single family of individuals over a period of years. Such an individual probably evidences a marked lack of Satisfaction motives. It is interesting to note that New Englanders whose behaviour in the thrifty saving of money, gloating over antique furniture, and emphasis upon the family tree is clearly motivated by Satisfaction, are usually extremely loyal and constant in their family relationships. Gratitude also would seem to be a motive compounded of Satisfaction and Submission toward persons who have benefited the grateful individual.

Passion.

We have previously mentioned the importance of Passion motivation in connection with the development of Submission motives which differentiate law-abiding behaviour from habitual criminality. This previous mention of Passion motives may serve to emphasize the fact that although Passion is an erotic response, its influence is not limited by any means to love affairs between the sexes, though its natural origin and development are closely connected with the erotic drive.

Love behaviour, which consists primarily of eager surrender of one's self to a lover, is motivated by Passion. Though both sexes manifest this type of behaviour, Passion would seem to predominantly motivate male love behaviour because of bodily structures and mechanisms described elsewhere at some length.[1] The behaviour of a man who becomes erotically fascinated by a beautiful woman and devotes the major part of his time and attention to the task of winning her favour, is motivated by the unit response of Passion. Passion would appear to be the natural and efficient male motivation in love affairs with the opposite sex.

Female love conduct may, of course, be similarly motivated by Passion. Young girls experience " crushes " for older girls and men. Mature women frequently become helplessly fascinated by the love attraction of a handsome man. Under the influence of such an attraction, motivated by Passion, the woman may obviously seek to attract the man by trying to yield herself to him. She may, in the phrase of an older generation, " throw herself at a man's head ". This type of obvious self-surrender on the woman's part, however, is seldom efficient in its effect upon the male. A man's vanity (i.e. his Inducement-Dominance) may be flattered temporarily, but his erotic responses are not evoked to any considerable degree unless the woman's conduct is motivated by Captivation rather than Passion. True Passion motivation therefore, would seem to play a comparatively small part in female love behaviour of this type.

Occidental customs and social conventions largely taboo behaviour motivated by Passion. Therefore, the development of Passion motives in natural sexual love behaviour of both sexes is definitely minimized. Passion, nevertheless, represents one of the most powerful springs of human conduct and when it is diverted from its natural type of behaviour expression it tends to express itself in various disguised and indirect ways emphasized by Freud and the psychoanalysts.

Possibly the type of human behaviour most clearly motivated by Passion is religion. Of course a great deal of our modern Christian religion has become formalized and is motivated largely by Compliance with business and social necessities. Nevertheless considerable numbers of people, especially of the less educated classes, experience the spontaneous urge to surrender themselves passionately to a personal Saviour and Redeemer. Such religious self-surrender seems definitely

[1] W. M. Marston, *op. cit.*, pp. 317 ff.

motivated by Passion. The religious rituals of kneeling before the altar, bowing the head, rendering blind and unquestioning obedience to a beloved master, and especially confessing all the innermost secrets of consciousness to a priest, represent carefully worked out forms of Passion motivated behaviour. An extreme of this Passion motive would appear to be responsible for the behaviour of the early Christian martyrs who joyfully sought and endured physical torture as a consummate expression of their passionate self-surrender to their master. Religion, on the whole, seems to be a system of behaviour-training designed to teach Passion motivation to its disciples without permitting the natural physical Passion behaviour. Because of this limitation it would seem that religious behaviour serves as an outlet for previously developed Passion motives more effectively than it acts as a stimulant to further development of Passion motivation. If the latter purpose could be accomplished religion would undoubtedly furnish a most important constructive influence in building up in the public at large the only completely pleasant motive for social Submission to authority.

Captivation.

As we have already noted in regard to love behaviour between the sexes, Captivation would seem to be an outstanding female motive as contrasted to the typically male motive of Passion. Flirting is a type of female behaviour clearly motivated by Captivation. Little girls frequently begin to flirt with persons of both sexes at about the age of three. Flirtatious behaviour on the part of women ordinarily persists until motherhood, frequently recurring once more in the mother's behaviour pattern a few years after childbirth.

Behaviour of both sexes which seek to attract and hold members of the opposite sex, is motivated primarily by Captivation. Exhibitions of the body or of bodily skill or strength are motivated by Captivation when these acts are performed in the presence of the opposite sex and for the purpose of attracting their admiration.

Female Captivation behaviour is likely to be more subtle than male behaviour similarly motivated. The female body seems naturally adapted to captivate men and, therefore, subtle inflections of the voice and female gestures and mannerisms even when not expressly motivated by Captivation, nevertheless tend to produce that effect. More subtle female Captivation therefore customarily conceals its true motivation under various disguises, but nevertheless retains its efficiency.

Women's interest in clothes seems primarily motivated by Captivation. The underlying Captivation motive may be very general. It is frequently complicated by admixture of other motives. For example, a woman may purchase expensive dresses to dominate women rivals at social functions. Or she may select garments whose colour and texture delight her. In such instances her behaviour is partly motivated by " æsthetic response " which seems to be an attenuated form of Satisfaction or Compliance response. Nevertheless, intermingled with these other, more specific motives there would seem to be a general Captivation motive nearly always present. Woman's attention to dress, in short, primarily seeks to beautify her person and render it more intrinsically attractive to persons of both sexes. Even though no other person were present, as in a desert island situation, Captivation motives might still result in female self-adornment. The existence of Captivation motives in such a case would be ascribable to woman's natural erotic drive as detailed in a preceding chapter.

Captivation may mingle with other motives of an appetitive nature to produce various types of attempted leadership and control of other people. We have already discussed ambition as a motive compounded from Captivation and Dominance. Religious leadership and leadership by sheer eloquence and charm of personality possibly represent types of behaviour rather specifically motivated by Captivation. Certainly a woman's " social charm " exerted upon her social guests or companions may be attributed in large part to Captivation motives.

Professional Captivation is found to a great extent on the stage. Chorus girls, dancers, and motion picture actresses who depend largely upon their physical attractiveness are carefully taught a type of behaviour which would express the purest Captivation motives, were such behaviour spontaneous. While the actual motivation underlying the stage performance of a successful chorus girl or actress may contain a considerable admixture of Desire for money and of Dominance in surpassing rivals, such behaviour nevertheless, by virtue of its very success, would seem to be motivated to a considerable extent by Captivation.

The social value of Captivation motives is very great. Every social group from family to nation must have its leader. And social leadership motivated by Captivation in as pure a form as possible represents by far the most pleasant and effective form of control. Political leaders such as Abraham Lincoln and Theodore Roosevelt seem to have been motivated largely by Captivation (and its component Inducement) in the considerable amount of their time and behaviour which they devoted to attracting and controlling public esteem and admiration.

Complex Unit Response Motives.

In completing our brief sketch of human motivation it is necessary to mention complex unit response motives. Many human personalities are probably incapable of acting under the influence of these motives for any considerable period of time. The reason for this seems to be that the unit responses in many personalities are not synthesized into complete creative patterns. In other words, many individuals have not developed their unit responses into unit personalities. Whenever a unit personality appears, however, it represents a synthesis of simple and compound unit response motives into the complex unit response motives of Creation. In closing this chapter, therefore, we may suggest briefly the types of behaviour expressive of the two creative motives—origination and transformation.

Origination.

Maternal origination in connection with conception and child bearing has been dealt with in a preceding chapter. The synthesis of unit response motives of Love and Appetite is accomplished in the mother's case by the natural procreative drive.

Original work of an economic or artistic nature seems more characteristic of male behaviour than of female. It may be that synthesis of the simpler unit responses into Origination when it occurs in the female personality, tends to express itself more or less exclusively in procreative activities. However this may be, we find that a great majority of the originators of new forms of art, new ideas, inventions and innovations of all sorts have been men. We must, however, allow for the fact that some of the ideas resulting in these original creations may have come in the first place from wives and women friends.

Our own case studies indicate on the whole that Origination responses motivate a greater proportion of male than of female behaviour.

Artistic creations such as the carving of statues, the painting of pictures, and the writing of stories, are motivated by Origination response variously combined with Transformation motives (using existing forms and materials of art to entertain or influence the public), and are also compounded with various unsynthesized unit response motives of Appetite or Love, such as Desire for money, ambition for fame, Passion for a loved woman and many other motives. Poetry such as that of Edgar Allen Poe seems to be motivated very largely by Origination. Modernistic and cubistic paintings, musical compositions like those of Cyril Scott and Debussy, and stories like those of O. Henry and Edgar Rice Burroughs give evidence of a high degree of Origination motive. More conventional and more highly commercialized forms of artistic creation such as a majority of magazine cover drawings, and motion picture productions, evidently are motivated less by Origination than by Transformation and by various types of appetitive unit responses.

Origination appears more frequently in art than in religion, commerce, social customs, or forms of government. Changes in these fields apparently represent a very slow and prolonged process of development by trial and error. Nevertheless, Origination motives may be traced in the appearance of new religious sects, radical changes in dress such as the short skirt and one-piece bathing suit, new social customs and conventions like Judge Lindsey's companionate marriage, and the occasional attempt to found a new political party like Roosevelt's Progressive Party, or a new form of national government like the Soviet government of Russia. In most instances these changes in group behaviour may be traced to the Origination motives of a single leader.

Mechanical and electrical inventions with which the present century is replete, probably represent the most clear-cut examples of Origination motives. While many improvements in existing machinery represent adaptations of previously existing devices to serve the requirements of users, there are many outstanding inventions which cannot be traced to sources of this kind.

Of course all original creations actually consist of previously existing units or elements put together in such a way that the combined creation possesses new properties or functions. Thus we may trace the invention of the steam engine to the inventor's casual observation of how steam lifted the cover of a tea kettle. But it is at precisely this point that the Origination motives of Isaac Watts begin to play an important part in the matter. Watts responded to this observation of the tea-kettle by combining steam and a movable container in such a way that a mechanical device with new potentialities and attributes was created. A million other people had doubtless observed steam moving kettle covers but lacked the Origination motive to invent a steam engine based upon this same principle.

Inventors would seem to be individuals whose entire pattern of unit response motives is synthesized rather completely into a single complex Origination pattern of motivation. It seems significant in this connection that inventors are seldom able to apply their own original devices to practical requirements of manufacture and commerce. A good mechanic notably lacking in Origination motives is far more efficient for such purposes.

Transformation.

The mother's behaviour in training and developing her children has already been mentioned as one of the natural types of Transformation activity. Paternal behaviour and attitude toward children and toward younger or weaker persons in general is motivated by Transformation response. Closely resembling this behaviour we may place that of the teacher, the athletic trainer, and the clinical advisor. The life work of these individuals is largely motivated by Transformation response. They perceive the shortcomings and potentialities of their pupils or clients and respond by attempting to train these individuals in such a way as to develop their personalities along the lines indicated.

We have already mentioned that a great majority of the creations of all the commercialized arts are motivated by Transformation rather than by origination. The average commercial story writer, for instance, recombines a number of previously successful story plots and styles of writing in such a way as to adapt his materials to suit the public. But his motives do not lead him to put these materials together in such a way that a truly original story or new literary form is created.

The combination of elements is not such that the combined unit possesses new attributes or functions, not previously possessed by the separate parts.

The activities of propagandists are motivated by Transformation response ; at least insofar as the propagandists are sincere in their wish to help humanity by teaching them a new truth. It seems to be the fact, moreover, that propagandists are always motivated to a considerable extent by Transformation response, even when their motives reveal marked admixtures of Desires for money, ambition for power, and destructively dominant response toward rivals or disbelievers in their doctrines. The firm and sincere conviction that humanity is wrong in its present state but can be redeemed by the proposed modification of behaviour furnishes conclusive evidence that a true Transformation response underlies the given propagandist's activities. Propagandists are seldom originators. The reforms which they offer are almost invariably originated by someone else long before, as, for example, in the case of prohibition propaganda, the teaching of Christianity and other religions by priests and churchmen, and the dissemination of socialistic and other radical political doctrines. By far the majority of teachers and propagandists are not interested in original creative activity but rather in the application of existing doctrines to fit what they believe to be the needs of their clients, and in the Transformation of these clients along the lines indicated.

Individuals whose motives are synthesized into an Origination pattern are much rarer in any community than those possessing some degree of Transformation motive pattern. But the latter are usually far more influential within their own social group or community.

The above discussion of motivation is, of course, only introductory. Although in the case of a given personality nhe motivation is usually extremely complex and only to be discovered by careful study over a relatively long period, tevertheless when we take a population at large the most important motivations seem to be Dominance, Compliance, Submission, Inducement, Desire, Satisfaction, Passion, and Captivation. Less usual but also important motivations are Origination and Transformation. The scope of our present discussion is too limited to include any but the most rudimentary and basic of human motives.

CHAPTER XII

Introductory

ALL integrative combination of separate unit responses into enduring patterns of human behaviour depends upon *learning*. It is necessary, therefore, that we take up the question as to how learning is possible.

An eight months old infant accidentally discovers his ear. He pulls and twists it until his attention is distracted elsewhere. An hour later he may voluntarily try again to locate his ear but is not successful. His hand hits his head above, below, and beside the ear many times. Sooner or later he may evolve a technique of hitting his head with his hand and contacting the ear by twisting his head, but it will be many weeks before he *learns* to locate his ear directly.

Putting his hand to his head is a very simple accomplishment compared to the many complex modes of behaviour that the baby must attain before he reaches maturity. Yet it remains a true instance of learning and contains just as many psychological problems as the mastery of calculus or the acquirement of engineering or architectural skill. There are many trials, many failures, many repetitions of the correct movement, gradual elimination of false motions, an increase of speed with each trial, and the final success. Once the skill is attained it is never completely forgotten and when well established can be recalled at will. As a result of great activity over a long period of time, a permanent change has been wrought in the infant's behaviour.

Preliminary Definition of Learning

Learning can thus be defined as a basic modification of behaviour built up by previous activities. Both these elements are necessary. As the baby grows older his cry becomes louder and his arms and legs more active. This behaviour is not learned, however, because, although there is plenty of activity, there is no real modification of the native responses. These have merely been intensified and strengthened by the genetically controlled growth and intensity increase of the stimulus mechanism.

On the other hand, if an adult seriously injures his foot so that he limps or walks with a cane or on crutches, there is a definite and irremediable modification, but it has been thrust suddenly upon the organism from the outside instead of being built up from the inside. In the case of the baby learning to locate his ear, both necessary elements are present in proper sequence, that is, a fundamental change in behaviour brought about by practice or experience.

Learning in this sense covers the whole range of acquired behaviour. We learn to fear the dark, cats, dogs, snakes, and rats, the sight of a Western Union messenger, or a tray of dental instruments. These are modifications of our emotional responses and are sometimes established after but one intense and prolonged experience with the conditioning object. We learn to play tennis and golf, drive a speed car or an aeroplane, cook an appetizing meal ; we can also learn the techniques that enable us to model a pleasing statuette, or paint a sunset. These are all acquired co-ordinations of hand and eye. Our habits are learned ; orderliness, honesty, neatness, punctuality or the reverse, hours of sleep, table manners, style of dress and the like. We memorize a poem, or the multiplication table, the number on the police box on the corner, a section of the Negotiable Instruments Law, and this is still another type of learning. We learn to be skilful engineers, advertising men, lecturers, we evolve new principles in our chosen field and we say we have learned to think, reason, or reach conclusions.

Where and How Learning Occurs

All these instances are modifications of original part-reactions which, because of their permanency when once established, change the total unit response of the individual. Modification takes place primarily in the integrative centres. That is to say, the tennis player's visual receptors are in no way modified as his play improves. He learns to keep his eye on the ball, to judge distances, and to hit the ball at a given angle. There is, correspondingly, no important change in his muscular capacity, though the neural connections between muscle and eye have been increased in number and greatly refined by bringing new facilitating muscular action into play. Nevertheless, neither the capacity nor the structure of the muscle has been fundamentally modified. Whatever basic modification takes place must occur, then, in the neurons and psychons connecting the incoming afferent impulses from the receptors with the outgoing efferent impulses to the muscles.

It is further thought that this change is not made possible by any principle of neuron activity but is of psychonic origin instead.[1] Changes taking place in the dendrite, cell body, and axone are for the most part fixed in nature and have to do with transmission within the neuron. Changes taking place within the psychon are motile and result in selection and retention which together constitute the functional bases of learning.

Selection, that is, the determination of the intricate details of synaptic behaviour which shall go to make up the newly learned activity, is due to the equilibrium of synaptic resistances at the time of the initial act. The customary motor outlet is blocked, when we are confronted with a new situation or when, for one reason or another, we are determined to change our behaviour. Fortunately our particular type of nervous system, in addition to the main pathways, is well supplied with collateral outlets, side-branchings, and interconnecting pathways which permit a crossing-over to other centres, and by this means form new outlets. The main pathways which provide for the customary behaviour are open as a matter of innate organization. The collateral or little used branchings provide the structure for learning the myriads of individual reactions which are developed in the course of a lifetime. New connections are also facilitated by the fact that " many different kinds of fibres may make synaptic junctions with a single neuron and further, that the axone of a single neuron may divide so as to distribute its excitation to neurons of two or more different functional types in centres far removed from each other."[2]

It is these two factors, varying thresholds of resistances in

[1] Herrick says, " The synaptic junctions are probably the critical points in such functional modifications of reaction patterns, for the junctional region is known to be especially susceptible to such functional factors." (*Neurological Foundations of Animal Behaviour*, p. 119.)

[2] C. J. Herrick, *op. cit.*, *Introduction to Neurology*.

the synapses under varying conditions, and a vast network of neural structure not yet taken up by the innate reactions and therefore awaiting development as the experience of the individual dictates, that explain the variety and range of individually acquired behaviour. And there is also a third factor in synaptic behaviour which explains retention.

When an impulse crosses over the synapse, that particular piece of neural protoplasm can never again revert to its former state of inactivity in regard to the newly set up response. *The excitation in crossing over leaves a mnemonic trace which thereafter becomes a permanent part of the neural structure.*[1] The exact nature of this change is unknown but is thought by most neurologists to be electro-chemical. It is the most important structural factor pertinent to the explanation of learning since its presence lessens the future psychonic resistance and makes it easier for excitations of similar rhythm again to pass the synaptic barrier.

Herrick explains this factor from the neurological standpoint. He says, " All functions of the nervous system are facilitated by repetition and many such repetitions lead to an enduring change in the mode of response to stimulation which may be called physiological habit. This implies that the performance of every reaction leaves some sort of residual change in the structure of the neuron systems involved. These acquired modifications of behaviour are manifested in some degree by all organisms and this capacity lies at the basis of all associative memory, whether consciously or unconsciously performed, and the capacity of learning by experience . . .

" The simplest concrete memory that can appear in consciousness is a very complex process and probably involves the activity of an extensive system of association centres and tracts. That which persists in the cerebral cortex between the initial experience and the recollection of it, is, therefore, in all probability a change in the inter-neuronic resistance such as to alter the physiological equilibrium of the component neurons of some particular associational system. What the nature of the change may be is unknown, but it is conceivable that it might take the form of a permanent modification of the synapses between the neurons which were functionally active during the initial experience such as to facilitate the

[1] S. T. Bok, " The Development of Reflexes and Reflex Tracts," *Psych. en Neurol.*, 1917, no. 1.

active participation of the same neurons in the same physiological pattern during the reproduction."[1]

Although the theory of permanent modification of the synapse has widespread acceptance among the neurologists, it has been challenged by some experimenters. Lashley, for instance, trained a rat in the Yerkes discrimination box with the left eye blindfolded and then tested for retention with the blindfold changed to the right eye. In the terms of the experimenter, the "transfer of learning with the right eye was complete". Lashley says in his conclusion, "It seems then that the theory of wearing down of the synaptic resistances is not applicable to this case of learning and we must seek for some other principle to account for the altered conductivity of the nervous system."

There are two possible objections to drawing this conclusion from the experimental facts as given. First, considering the response as a unit, the kinæsthetic clues may be quite as important as the visual. Their primary importance has been very definitely established in the case of maze learning which consists basically of co-ordinations of muscles of the kinæsthetic system. In the initial part of the learning process excitations from the eyes, the ears, the nose, the vibrissae, and the contact receptors serve as contributory guides, but control is rapidly transferred to the kinæsthetic unit. After learning is completed, the response pattern is almost entirely kinæsthetic, with occasional reliance upon contact in times of emergency. In the case of discrimination experiments, visual reception is a part-reaction involving only a fraction of the total number of synapses going to make up the unit response. It can be presumed that there will be very little resistance in the synapses of the visual centres since the animal has had considerable practice in seeing from birth. The resistance, if any, comes for the most part in the correlation centres which are the same for both eyes.

The second objection to Lashley's conclusion is that blindfold experiments as a whole have been taken to show that the training of both eyes proceeds simultaneously even though one eye is covered. If the right eye is focussed for middle distance left, the left eye will be similarly focussed in spite of the blindfold. The sensory part-reaction from the blindfolded eye, when it does take place, finds the paths already open in

---

[1] C. J. Herrick, *op. cit.*

the correlation centres. If this is the case, then the blindfold experiment is irrelevant to the issue and has no bearing upon the question of whether or not synaptic resistance is reduced by the passage of the nervous impulse.

The Learning Process

We have taken some pains to define learning as the permanent modification of behaviour as a result of experience and to show that the number of synapses and the nature of the synaptic tissue provide sufficient physiological plasticity for the myriads of modifications that are the end-result of learning. It now remains to study the learning process in detail and to discover whether or not the experimental facts as we know them, are explainable by further elaboration of this physiological explanation.

Animal Learning

Experiments in animal learning have been either of the maze type or the problem box type. The mazes ordinarily used are adaptations of the ground plan of the gardens of Hampton Court in England. The animal is placed in the maze at the entrance, the maze is locked, and the animal is left to find the exit. Proper motivation, of course, is important. If the animal has just been fed, it will probably lie down and go to sleep. Usually hungry animals or animals in heat are used. If the problem box type of experiment is conducted, the animal is placed in a cage from which he can escape by manipulating a simple lock.

Maze learning : White rats are more frequently used in the study of maze learning than any other animal. When first put in the maze they wander at random, exploring every cul-de-sac in turn, and only by chance reach the food box. The first trial is characterized by great energy and in about half an hour the rat may run thirty-six hundred feet At the end of thirty trials he traverses the distance from entrance to food box in half a minute or less, running a total of only forty feet.

Watson, who has investigated this type of learning in great detail, has shown that it is largely dependent upon proprioceptive clues. By conducting a series of experiments in which he eliminated successively vision, hearing, feeling, and contact receptors, he found that with the previously trained

T

rats there was no appreciable loss in efficiency and that untrained rats learned in the usual number of trials, nor was
their final speed any less than that of the trained rats.

Problem box learning : Many types of animals have been
experimented with in the problem box, including cats, monkeys,
racoons, birds, and dogs. Cats are more frequently used
than any of the others. When the animal is first put into
the box, it races around, paws at the bars, and enters upon a

HAMPTON COURT MAZE

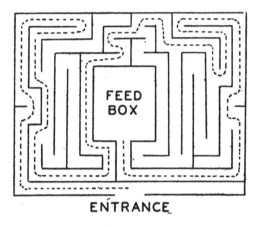

FIGURE 39

period of furious activity. The bars continually repulse the
animal but the lock gives way slightly, so that the attack is
gradually focussed upon the lock, until a chance movement
frees the animal. On succeeding trials the animal frees itself
more quickly, until finally the problem box has been learned.

Basing our analysis upon these two types of learning, we
can say that learning is primarily the building of a response
through a gradual integration of isolated part-reactions.
These part-reactions have all been experienced before, but
now they are gathered together in a series, the sequence of
which is dictated by the conditions of the new problem.

The building up of this sequence is characterized by three
periods of activity : (1) a phase of random, sporadic, and
useless activity with slight serial connection in a few segments,

but for the most part unintegrated; (2) a second phase characterized by the gradual elimination of false movements and the fixation of efficient movements; (3) the final period of welding the efficient movements into a unit response pattern. It should further be noted that neither the substitute stimulus nor the substitute reaction appear in this typical learning situation. We shall comment further upon this fact in our later discussion of the conditioned reflex as an explanation of retention.

Human Learning

Can human learning be equally simplified? Experiments with the pencil maze and with mechanical puzzles show that human behaviour while learning is very similar to that of the animals. There are many random, exploratory movements at first, which are gradually lessened as the experience is repeated. The human being is just as unable to eliminate the cul-de-sac at the end of one trial as is the animal.

There are three differences, however, that can be demonstrated. The first is that the human being profits by recall of past errors, that is, a clue institutes an ideational or verbal trend that permits him to run the cul-de-sac in his head instead of with his hand. In the second place, the human being profits by insight, that is, he can get at the principle of the problem by verbally or ideationally utilizing past experiences of a similar sort; and thirdly, he can utilize the learning of other human beings by imitation. Some animals have been shown to have done this also, but they are the exception rather than the rule.

These variations, although they short-cut the time required to establish the new response, do not change the fundamental trial and error procedure. No one in learning tennis can imitate the instructor's motions immediately. A long period of practice will ensue before the model can even be approximated. Whether in the long run similar perfection of form will be attained, depends on the pupil's native equipment. His physiological limit may be attained long before he reaches the professional's excellence or he may in time exceed his teacher. Having a model, however, is expedient. It ensures a maximum of correct responses in as short a time as the native equipment of the learner will permit.

Recall and thinking as aids to learning are also time savers.

Recall means doing a single part of the problem in your head and thus eliminating physical activity. In thinking out the principles of a problem, there is a great internal activity, considering this possibility and that, rejecting this solution, retaining a part solution here and a part solution there, until the problem is solved. Even though this type of activity is substituted for running to and fro, very few people are able to get all the facts and reach correct conclusions. There is usually a period of physical trial and error also.

In spite of these helps then, the fundamental problem for humans remains the same as it is for animals. By what means is retention established? How are false moves eliminated and successful ones retained?

Retention

There have been many answers to the problem of retention. The tendency is with most theories, however, to isolate one single aspect of behaviour and make this single factor account for the whole learning process. The learning process, on the other hand, is a complex affair dependent fundamentally upon synaptic modification. How and why these synaptic traces are effected in the first place, and further how some are cancelled and others reinforced by projected neuronic connections, is a matter of many factors working together toward a common end, rather than the resultant of a single isolated experience. In other words, there is a fundamental, inescapable process which occurs in every type of learning and results in permanent modification. It is not a simple process but is, rather, exceedingly complex and must be explained as such.

Factors in Behaviour which Make for Retention
1. Frequency

In establishing a new and permanent type of response it is first necessary to overcome resistance at the synapses along the constituent conduction paths. In his first attempt to accomplish this result the animal and the human being by random and sporadic movements, open up every possible type of response which might directly or indirectly contribute toward the end result. With each repetition of the journey certain responses are repeated, not as isolated units, but in series, as parts of a larger unit.

With each repetition the series of neuronic connections will be more and more extensive. Suppose the series for the proper pathway consisted of A, B, C, D, E. The rat in the early process of learning might run from A to B, then down a cul-de-sac and back along C, down another cul-de-sac and back to D·and E. Eventually the goal is reached and the total process completed. When the next trial occurs the physiological foundation for the serial unity of A and B is already laid and is merely reinforced by this second running. The moves which fill the gap between B and C are mutually conflicting and inhibitory. The mnemonic traces formed for the movements in one direction are broken up by those of equal power in an opposite direction. Now it is conceivable that when the rat stood at the end of the second path and was confronted with the possibility either of entering the cul-de-sac or of passing along path C, that a conflict of tendencies took place. But the tendency to enter the blind alley being stronger, the animal took that path. There still remains, however, the tendency toward the alternative and correct pathway along C. In other words, the start of the serial connection between B and C is already laid so that when the animal takes the correct path either by chance or because he would avoid the conflict set up by the cul-de-sac, he is reinforcing the initial tendency in the right direction. In any event the right path, once traversed, adds another increment to the serial pattern, carrying with it an increase in the total facilitation of impulses. This facilitation drains into its pathway any impulses from weaker reflexes and its strength, coupled with the weakness of the mutually inhibitory paths in the cul-de-sac, brings about the elimination of incorrect moves and the establishment of correct ones.

As the number of trials continue, the correct movements are repeated again and again in the same series. Each additional trial means a more unified pattern of response which continues to be repeated as a unity, whereas the incompleted portions (and by incompleted we mean sporadic, isolated movements having no unity one with another and not directed toward any one channel) will never occur twice alike in the same sequence and, therefore, can never be said to be precisely repeated.

With each trial the unbroken stretch of the unified series becomes longer, and in time a final successful response eliminates all false moves and includes the whole correct path. Frequency in this sense, that is, repeated repetitions of unit wholes, is probably the most important single factor in the learning process. If taken, however, to refer to the repetition of isolated movements, as Watson used the term, then it is without significance, for the reason that certain isolated, incorrect movements are sometimes repeated more frequently than single successful movements.

The frequent repetition in series also affords an explanation of Thorndike's law of exercise. Thorndike used the analogy of the muscle to explain the stamping-in part of the learning process. A muscle which is used frequently, is built up to greater strength with each repetition. A muscle which is disused atrophies. Applying this law to learning, frequent repetitions of the correct response increase the effectiveness of the physiological mechanism and, by so doing, result in stamping-in the response. In the same way the incorrect motions are lost through disuse. It should be pointed out, however, *that the physiological basis consists of connecting up unit responses in teams, with a mnemonic trace of each connection left on the integrative tissues, or psychons.*

2. Recency

Under ordinary conditions, the most recent association is the one to be first re-established. If the last time we motored to town, we turned left at the cross roads, we shall tend, other things being equal, to make that same left turn on our next trip also. The mnemonic trace most recently established is stronger than a connection of similar strength but of earlier origin, unless the earlier connection has become permanently established physically on account of many repetitions. If during childhood we are taught to pronounce progress with a long " o " and later are sent to a school where the students pronounce the word with a short " o," recent hearing of the short " o " may make us tend to use it occasionally, but on the whole, by and large, we shall tend toward the earlier pronunciation. We are forced to conclude then that while recency may play an important part in fixation, it is only occasionally a decisive factor. In the long run, frequency will outweigh recency unless the time interval is very short. Presumably, in the case of learning, the two factors are working to facilitate each other, that is, the already established segments of the unit response are repeated with each trial. They therefore occurred in the last trial and are both the most frequent and most recent. In the case of an incorrect part-reaction, recency may tend toward repetition but only until the momentum of the total reponse gets under way.

3. *Intensity*

Intensity is also a factor which co-operates with frequency. It may be said to help, if not determine, fixation. Propagation of nerve impulses which lead to the correct responses, means the directing of all the animal's drive or tendency to action in one closely integrated neural pattern. As the integration becomes more unified the true response becomes more vigorous and intense. The main path is run rapidly without any break with a free flow of energy along the neural paths. At the same time the impulses governing the incorrect responses become weaker and less intense and finally decline altogether.

4. *Congruity*

The fixation and elimination of new responses have been explained on the basis of congruity. That is, all acts which harmonise are retained and reinforce each other, whereas all acts which inhibit or conflict with each other are cancelled out. The reflexes which make up the correct response must be in harmony both with the self activity of the organism and with each other. In the cases of maze learning which we have been using as an example, the self activity of the organism is focussed usually upon finding food. The stomach is in a violent state of activity, the ensuing hunger pangs send afferent impulses to the cortex, which arouses the skeletal muscles and precipitates chemicals into the blood stream, and also sets up general activity of the organism. Under these conditions almost any sort of random activity will be in keeping with the inner condition. This would not be so, as we pointed out before, if the animal or human had just had a good meal. It is only with quite an effort that violent skeletal activity can be engaged in when we are completely satisfied and in the process of digesting a good dinner. It would be quite futile to attempt to get an animal to learn to run a maze under such conditions, so that it may be said that the more congruous the new reactions are with the self activity pattern or actions of the organism, the more they will be enabled to get through to motor outlets and so leave synaptic traces.

It is also true that the part-reactions which go to make up the successful unit response must be in harmony with each other and particularly must each part-reaction harmonise with that which immediately follows it. This congruity of parts is involved in the unity of the basic pattern and in the elimination of conflicting and non-essential part-reactions. The less conflict there is between part-reactions at a given stage, the greater the freedom of outlet that will ensue. The rat which has his free running activity abruptly blocked by the physical presence and incoming sensations of a terminated cul de sac, experiences a complete inhibition of motor outlet. The paths will have to be re-established before general facilitation and congruity of action will occur. And while it may be that the initial elimination of a cul de sac is a matter of sheer chance, yet it is quite true that the unity and congruity of the resulting response will so effectively reinforce the neural pathway and so permanently modify the synapses involved, that the incorrect movements cannot under normal circumstances be established. It follows as a corollary of these two propositions that the more incongruous two actions or reactions may be, the quicker the weaker of each incongruous pair of groups will be eliminated from all synaptic trace or learning. This result ensues because its synaptic antagonist or opposite will form a trace in an opposite inhibitory synaptic direction. The points of contact from each synapse will be opposite and they will be organised against each other and will therefore cancel out.

Some practical aspects of the problem of retention.

The integrative explanation of learning that we have endeavoured to set forth in these pages, makes it possible to understand some of the practical findings that have been made in regard to efficient fixation.

Most experimentalists agree, as between one long session of practice and two short sessions a day, that the shorter sessions are more efficient than the one long one; in other words, that spaced learning is more productive of results than unspaced learning. Such a conclusion is consistent with the process of synaptic modification that must ensue before the new response can be established. The number of synapses excited and the amount of synaptic modification that can be accomplished at any one time is limited. Spaced learning permits a maximum of modification with a minimum of fatigue and gives the mnemonic traces left by one short practice period a chance to become permanent before more learning is attempted. Spaced learning also gives ununified reactions a chance to disappear.

There is great individual variation in the matter of the effectiveness of whole versus part learning. Where the serial arrangement of the response is a factor, then the whole method is better because it permits a maximum facilitation of impulses with greater resultant intensity into a unit motor path.

In the mnemonic factor also can be found a contributory explanation of the plateaus which are so frequently found in learning curves. A typical curve shows negative acceleration, that is, most people learn much more during the first trials than they do after they have been practicing awhile. Very often in the middle of such a curve will be found a level portion where apparently no progress at all was made. This is called a plateau. Plateaux may sometimes be traced to discouragement, lack of interest, fatigue, illness, or other similar conditions. At other times learning apparently ceases from no obvious cause and is usually followed by a sudden spurt. In such cases it is thought that the previously formed synaptic modifications require time to set. The electro-chemical change is still operative, is functioning to unify the whole pattern, and further change cannot take place until the initial modification is completed.

Transfer, if it does occur, is only possible physiolcgically by the utilisation of identical serial response units by two different types of learning. If there are no such common elements, then the transfer will not take place.

Individual differences in learning capacity are due to differences in number and type and degree of synapses capable of modification. With some individuals, the synaptic tissue is more highly sensitized, the whole integrative organism more plastic, and the individual can therefore learn more than his fellow of poorer native endowment.

Successful Completion of Actions or Reactions

It is generally held that successful completion of an act has

a very important effect upon establishing the neuronic connections which go to make up the new response. An old
theory involving this point held that an act successfully
completed was pleasant whereas the unsuccessful act was
unpleasant, therefore the right act because it was pleasant,
would be stamped in whereas the response that brought
annoyances would be eliminated. Such an explanation leads
us round in circles since it amounts to saying that the completed act results in pleasantness and then turns round and
brings about that which had already occurred, namely successful completion. In light of our integrative explanation of
learning it may be clearly seen that successful completion
greatly augments all the factors previously enumerated, that
is, the uniformity of pattern built up by frequent repetition,
the free flow of impulses that constitute intensity, and the
greater harmony resulting from increasing congruity. This
result is accomplished by the strengthening and intensifying
of the general motor outlet for the many part-reactions that go
to make up the completed response, through the final transfer
of the total unit of neural energy activating the just completed
response to another completely different pattern of activity.
All these factors cause greater alliance of motor impulses,
and this alliance actually *is* pleasantness, according to the
integrative theory.

Hunger, it will be remembered, is characterized by a great
intensity of sympathetic innervation which sends impulses
to the skeletal muscles, increases the supply of adrenalin,
and increases the blood supply to the surface of the body.
At the sight and smell of food which occurs with a successful
run of the maze, what happens ? The balance of power switches
from the sympathetic to the vagus centres, blood supply to
the muscles is decreased, impulses to the viscera which speed
up the salivary and gastric flow and otherwise facilitate
digestion are increased, energy is drained from the old response
into the new. By operation of the principles of facilitation
and drainage this transfer focuses all bodily activity into one
channel and in so doing tends to bring all the straggling
impulses in the food-seeking response into line. Those stimuli
with connections to both the correct and the incorrect motor
outlets will tend to be drained into the correct pathway on
account of its comparatively greater strength. At the same
time those stimuli which have connections to the right path-

way but are subliminal, that is, they would not of themselves be sufficiently strong to innervate the final motor path, are re-enforced by other stimuli which are sufficiently powerful. The impotent stimulus is rendered effective and the excitation of the correct response is increased. It is quite true that this increased facilitation is pleasant but it is also true that the pleasantness is an effect rather than a cause, a point which is explained in detail in the chapter on Emotions.

In this manner successful completion accentuates and enhances the effect of all previous facilitations. By opening up a wide motor path it exerts a general fixative effect on the sensitive psychonic tissue and thus insures the later duplication of the correct response.

After all is said and done, however, the crux of the learning process is the stamping-in of integrative connections between parts of the successful response and the integrative elimination of useless part-reactions. Our view that this is primarily due to the repetition of the correct part-reactions *in their correct order and integrative relationship*, is worth emphasizing here.

The physiological basis of learning is thus the strengthening of the proper synaptic modifications by repetition. The correct pattern of part-reactions is strengthened in this fashion because it is the only series *ever repeated as a series*. Isolated mistakes may be repeated again and again, but they are not repeated twice in the same order, whereas the correct part-reactions that go to make up the total response are *always* repeated in the same order, or integrative relationship to other part-reactions in the successful unit response, since it is their order that makes them the correct part-reactions. *What is really learned is not a number of part-reactions but the integrative relationship of these elements.*

The Conditioned Reflex

The conditioned reflex was originally used by Pavlov to refer to the substitution of a neutral stimulus for a natural one in bringing about a reflex response. Pavlov, noting that the sight and smell of food excites the salivary flow, set out to discover whether or not some other neutral stimulus could be made to have the same effect. He used dogs as subjects and worked chiefly with the nutritive and reject reflexes. By sounding a bell and keeping it ringing until after the food was presented, he found that after thirty trials the salivary flow occurred if the bell alone was sounded. He called the new reaction a conditioned reflex.

Technique for Integrating Substitute Stimuli

In developing a new reflex there are three possible ways of combining the neutral stimulus with the natural stimulus. The bell may be started before the food is shown, or started simultaneously with the presentation of the food, or it may be rung after the food is put before the dog. Only the first two methods are effective in bringing about the desire response. To test the third possibility one experimenter made 427 presentations of vanillin, five to ten seconds after the mouth was stimulated with acid, without result, whereas only one trial in the reverse order was necessary to bring about the response.

Although it is best to have the excitation of the neutral stimulus overlap that of the natural stimulus, successful experiments have been conducted allowing quite an interval of time between the two. The longest elapsed time reported has been 30 minutes. In such cases the final response is due, not to the neutral stimulus itself, but to its trace left in the central nervous system.

Substitute Response

When American experimenters began to work with the conditioned reflex they proceeded to apply it to more complex conditions. Children naturally afraid of only loud noises and falling could be made to fear the dark, animals, insects, or anything else. By operation of the same mechanism these fears could be removed. The resulting change was known as the substitute response. To cite a simple instance, an electric shock in some parts of the body will combine with food and incite salivary flow instead of withdrawal. If the shock is given in other parts of the body, the shin bone for instance, the conditioning will not take place. It will be seen that this procedure removed the experimentation from the field of simple reflexes to the control of quite complex, though native, forms of response.

Popular Usage

In addition to the wider application of the concept in scientific circles, the term conditioned reflex has received a wide-spread popular usage, wherein it may mean any kind of modification regardless of the underlying mechanism.

Objections

With this background of what the conditioned reflex started out to be and what it has now become, we shall try to discover whether conditioning can legitimately be used to explain retention. Let us first take the objections.

1. Even when strictly used the term has been objected to because the conditioned reflex is not a true reflex. Lang and Olmstead[1] conditioned the salivary flow to the beat of a metronome. They then cut the salivary receptor tract leaving the effectors intact. Nevertheless, when the metronome was started, the new response did not occur. This fact demonstrates that the beat " reflex " was dependent upon a second neural mechanism, namely, the salivary reflex, for its potency, which could not be the case were it a true reflex.

2. The integrating of a substitute stimulus, if it can be called learning at all, is learning of a very low order. It will be recalled that we have defined learning as a permanent modification of behaviour due to experience. From one point of view any new integration might come under this definition because it is a change in behaviour. But even if this point be granted, the substitute stimulus can hardly be compared with a complex behaviour pattern built up after much practice and permanently established. In some instances integration with the new stimulus cannot be brought about at all, and when it is successful it never lasts. This is not consistent with true learning, in which permanency is a basic factor.

3. The use of the term substitute response is not well founded neurologically. On a previous page we gave a short description of the conditioned response, using the electric shock and food reflexes as examples. A careful analysis of the integrative principles involved will show that the final result is either another substitute stimulus or else just the normal reflex. To explain this situation by diagram,

Food —> Salivary Flow.
Harmless shock —> Withdrawal.
Noxious shock —> Greater Withdrawal.

[1] J. M. Lang and J. M. D. Olmstead, " Conditioned Reflexes and Pathways in the Spinal Cord," *Amer. Jour. Physiol.*, 1923, 65, 603-611.

An attempt is made to condition salivary flow, first to harmless shock and then to noxious shock. If the harmless shock is presented a sufficient number of times together with food, its natural withdrawal response is inhibited and the shock alone induces salivary flow. But why should this result be called a conditioned response? It is the salivary reflex that is being conditioned and it is the salivary reflex that becomes integrated with a new stimulus. Being biologically the stronger of the two original reflexes, it inhibits the natural response to harmless shock and then drains off the excitation of the shock to reinforce its own motor path. Later, when the harmful shock is used, the shock reflex becomes neurologically supreme, the connection with the food reflex is wiped out in toto and the withdrawal response reinstated. The same thing happens in building or eliminating childish fears. The prepotent reflex always dominates. The loud noise, being stronger, integrates the rabbit as a substitute stimulus. To reverse the situation and say that the rabbit has integrated a substitute response is only confusing, because such a concept gives an integrative potency and dominance to the rabbit that it can never at any time possess. This situation seems to go to the heart of the matter. The natural stimuli and their natural responses are so firmly rooted in the physiological mechanisms of the organism that they always tend to re-establish themselves in their natural state. The substitute stimulus is only potent in so far as it is a real substitute or signal for the natural stimulus —some physiologists go so far as to say only in so far as it has meaning. As soon as this relation ceases, the new reflex is broken up. Some reflexes, like the knee jerk, cannot be conditioned at all. The pupillary reflex, after taking 400 trials to establish, is lost in three. In view of these facts, it would seem that the conditioned reflex instead of being cited as a fundamental type of learning, might afford an excellent argument against all possibility of ever learning anything at all.

What is there, then, in this situation that makes people feel as if the conditioned reflex were somehow basic to the phenomena of modification? Probably this feeling arises because the conditioned reflex, when it is actually brought about, affords a simple and clear-cut illustration of one fundamental type of integration, namely, the drainage of the lesser reflex into the more powerful one. If we are to use conditioning in this sense we should say so and cease from any further reference either to reflexes, substitute stimuli, or substitute responses. For it is in this sense and this sense only that conditioning can be said to be basic to learning.

Recall

We must now take up the problem as to how a learned response becomes subject to the recall process. After the new response has been correctly learned and fixed with some degree of permanency, its future use to the organism will depend upon the readiness with which it can be reinstated or recalled. There are, for the sake of analysis, three types of recall. The first refers to the unverbalized motor responses that are built up after a long period of practice, such as walking, swimming, and skating and so on. This class might be termed simple sensory-motor recall. The second class might be termed associative memory or associative remembering. This class of behaviour is sometimes reported upon as if it were in a category by itself, but allowing a dividing line to be made between learning and remembering, the two still have in common the need for fixating some materials and eliminating others. The main difference is that in one case a purely motor behaviour pattern is acquired while in the other a series of verbal symbols is impressed upon the neural tissue. The second difference is that in the case of associative memory the emphasis is upon the ability to reproduce the original material more or less exactly in its original sequence. A third type of recall can properly be designated as emotional, since it consists in the reinstatement of the original motor-centre portion of the learned response (as we will show later, this part of the response is closely connected with feeling and emotion). In human beings complete recall will involve all these three elements. In most cases recall is not complete because one or another of the three elements is partially or wholly lacking.

There is also another aspect of recall that frequently causes confusion in the estimation of its completeness, especially in regard to the recall of incidents in testimony. This is the fact that only what has been perceived (consciously) can be recalled ; much incompleteness of testimony is due to incompleteness of original perception rather than to incompleteness of recall.

This was suggested by an experiment at the American University, Washington, D.C., conducted by one of the writers. At this experiment an incident was portrayed before two classes of lawyer witnesses, one class not expecting the experiment and the other knowing it would be made. The differences in the results between expectation and non-expectation were much smaller than would be supposed, but the most striking result was that in both cases only one-quarter to one-third of the incident was recallable by the witnesses. It was impossible to say with confidence how much of this meagreness was due to failure of original perception and how much to weakness in recall processes ; but the evidence adduced suggested that much of it was due to actual lack of original perception.[1]

The Synaptic Process of Recall

Our subject now, however, is the recall process itself. What may we suppose to be the basis of this process when it does take place ? In the first place what is recalled is what has previously been learned, and we have said that learning is a process of synaptic modification whereby a certain series of part-reactions becomes unified in a special response pattern. The question of recall is the problem as to how this pattern is reactivated either in whole or in part.

We may note at once that such reactivation always occurs as the result of a *clue*. This is true both in voluntary recall and in the involuntary (unconscious) recall so largely used in psychoanalysis. It is also true with regard to all three classes of recall, sensory-motor, verbal, or emotional. It must be noted, however, that so far as concerns human beings, almost all recall is initiated in the correlation centres and thus begins as a process of intellectual (usually verbal) recall, even when it is a question of taking up bicycle riding again after a lapse of years, or of similar muscular activities. Remembering, in fact, is the overwhelmingly usual type of human recall.

We must remind ourselves that synapses are real things and that among other attributes, they bear actual spatial relationships to one another. This means that the successive

[1] W. M. Marston, " Studies in Testimony," *Journal of Criminal Law and Criminology*, vol. XV., no. 1, May, 1924.

or serial synaptic modification that is the learning process, establishes a certain pathway among the synapses involved. Suppose such a synaptic pathway has once been established but is not, at the moment, serving as a channel for nervous impulses. Let us now suppose that a clue (a group of such impulses from some exterior or interior source) impinges upon it. The result will be that the clue impulses enter the synaptic pathway wherever they strike it, and will then follow this pathway itself because, due to the fact that it represents a learned response, it offers the lowest synaptic resistance of any further pathway from that point.

We may note in passing that the clue must be congruous to the process to be recalled. From our point of view this subjective statement adds no difficulty necessitating a long explanation. It really means that the impulses representing the clue must have a special pattern, such that this pattern insures the entrance of the impulses into a particular, pre-established pathway (the thing or process to be recalled), if they are to enter and activate any pathway at all. In other words, the attributes of the clue impulses are such that if they are to produce any definite, unit effect upon the organism, they must produce this effect by entering a particular, previously established pathway. They may be likened to a special series of radio waves which can be effectively picked up only by the instrument that is tuned to receive them. To us this appears to be the essence of the congruity of the clue.

There is, however, one difficulty to be met. It is obvious that many different clues may suffice for the same recall. The essential differences between these clues are the differences between the various parts of the original learned process to which they apply. Within limits it would seem that a clue congruous to any part of the process to be recalled, is adequate for the recall of the entire process.

If we may divide the original learned process for convenience into pathway stages, A, B, C, D, E, how does it happen that the clue impulses impinging upon this pathway at C not only arouse the series, C, D, E, but also the whole process, A, B, C, D, E, including A and B, which are previous to the point of entry of the clue impulses? We know that the impulses cannot spread backwards along the synaptic pathway, because synaptic conduction is one-way conduction. Of course it is generally supposed, in most learned patterns, that integrative cross-connections exist, leading backward in serial sequence as well as forward. Thus it is highly probable that integrative paths have been formed leading from C to B, as well as from B to C.

But there may exist special cases where integrative cross-connections in reverse direction have not been made. In such case it would seem that we must look to the phenomenon of neural drainage or to a kind of electrical suction for an explanation here. It would appear to us that this phenomenon almost surely takes place in the case under consideration.

We have an open channel, A, B, C, D, E, represented by lowered resistances among the synapses along this pathway ; and we have the activation of C, D, E, by the clue impulses. In the correlation centres as a whole there is always a considerable amount of energy present, represented by impulses continually crossing these synapses from outer or inner sources. If we may suppose that some of this energy, at any rate, will be drawn toward the activated part-pathway, C. D, E, by the relatively intense activation there present, then it is plain that it will be drawn there primarily over the part-pathway, A, B, since this is the line of weakest resistance leading to C, D, E.

In this manner the activation of A, B, D, D, E at C (or at any other point) will lead to the resulting activation of the whole pathway, A, B, C, D, E. Such activation is a repetition of the original learned process, and such repetition *is* recall. To sum the matter up we may say that learning is the process of synaptic modification in a special series or a particular order, and that recall is the reactivation of the synaptic pathways thus established, by means of an entering group of clue impulses.

Intelligence

Another phase of human behaviour arising from the plasticity of the nervous system, or more exactly the synaptic tissues, is the capacity to react quickly and efficiently to new situations. While acquiring and retaining are based upon the ability to overcome synaptic resistances in one particular situation and the retention of an ineradicable trace once the pattern is laid down, intelligence seems to depend upon a more general plasticity of psychonic tissue which carries with it the ability to throw whole series of rearranged part-reactions into an action pattern which will meet the new emergency. It consists apparently of a native factor and the realignment of later acquired habits.

What is Intelligence ?

There is no general agreement among psychologists as to the nature of that factor in behaviour known as intelligence. The disagreement is just as varied whether the argument starts with an *a priori* definition based upon the customary use of the word by ordinary people or whether it starts with intelligence tests and an attempt by their originators to describe what they measure. Among the definitions to be found are, " the capacity to learn ", " the capacity to perfect and acquire new modes of responses ", " ability to catch on ", " good sense ", " intellect plus knowledge ", " ability to carry on abstract thinking ", " ability to adapt to a novel situation " and so on.[1] The definition which meets with the greatest approval in all quarters is one derived from Stern, the German psychologist, " General intelligence is the ability of the organism to adjust itself adequately to new situations."

An analysis of these definitions chosen at random from our foremost psychologists, shows a stress on three elements. Intelligence is general ability to learn, or to reason, or to adapt, that is, intellectual capacity receives the greatest stress, emotional capacity, (adaptation), the next, while sensory capacity is left completely out of the picture. Woodworth by indirection may be said to recognize the presence of the sensory factor when he lists curiosity as a necessary aspect of intelligent behaviour and when he mentions the ability " to see the problem ".

Intelligence then becomes a general ability to use our brains in responding effectively to a new situation. This general ability has a stated value which is applicable to all situations. It has a low value in those people who are able to meet only the simplest situations and a high value among those who react efficiently to the most complex problems. It is a basic factor prevading all our psychic activities, just as rate of metabolism is a basic factor pervading all our physiological activities.

[1] " Symposium : Intelligence and Its Measurement," *Jour. Educational Psych.*, vol. XII, no. 3 and 4, pp. 123–147 ; and pp. 195–216.

Approaching a definition from a study of test results, we have " Intelligence is what the tests measure "—a very satisfactory answer for those who wish no further understanding of the matter. Pushing farther to discover what it is that the tests measure, we find that some psychologists say the tests measure " the speed with which an individual takes on a new mode of response," and if experience in giving group tests may be used as a basis of interpretation, they measure " the capacity for quick and accurate sensory-motor reactions, with a minimum of intellectual activity intervening." What can be the matter with our main proposition and its corollaries that there should be such a discrepancy between the analytical definitions and the practical reactions ? In terms of our unit response psychology the trouble does not lie so much with our definition that intelligence is the capacity to dominate our problems quickly and efficiently but rather with the further assumptions that we attach to this statement.

In the first place, why should there be general intelligence rather than a great many separate types of efficient responses, which can be called upon as needed to solve the particular problem at hand ? If there are a great many types of intelligent behaviour as yet unanalysed, how can we hope to get at an index of their efficiency with a test limited at best to some ten types of response ? Spearman meets this problem by saying that, in addition to a general factor, there are many specific factors which go to make up an intelligence. Thorndike, after a lifetime of devising and applying tests, is of the opinion that there is no general, measurable factor which can of itself be called intelligence. Intelligence is a way of acting, that is, acting efficiently on the basis of the facts or other stimuli before you. Such a response may occur on three possible levels—the abstract or verbal, the sensory-motor which involves close co-ordinations of hand and eye, or the emotional which involves the ability to get along with other people. On each level, native equipment and past experience may limit intelligent responses to very simple situations or they may permit the efficient handling of very complex problems within the same category. Your range may be limited, on the one hand, to wiring an electric bell or, on the other, to taking command of the control room of a battleship ; or in the category of abstractions you may be able to add up the amount of last month's grocery bill or to recast the universe in terms of the geodetic line.

Thorndike's idea that there is no such thing as general intelligence, is more in accord with the principles laid down in this book than is the thesis of continuously operative general intelligence.

In a later chapter on Personality we hope to make it plain that certain types of persons are directed or oriented in particular ways ; that is, some are predominantly sensory in type, others are emotional, and others intellectual. Each type will respond most intelligently in those situations that are closest to their native capacity and experience, but not so well in problems quite foreign to their outlook. Thus Edison, representing the sensory type, would perform very intelligently in the laboratory but he wouldn't necessarily be on time for dinner no matter how important the guests might be. Bertrand Russell might do rather well with a theory of knowledge but wouldn't be so good in a nursery. Clara Bow might register effectively in an emotional situation, but would she ever bother to keep her cheque book balanced ?

A person who had organised his behaviour in all three major types of unit response and on many levels for each type, might be said to be generally intelligent, but only because he possesses a great many intelligent responses and not because of any such factor as general intelligence.

This brings us to our second point ; how can tests which deal with random selections of response situations, mostly of a sensory-motor sort, be used as an index of general adaptability, there being so many types of situation not represented in the test ? The answer is that the I.Q. can only be an index of a person's relative standing among people of similar experience. The Indian child does poorly, the white child well, but the Chinese child does best in certain types of tests involving memory and other scholarship factors. But suppose the tests had to do with saddling a pony, detecting hidden beasts of prey, finding signs of a water hole, and so forth. The I.Q.'s would probably be in reverse order, the little Indian heading the list with no great trouble. It is not surprising, either, that the Chinese children should lead the American children in tests based on responses derived chiefly from the teacher-child situation, since the Chinese system of tutelage stresses accuracy of original perception, forced upon the child by inflections of spoken Chinese, or again by the many characters of the written or printed Chinese language. The Chinese child is also especially trained in compliance, as is evidenced by an elaborate system of etiquette, respect for elders and betters, a careful technique for poetical forms which must be mastered, admiration for calligraphy, and so on. The hard memory training derived from the classics the encouragement in learning foreign languages, and the age-long emphasis upon scholarship are also elements favouring the Chinese child.

Speed, except in such tests as Thorndike's[1] C.A.V.P., is also too greatly emphasised. This is a practical necessity. No one wants to take all day to give a test, even though the rating of a great many people is involved, nor do they wish to take a month to correct the tests after they are given. Speed is therefore of the essence in giving and taking tests. Nevertheless, speed of responding may or may not be intelligent according to the individual situation. The little Indian who, after studying a Healy performance board very carefully, arranges the pieces very slowly but with no error is more intelligent for his type of life than is the grade school child who flips the pieces about making a couple of false moves for each, but getting the whole problem correctly solved long before the Indian child. A slip would be fatal to the Indian in choosing edible mushrooms, but the city child can easily remedy a mistake in calling a telephone number.

Under ordinary conditions the stress on speed is favourable for most of us rather than otherwise. We live in a fast age in a rather catch-as-catch-can manner. If we miss the limited, there is always the transcontinental air transport. If we don't speed, we lose our jobs, get run over by automobiles, or lose a big order, so that a test for speed is rightfully included in any measure of modern effectiveness. But we should really designate the particular brand of effectiveness of response, or intelligence, that we are testing: as, for example, "New York intelligence," "London intelligence," "frontier intelligence," "1930 intelligence," and so on. Pericles was rated as a brilliant man in his day and age ;

[1] The only comment one hears against the Thorndike tests in higher levels, does not concern its efficacy as a measure but rather laments the time lost in giving the test and scoring it.

but if he took time for intellectual reflection in the midst of an Army Alpha intelligence test, as he is reported to have done in solving the problems of ancient Athens, his resulting test score would doubtless prove him a moron. Or if Socrates instead of responding promptly with the routine answer, in the Stanford-Binet test, to a question concerning the differences between a king and a president, began to question the tester in approved dialectic fashion for the purpose of bringing out his questioner's ignorance of the metaphysical meaning of the terms involved, he would undoubtedly be rated at an I Q below 50.

Tests have been most useful in rating pupils for ability to acquire schoolroom learning. They are also effective in the army in ruling out the incompetent and selecting the most capable for training as officers. From these two instances one cannot help but surmise that the tests of general intelligence so far derived, are tests of special ability rather than a test of general capacity to survive under all conditions of life. Furthermore, if general intelligence does not exist, the most any test can do is measure a few of the many possible unit response types. The mental test is probably no exception.

Despite our willingness to accept the definition of intelligence set forth above, we doubt if those people who define intelligence as general efficiency really mean what they say. We think they probably mean the efficiency of the retention and recall powers of the organism as applied to the present unit responses. For instance, in the ordinary meaning of intelligence, would a response be regarded as intelligent if it were a simple, sensory-intellectual-emotional reaction gone through for the first time, without any modification by previous experience? We doubt it. Such a response might be termed "highly efficient," or "intuitive," or "instinctively correct," but it probably would not be called intelligent. We believe intelligence in its current meaning always refers to the use which an animal or human being makes of its past experience in relation to the present reaction. Therefore, according to this usage of the word, intelligence depends on the retentive capacities of different parts of the individual's nervous system.

This will differ greatly in sensory, intellectual, and emotional capacity as above indicated. The facility and efficiency with which the present reaction is able to furnish clues for the experiences retained will also regulate, to a large extent, the degree to which it is effective in modifying and improving the present response.

We do not say that intelligence *ought* to mean this; only that this is what current use of the term actually does mean.

We suggest that perhaps intelligence ought to refer to the simple efficiency or success with which the self activities of the organism shape incoming stimuli into unit responses maximally favourable to the development and organisation of the self activities. Under this definition of intelligence, retention and recall would have equal importance with the original strength of self activities, drives, and perfection of the integrative machinery used by the self activities to form incoming stimuli into unit responses. The five variables in intelligence would then be self activities, drives, integrative machinery, retention, and recall.

CHAPTER XIII

THE PLACE OF CONSCIOUSNESS IN UNIT RESPONSE PSYCHOLOGY

Subjective Considerations

WE now come to a subject at the heart of psychological theory, a subject which has caused, and still causes, endless discussion and controversy even among psychologists, the subject of consciousness. Up to the present chapter we have scarcely mentioned consciousness at all; we have been concerned solely with giving an objective (that is, an exterior) account of the behaviour of the human organism as investigated by psychologists, that is, from without. This psychology of " You " we do not now propose to abandon; yet since psychology must sooner or later face the problem of consciousness (indeed this problem is within the psychologist's special province), it becomes necessary to allude for the moment to certain subjective considerations.

The problem of consciousness arises, in the first place, from our own subjective experience. Except for this initially private experience of our own, we should never imagine that other human beings (and perhaps animals) possess any such attribute as consciousness; but indeed, all science and all " voluntary " activities rest upon and presuppose the fact of consciousness. There are some psychologists, frequently classed together as Introspectionists, who maintain that the classification and investigation of the subjective states of consciousness directly, by a sort of " turning inward of the mind upon itself ", constitute the entire field of psychology. With these psychologists the present writers do not find themselves in agreement; nor, on the other hand, can they join with those who escape all difficulties by the simple assertion that the whole human race is quite mistaken and that no such fact as consciousness has any reality. We are prepared to admit the fact of consciousness and that the psychologist is legitimately responsible for some account of it. In the present chapter we propose to offer such an account from the view-point of a psychology exterior to its subjects ; a psychology, in the contemporary usage of the word, which is objective.

Consciousness as a Part-Reaction

It will be necessary here, even at the expense of some slight repetition, to remind the reader that the present book hopes to emphasize the importance, for psychology, of the *Unit Response*. It is this whole response of the integrated, dynamic organism which is the determinative factor in the psychology of human beings and of the higher animals.

The Gestalt school of psychology, which has had its rise in Germany, emphasizes this same aspect, especially in regard to the external stimulus situation and the resulting internal pattern of consciousness, which is viewed in a mysterious, vitalistic fashion. The true total response, however, and particularly its efferent and effector portions (without which the response becomes but a mutilated section of the total response) seem to be left entirely out of consideration. Furthermore, the Gestalt position appears to contain the fallacy of over-emphasizing the whole to the exclusion of everything else, and from our point of view fails to evaluate properly the importance of the *parts* which are included within the whole. There is not only the whole which is primarily determinative ; there are also the parts, which, within the whole, possess varying degrees of importance.

Within the *Unit Response* there is sometimes a part-reaction which is of the nature of consciousness. This may not be always so, for there are some activities of the organism that perhaps are not conscious at all. However, there are a multitude of others of which it is said that they are " accompanied by consciousness ". This consciousness is a part of the particular *Unit Response* in question, and on different occasions has a greatly varying importance in its bearing upon the entire response. Moreover, this special part-reaction is very important for psychology, since psychology is the only science that is directly concerned with the phenomena of consciousness. Before considering the explicit nature of this conscious part-reaction, it will prove useful to review briefly the several leading theories of the nature of consciousness, now held by those within whose province the subject of consciousness falls.

Various Views of Consciousness

In the first place there are the *Vitalists*. They include both psychologists and philosophers ; they are of many different schools, various theories and doctrines prevail among them, but they hold the following view in common ; they are agreed that the phenomena of consciousness are of a *different order* of phenomena than those of physics, physiology, biology, or any of the natural sciences. The subject-matter of all these sciences is objective in character but consciousness, they say, is essentially subjective in nature ; it cannot be investigated by the same means used in other sciences, but a special, subjective technique must be employed, comparable to the subject-matter investigated. It is possible, of course, that some such type of consciousness as is here referred to, actually exists, but the vitalistic proposal for its investigation goes far beyond the limits of the present book. We do not by any means feel that the phenomena of consciousness are inaccessible to an investigation from without ; the purely objective account of consciousness that we intend to give, possibly may not be a completely final account, but we believe it will suggest the limits within which an objective investigation can be made and that it will deal adequately with the subject from the standpoint of an objective psychology that proposes to employ the same methods as are used by the other sciences.

Somewhat similar to the vitalistic view, is that of many *Physiologists*. They seem prepared to admit that there is a consciousness apart from, but connected with, the organism, and they seek to ascertain some anatomical region within the organism through which the connection is made. For this purpose they have picked out certain hypothetical brain cells ; their theory is that whenever these cells are stimulated as a result of the interior activities of the organism, the necessary connection is made and consciousness results. Other physiologists, who also embrace the brain-cell theory, feel that the stimulation of such cells in itself constitutes consciousness, thus doing away entirely with the necessity of any subjective consideration. However, no actual cells have been found as yet which give evidence of fulfilling the functions postulated by this theory; it remains simply an hypothesis dictated by necessity and lacking in verification.

The *Neurologists* are disposed to believe that consciousness is connected with the electric field surrounding the nerve-impulse during its ordinary propagation along the nerve trunk, during the process, that is, of nerve trunk conduction. We have already dealt with the nature of this phenomenon as a sort of progressive series of minute explosions, electro-chemical in character, and, of course, during this progress, an electrical field exists around the nerve trunk in question. This hypothesis is also wanting in any special proofs; it seems to spring from the same necessity of taking some account of consciousness and of finding within the organism some mechanism sufficiently subtle to possess an initial comparability with the complexities of conscious phenomena. The neurological hypothesis is also held by some psychologists.

Finally we have, among psychologists, those *Behaviourists* who believe that an adequate account of everything occuring in the organism can be given without any reference to consciousness whatsoever. Commencing with that proposal, they have achieved a success so considerable that they have been emboldened to proceed to a quite different position, the position that the term, consciousness, in fact refers to nothing real, but is simply an illusory concept originally carried into psychology from religious sources and confirmed in a conspicuous position by the introspective technique which has held so prominent a place in psychology in the past. Their criticism of introspection as being subjective, prejudiced, and unreliable, and thus an inadmissable tool for any objective, scientific investigation, has been carried over to the fact of consciousness itself, since, as they say, all the evidence for its existence derives ultimately from introspective grounds. Their position is that consciousness is not a real fact, but only a kind of hallucination centring around the verbal response.

There are several reasons why the writers of the present book cannot find themselves in agreement with this behaviouristic view. In the first place, there is the extreme violence done to the *universal* human experience of consciousness. There are many prejudices in the world, but one of the leading characteristics of prejudice is precisely that it is *not* universal in any given instance; to challenge so fundamental an attribute as consciousness, which is the possession of all men of all prejudices, already suggests an over-exaggerated view-point. Furthermore, no investigation, not even a behaviouristic one, can be initiated except on the premise that the investigator and his assistants possess organisms capable of responding not only mechanically and chemically, but also (which is quite another matter) *consciously*, to the subject-matter under investigation. No mechano-chemical robot will ever be able to initiate novelties like behaviourism.

Another consideration which should cause us to regard the behaviouristic position with some suspicion is the ease with which it escapes the necessity of a difficult investigation. The phenomena of consciousness are complex and baffling ; they comprise perhaps the most subtle problem that comes under scrutiny in any of the sciences, and it cannot be denied that they fall within the special field of psychology as a particular department of science. No other science is obligated to deal with them directly ; psychology is so obligated. We most certainly do not mean to suggest that the behaviourists have devised their position for the purpose of escaping responsibility ; nevertheless, that is the plain result achieved by behaviouristic theory, and our own experience is that no difficult problem has ever been successfully solved by the simple expedient of denying its existence. We do not believe that psychology will be a complete science, even in outline, until the problem of consciousness is admitted and solved.

On the other hand, we agree entirely with the behaviouristic objection to the subjective technique of introspection. Not only is it theoretically a prejudiced and unscientific technique, but its results, embodied in thousands of pages of psychological literature, prove it, in our opinion, to be as self-contradictory and unreliable as it is charged with being. In other words, we agree that an objective science must employ objective methods of investigation. The present book has kept, so far, to the objective (exterior) view-point of the behaviourists in its account of the human organism. We now propose to give an objective (exterior) account of consciousness from the standpoint of an objective psychology, a psychology of " You " as seen from without.

Where are we to find in " You," in the human organism, anything corresponding to the subjectively known phenomena of consciousness ? A delicate and complex mechanism must be looked for, and at first glance the physiologists' nerve trunk conduction theory has some *a priori* plausibility. But unfortunately the phenomena of consciousness, as subjectively known, do not correspond with the phenomena of nerve trunk conduction, but rather with those of reflex arc conduction. It is possible, of course, that the action of the field surrounding the activated nerve may differ from that of the nerve itself, but there is no reason to suppose so in regard to the general principles of its activation and every reason to suppose the contrary. Also, to take leave of the nerve itself and retire into a surrounding field, seems a little far-fetched.

It may be well to consider several further objections to which the nerve trunk conduction theory is subject. Thus (1) the same nerve trunks are used for several purposes in the organism ; for example, pain, cold, auditory impulses and so on may all be conveyed over the same nerve trunks. (2) Conversely, different neurons, that is, different nerve cells, must be involved in processes that yield the same elements in consciousness, for example, a centrally and a peripherally aroused sensation of red, as in a visual image of the colour and in its direct perception, cannot involve the same nerve trunk. (3) The phenomena of conduction that correspond to those of consciousness are not nerve trunk, but rather synaptic, phenomena. (4) What must correspond to the continuity of consciousness takes place, not along the nerve trunks, but at the synapses. (5) Only on the James-Lang theory of emotions can the nerve trunk theory account for emotional consciousness. But Sherrington's transection of the vaso-motor nerves in the dog[1], Goltz' work on emotional patterns,[2] and Cannon's investigations of bodily and visceral changes during emotional states, have shown conclusively that emotions cannot be either visceral sensations or the sums of such sensations. In view of such an impressive list of serious objections we cannot well do otherwise than abandon the nerve trunk conduction theory of consciousness.

[1] C. S. Sherrington, "Experiments on the Value of Vascular and Visceral Factors for the Genesis of Emotion," *Proc. Roy. Soc.*, 1900, LXVI, 390.

[2] F. Goltz, " Der Hund ohne Grosshirn," *Arch. f. d. gesam. Physiol.*, 1892, LI, 570. W. B. Cannon, *op. cit.*

Attributes of Consciousness (Subjective).

In looking further it will be well to have in mind a more definite conception of what, in fact, we are looking for. For this purpose let us see if we can construct a list of definite attributes of consciousness, correspondences to which we shall search for in the organism. We may put down the following attributes of consciousness, immediately recognisable in everyone's experience :

First Attribute : The greater the consciousness of a given experience, the greater is the slowing-up of the reflex action involved in that experience. For example, let us take the case of a person already practised in the technique of playing the piano, to the extent that reflexes have been established between his hand and arm muscles and the visual impulses that originate from the printed notes of sheet music. These reflexes are the basis of what is called " reading music ", and they permit of the transfer into sound, by means of finger movements striking the piano keys, of the musical notations upon the printed score. We observe that when this player is learning a new piece, his movements are relatively slow ; he hesitates during his progress through the score and even when not puzzling over matters of cadence and expression his fingers descend upon the keys with an unaccustomed deliberation. At the same time, he informs us that he is subjectively in a high degree of conscious concentration ; the more difficult the piece, the more intense he affirms his concentration to be, and the more slowly, we note, he plays.

But now we ask this same man to play for us an old piece of his, a favourite composition. Immediately he places a different score upon the piano rest and commences to play with an entirely new verve and celerity. More, during this rendering he replies to our questions, tells us why he likes this particular piece of music and enters into a recital as to how he became acquainted with it in the first place, all without the slightest interruption of his playing. When we later inquire how he is able to do these several things at once, he informs us that the playing itself, so accustomed is he to that composition, took practically none of his conscious attention, thus enabling his consciousness to be concerned primarily with our conversation. It seems clear that the more his consciousness is involved in the playing itself, the more slowing-up takes place in the reflex movements concerned.

Second Attribute : The greater the consciousness of a given experience, the greater the after-discharge, or hangover, involved. We may here consider the situation that arises when one undertakes to answer a difficult examination question. One ponders, considers various points associated with the question, thinks of several possible answers, strives to recall further information bearing upon the subject ; altogether a considerable amount of consciousness is involved. We may suppose that eventually a reply, considered satisfactory by the subject, is set down, and he passes on to the next question. It is a common experience, however, that the matter is not so easily to be dismissed. Alas, there continue to return to him recollections of the points he has just been considering ; they intrude upon his reflections concerning the new problem, his attention is distracted by some fresh point he has just remembered and by doubts concerning the accuracy of some detail or other referring to the former problem. It is further noticeable that the more difficult that former problem was, the less easily it can be dismissed and the attention centred upon the one now in hand.

With this we may contrast what happens when one replies to the conventional inquiry, " How do you do ? " Here also is a question, but one answers immediately, and more by habit than accurately, " Oh, I'm fine, thanks," ; the next moment all recollection has vanished and one cannot recall, even with some effort, in what form the reply was made. In the first case, a large amount of consciousness was involved ; in the second, almost none, and plainly when there was more consciousness, there was also much more continuance or reverbration of the response, after the response itself had ceased.

Third Attribute : The greater the consciousness of an experience, the greater the difference between the rhythm of the stimulus and the rhythm of the response. This particular effect is noticeable, among other instances, in the game of tennis. We observe a good player, faced by an agile opponent, and we note that the rhythm of his forehand drive, for example, is little affected whether the ball is being returned to him swiftly or slowly ; in either case the swing of his arm, the movements of his shoulder and wrist are approximately the same. We find, surely, that his responses vary ; sometimes he executes a hard, quick movement, sometimes a slow, delicate one, but it is evident that these changes occur in accordance with his intention as to the placing and effect of his shot and very little in accordance with the nature of the ball he is receiving, since he can, and does, return in these various ways the same kind of received ball.

The next morning, however, it chances that we see the same player engaged in returning the ball against a practice wall. In this case it comes back to him always in the same way, and we cannot fail to notice how inevitably his response tends to become an even, uniform swing, almost exactly corresponding to the rhythm of the stimulus (the ball). The man himself informs us that in the first case there was much consciousness, in the second little. We can therefore conclude that the correspondence between the rhythms of the stimulus and of the response varies more greatly with a greater degree of consciousness.

Fourth Attribute : The greater the amount of consciousness the greater the amount of temporal summation involved. Let us suppose that in order to cross a given threshold, an amount of stimulus denoted by the figure 10, is necessary. There is present a stimulus amounting only to 3 and the threshold, therefore, is not crossed. Later, however, another stimulus of the same kind, equalling 2, is received ; and later still, others in varying amounts. Temporal summation is the process whereby these successive increments are stored up and added together as they occur, until the adequate value is reached, in this case 10, and the threshold then crossed.

An illustration of this effect may be seen when, for instance, we break a fountain pen and make note of the fact that we must purchase a new one. Of course we promptly forget about this in the press of our important affairs ; but presently happening to pass on our way down a street containing several shops offering pens for sale, we enter one of them and make our purchase. Returning later by the way we have come, we notice with some surprise that, before we had bought our new pen, we had already passed two or three shops where it might just as well have been had as at the one we finally patronised ; we can even remember having seen these shops and having been vaguely aware that we should have been reminded of something at the time. The suggestion is that the successive stimuli represented by the sight of the pens displayed in the recurrent windows, finally crossed the necessary threshold. We were reminded of our intention, let us say at the fourth repetition, and then made our purchase. On the other hand, there were many other articles successively displayed in the windows on the same thoroughfare, for which we had no conscious want whatsoever. These displays could have been repeated very many times before any effect of temporal summation would have occurred in the absence of a conscious impulse toward them, although were they to be continued long enough, the articles on view would eventually elicit an overt response in spite of the preceding impulses toward this response having been unconscious. Still, again, had we gone out with the express purpose of getting a pen, the maximum consciousness possible in the given situation, we should have entered the first shop where they were on display, other things being equal. From one point of view, this is the greatest temporal summation possible, and we see that the more consciousness there is, the greater is the temporal summation effect.

We may note in passing that one of the principles of modern advertising consists in taking advantage of the effect of temporal summation in regard to the suggestibility inherent in repeated admonitions to buy this or that usually useless article. This process of insisting and insisting that people want something or other, until finally they begin to wonder if perhaps after all they do want it, eventually produces a conscious desire for the object advertised by means of temporal summation. The process is frequently misnamed " creating a want "; it might better be called " hallucinating " one. Such achievements as that of " making America garter-conscious " are accomplished along these lines.

Fifth Attribute : The greater the amount of consciousness the greater the amount of fatigue. It is, of course, the experience of every student that the mastering of a theory new to him, an operation involving a considerable amount of consciousness, brings about more mental fatigue than the mere recalling and repetition of ideas with which he is already acquainted. In the case of original research, where it is necessary not only to familiarize oneself with a novel point of view but actually to work out and devise details of procedure, if not the hypothesis itself, more consciousness than ever is called out, and the corresponding fatigue is greater still. The same situation holds for the piano player considered under the First Attribute above. An hour spent in learning to play a new composition is much more fatiguing than an hour occupied in simply running through a series of pieces already familiar. And in hundreds of similar instances it is very plain that the greater the demand upon consciousness the greater will be the resulting fatigue.

Sixth Attribute : The greater the consciousness the smaller will be the correspondence between the intensity of the stimulus and the intensity of the response. We are all acquainted with the surprising results occasioned by a remark which the recipient believes to be of an insulting nature. The offending remark may be made in a casual manner and in a low tone of voice ; in this case the stimulus consists of a few sound waves of very little intensity. Yet the result includes a flush spreading over the countenance, a tightening of the musculature generally over a wide area of the body, a verbal retort of obvious intensity, perhaps a fiercely aggressive, physical attack upon the speaker. In other cases where these overt responses are reduced to a minimum, the stimulus nevertheless evokes a highly disproportionate interior response, setting up energy sequences within the organism which will continue for hours or years or even during the remaining lifetime of the organism. These energy trains, moreover, will thereafter be waiting and prepared for some future opportunity of overt reprisal. In both these instances a high degree of emotional consciousness is present, out of all proportion to the intensity of the original stimulus.

But a casual remark of an inoffensive nature, which therefore arouses no such intensity of consciousness, likewise brings no such result in the response. Here the reaction varies much more closely with the actual intensity of the stimulus ; a greater response is evoked, the louder the tone in which the stimulus is conveyed. The response has also other points of comparability with the stimulus ; for example, it is likely to pass out of mind at about the same time that the remark which occasioned it, is forgotten. Thus we see that when the stimulus arouses a higher degree of consciousness, the correspondence between this stimulus and the response it evokes, is respectively less as regards intensity.

Seventh Attribute : The greater the consciousness the greater the ease of inhibition. For the purpose of observing this principle in action let us go to a summer camp or other resort and watch a pair of canoeists out on the lake. We note that one of these canoeists, let us call him A, is just learning the art of paddling ; his movements are slow and deliberate ; he appears to be taking great pains with the process of propelling his craft and occasionally dips his paddle into the water at an entirely incorrect angle, almost causing an upset. Mr. B, on the contrary, is an old hand at the game ; he slips his canoe through the water with little apparent effort, his movements are smooth and rhythmical. We have previously pointed out that in these circumstances A's consciousness is relatively much higher than B's in respect of the paddling activity.

We now make a little experiment. From our position on the shore we raise a sudden shout, sufficiently loud to attract the attention of both canoeists. At once they turn their faces in our direction and seek to ascertain the cause of the disturbance ; it is evident that we have been heard by both. We note, however, that there is a difference in their behaviours ; A's activity has been totally interrupted and he has shipped his paddle, while he sits holding to the sides of his canoe and looks inquiringly toward us. B's attention is also fixed upon us, but he continues to paddle along without interruption. This characteristic effect may be observed in all sorts of situations ; the effect whereby a relatively unconscious activity remains uninhibited by an outside disturbance and a relatively conscious one is immediately inhibited.

Eighth Attribute : The greater the consciousness the greater the ease of interference or interruption. This attribute, while quite similar to the last one mentioned, differs in that we are not considering, under this head, the inhibition of a series of part-movements, but an interruption of the entire integrated activity of the organism in question. Such an entire activity may be the composition or even the copying of a poem. Let us look through the doorway at a poet engaged in devising an original sonnet. His work appears to be getting along very well ; alternately he appears to be thinking over the next detail of his poem, then setting down a line or two, perhaps looking it over and revising a word here and there, then progressing further. But an office building is rising nearby and suddenly the riveters break into a chorus of operation with their machines. For a little longer our poet continues at his task, but presently he throws down his paper with a gesture of disgust, cries out a well-chosen oath, and abandons his work. For a short time he paces the floor and seems to be considering what to do. Then he sits down once more at his desk and, drawing out some already completed poems of his, commences to copy them into the manuscript of his new book, the while the riveters continue busily in their occupation.

In this instance we see that a distraction, the noise of the riveting, is sufficient to interrupt the progress of a highly conscious activity, although a similar activity, lower in degree of consciousness, is enabled to continue in spite of it. And we conclude that the greater the consciousness involved in an activity, the more easily can that activity be interrupted.

Ninth Attribute : The greater the consciousness the greater the ease of interference by drugs. In illustration of this principle we take the use of alcohol, although perhaps in the strict sense of the term it is not a drug. However, some of its effects upon the organism render it suitable as an example in the present instance, and its use in beverages is so widespread that it will better serve our purpose than a less familiar substance. For our experiment, then, let us select a marksman of our acquaintance and accompany him to the target range. We watch his performance and observe that he makes an excellent score, say 90 out of a possible 100. In order to establish that this is no fluke on his part we let him continue until we are convinced that this is indeed his average score. Now, in between his performances with the rifle, we offer him a succession of drinks containing alcohol. Presently we note that his scores are changing ; they descend from 90 to 85, from 85 to 70, then to 60, to 30. At this point we deem it advisable to suggest that he give up the exercise until the next day. He is an agreeable fellow and consents to do so.

On the way home we remark that although his marksmanship became progressively worse the more drinks he took, we had failed to notice the slightest difference in the efficiency with which he raised the glass to his lips, as between the times when his score was 90 and when it was 30. " Of course not ", he says, " but raising the glass is simply a habit ". We ask him if his shooting is not also a habit since he engages in it so often. "Perhaps you might say so," he replies, "but habit or not, it always takes a great deal of conscious attention on my part to make a good score at it."

In further illustration of the same effect we might add an even more typical instance that recently took place. Four or five men were engaged one evening in a discussion of the relativity theory of Einstein and its bearing upon modern physical conceptions. They were all well-informed and competent to take part in such a discussion, but it soon developed that each was advancing a slightly different view based upon his personal approach to the question. This situation necessitated the most careful distinction between the terms used, accurate formulations of the complex conceptions involved, and a relatively high degree of accurate mental consciousness.

All went well until, as the evening progressed, the consumption of high balls continued to mount. The first effect seemed to consist in the blurring of the formerly accurate distinctions employed; it became increasingly difficult for each to understand his companion's special point of view or to find those common denominators of concept by which the discussion could advance. Later still the concise understanding of the relativity principle itself, which each of these men had undoubtedly possessed earlier in the evening, became confused and vague and they began to attach to it implications which certainly the theory does not contain. It was obvious that the rather severe type of mental consciousness had been seriously interfered with. At the same time there was no drunkenness in the usual sense of the word; all continued to walk about, to mix their drinks and manipulate their glasses with steady hands.

In all such instances it is plain that the conscious reaction is what the drug has interfered with; as between a more and a less conscious activity, it is the former which is interfered with first and most disastrously.

Tenth Attribute: The greater the consciousness the greater the degree of variability of the responses. Here, let us take the case of a man before whom a serious practical problem has arisen. We will say that he is called upon to decide whether he will move with his family to a distant city in order to take over a new business position that has been offered him. It is impossible for us to predict what he will do when this question first faces him. He may sit quietly at his desk thinking over the proposition. He may rise and pace the floor, he may telephone to a friend to seek his advice or to tell him of the offer, or he may seize his hat and depart immediately to confer with his wife on the matter. All of these things he may do, or none ; there are probably thousands of responses which will occur, and even the order of them will be extremely variable.

Contrast with this the situation when a friend calls him up at noon and suggests that they lunch together. Supposing that no circumstance interferes and thus occasions an unusual amount of consciousness, he will say, " Surely, I'll meet you at such-and-such a restaurant in fifteen minutes," put down the telephone, rise, get his hat, and leave the office. Other circumstances remaining the same, this will be the pattern of his response whenever the stimulus is repeated. Obviously, in the first instance we gave there was involved much more consciousness than in the second ; and we see that the greater the consciousness the more variable and thus unpredictable will be the response.

Let us now recapitulate the above important attributes of consciousness, as viewed subjectively. We have found that the greater the consciousness :

1. The greater the slowing-up of reflex action.
2. The greater the after-discharge or hang-over.
3. The greater the difference between the rhythm of the stimulus and the rhythm of the response.
4. The greater the amount of temporal summation.
5. The greater the amount of fatigue.
6. The smaller the correspondence between the intensity of the stimulus and the intensity of the response.
7. The greater the ease of inhibition.
8. The greater the ease of interference or interruption.
9. The greater the ease of interference by drugs.
10. The greater the degree of variability of the response.

Here, then, we have what approaches a descriptive definition of consciousness from the side of subjectivity and our task, from being vague and nebulous, becomes concrete. If we find these ten definite attributes somewhere in the operation of the hidden machinery of those responses that are accompanied by consciousness, we shall be close to that part of the response where consciousness resides.

There is also, of course, another point that can aid us in our search. We should naturally expect to find that whatever energy within the organism is associated with conscious phenomena, would be of a more intense degree, or of a higher vibration-rate, than those energies that are associated with less complex organic activities. Mechanical and chemical energies, even the electric energy of the simple nervous impulse, all take part in unconscious activities; from this very fact it is doubtful whether they can be primarily concerned with consciousness. But if, in connection with the attributes just listed, we succeed in finding a type of energy more complex than the other forms of energy within the organism, we can be almost certain, it would seem, that we are on the right track.

The Corresponding Attributes of Synaptic Conduction.

We have already found, in considering the nerve trunk conduction theory of consciousness, that consciousness corresponds to the phenomena of reflex arc conduction rather than to those of ordinary nerve trunk conduction. What distinguishes these two kinds of conduction neurologically, is the presence in the reflex arc of various *synapses*. The presence in the arc of these synapses introduces into the principles of nerve-impulse conduction certain modifications, listed by Sherrington, a neurological authority, as follows :[1]

1. Latent period.
2. After-discharge.
3. Loss of correspondence between rhythm of stimulus and rhythm of response.
4. Temporal summation.
5. Fatiguability.
6. Interference with grading of intensity.
7. Inhibition.
8. Variability of threshold value of the stimulus.
9. Susceptibility to drugs.
10. Mutual facilitation and conflict of impulses.

[1] C. S. Sherrington, *The Integrative Action of the Nervous System*, 1920, p. 14.

It will be seen at once that the influence upon nerve-impulse conduction exercised by the synapses corresponds, point for point, with those characteristics of consciousness for which we have been searching. The correspondence, in fact, is so close as to be astonishing when it is first realised.

What, then, is the form of energy manifested at these synaptic points in the reflex arc where modifications, so characteristic of consciousness itself, are impressed upon the phenomena of nerve-impulse conduction ? In this connection we must remind the reader that, during its propagation across the synapse, the nerve-impulse itself must undergo fundamental changes in the form of its energy. We have earlier in this book explained the two theories of synaptic conduction, which we have called the sheet-electrode and the tungsten-filament theories. Whichever of these theories may eventually be established, it remains clear that the energy involved in the passage across the synapse is of a quite different character than that which arises during the passage of the impulse along the nerve-trunk proper ; it will be a more intense, and perhaps a more complex, type of electro-chemical force.

In the cases of the electrode and the filament, it is true that the energy remains electrical, as in the rest of the circuit. But at these points in the circuit it becomes more intense, more highly concentrated. This happens, as regards the electrode, because of the banking-up of the energy that takes place before a sufficient potential is achieved to cross the threshold introduced by the electrodic gap in the circuit. In the case of the filament we have a conductor of much smaller dimensions than obtain in respect of the rest of the circuit ; it is as if we forced through a very narrow pipe the same amount of water per second as had previously been carried along in a larger pipe. In both instances the energy at these crucial points is much more intense than elsewhere.

Psychons.

That part of the synapse that is energised during the passage of the nerve-impulse we have proposed to call a *psychon*. In the psychon we have a mechanism which furnishes a type of energy different from, and more highly organised than, the other types of energy to be found in the organism. At the same time, the action of this mechanism impresses upon the conduction of the nervous impulse just those characteristics by means of which subjective consciousness is definitely to be described. We suggest, therefore, that from the point of view of an objective psychology, exterior to its subjects, *this psychonic energy is consciousness*.

As we have already mentioned, there exist in the organism three general types of psychon, each differing from the others physiologically. There is no doubt whatsoever that the psychons in the sensory system differ from those in the motor centres; as to the psychons in the correlation centres there remains considerable doubt as to their exact nature, and perhaps the most plausible hypothesis is that, in this region, the brain cells become successively less sensory and more motor in character as we progress from the sensory side of this sub-division to the motor side. The typical correlation centres would then be made up of a mixture of sensory and motor cells; and it must not be forgotten that such a *combination* structure must inevitably possess a series of attributes very different from those of either the sensory or the motor systems, out of whose characteristic cells it is composed. This theory is not established, however, and we only mention it as a plausible hypothesis; but if it is not true, then almost certainly the cells of the correlation centres are of a kind different from the types of those composing the other two major divisions of the brain.

If our theory of consciousness is correct, we should thus be led to expect that three somewhat different kinds of subjective consciousness exist; and this is in fact the case.

For example, we find a mental type of subjective consciousness, the consciousness arising in the correlation centres just discussed. Of this type are such conscious operations as perception, association, conception, and so on; it may be that all of these various mental activities can be reduced to a least common denominator that can be described as the awareness of relationship.

As contrasted with this kind of consciousness, we can clearly distinguish the other two types of sensory and emotional consciousness. In the past, one of the main stumbling-blocks of emotional theory has been the hasty attempts to connect these two quite different kinds of consciousness with each other, to suppose that emotional consciousness consists of some sort of sensation, for example, of visceral sensations, or that it is composed of some delicate combination of sensations in balance. But it is obvious subjectively that there is as great a distinction between sensory and emotional consciousness as there is between sensory and mental. The " taste " of the various sensations is easily discernible in experience, and the common " taste " of all sensation as such is even more simply to be distinguished from the conscious qualities of both emotion and thought. It is a commonplace of observation that the very same sensation can, on different occasions, be associated either with pleasantness or with unpleasantness, or with any one, apparently, of an extensive list of emotions. It is evident here that the connection is one of an association, not between different kinds of sensation, but between sensations and emotions, which latter are entirely different qualitatively in subjective experience.

The work of Sherrington, Goltz, and Cannon, referred to earlier in this chapter, has successfully disposed of the theory that emotions are visceral sensations ; no further suggestions have been made that are sufficiently plausible to warrant serious research, and in view of the points brought out in the preceding paragraph, we do not believe that there exist *a priori* reasons for searching further for these elusive and contradictory " sensations of emotion ". Nor, on the other hand, are we greatly impressed with the frequent suggestion of psychologists that " emotion " is really but a verbal label which has become attached to specific types of responses or of overt behaviour, which, when examined, turn out to be describable in the cognitive or sensory terms employed in descriptions of phenomena other than emotional. This strikes us as merely begging the question ; the fact that as yet we have no objective description of emotional phenomena as such, does not argue the non-existence of such type-phenomena ; it merely means that a most fundamental task still lies ahead of us. Our own suggestion is that sensory consciousness is the psychonic energy manifested at the psychons of the sensory system and that the energy manifested at the motor psychons is emotion. One of the special virtues of the psychonic theory is thus that it offers *three* different types of organic activity to correspond with the *three* obvious divisions inherent in subjective consciousness. We have sensory, correlation, and motor psychonic energy ; and we have sensation, thought, and.emotion.

We believe that psychonic energy, although at present it remains beyond the possibility of objective measurement by laboratory apparatus, will sooner or later become directly measureable by such means ; we also believe that in describing the behaviour and functions of psychonic energy we have an adequate, preliminary account of consciousness from the objective view-point. We will take up in greater detail the manifestations of the three different kinds of psychonic (conscious) energy in the chapters on Sensation, Thought Processes, and Emotion, to follow.

The Place of Consciousness in the Unit Response

We have already reached a point, however, where we can discriminate where and how consciousness enters into the unit response. It will be recalled that we divided the entire unit response into no less than eleven part-reactions, earlier in this book. At this point it will be well to review that division, since it is just in certain of these constituent part-reactions that consciousness arises. It will be remembered that the part-reactions making up a typical unit response are as follows :'

 (1) Bodily tissues react, mechanically or chemically, to an external stimulus ;

 (2) The appropriate receptors within these tissues, react ;

 (3) The afferent nerve cells leading inward from the receptors, react ;

 (4) The psychons within the sensory centres to which these nerves lead, are activated ;

 (5) Connector nerve cells react ;

 (6) Psychons in the correlation centres to which the connector cells lead, are activated ;

 (7) Connector nerve cells, leading away from the correlation centres to the motor centres, react ;

 (8) Psychons in the motor centres are activated ;

 (9) Efferent nerve cells, outward bound from the motor centres, react ;

 (10) Effector organs (glands and muscles) react ;

 (11) Bodily parts or tissues connected with the effectors, react.

Under the heads (4), (6) and (8) above we have the psychonic parts of the unit response in question, the three places where consciousness enters into the unit response.

It is at the psychons of the sensory system that the external stimuli are first forced to combine themselves with the already proceeding self-activities of the stimulated organism. This effect is brought about by the function of mutual facilitation and conflict of impulses which the psychon exercises in regard to the conduction of the nervous impulses that pass over it ; some impulses will pass unhindered in the same order and degree in which they arrive from the afferent nerves, others will be modified in the sensory psychons, still others may be inhibited entirely. Much "sensory hallucination" may probably be due to this psychonic effect, as for example when a person fails to see some object for which he is searching and which happens to lie directly before him on his desk. It is impossible to suppose that the visual stimuli from this object do not affect his roving eye ; yet at some point before they reach the correlation centres concerned with perception and meaning, they are obviously inhibited. We do not believe it necessary to descend into dark theories of libidos and censors in order to elucidate such phenomena ; it seems evident that either in the sensory centres or in the correlation centres themselves, the psychonic condition is such that these appropriate and entering optic nerve impulses are damped.

At the psychons of the correlation centres an immense amount of co-ordination and selection of the entering impulses, is brought about ; here those psychonic phenomena underlying perception, conception, etc., take place, and it is determined how much of the external stimulation of the body at any given moment will come into mental consciousness ; and not only how much will become conscious but *how* it will become conscious, that is, what combination of sensations shall compose the resulting perception. Finally those combinations of environmental and self-stimuli are selected which are to be carried further in the organism to the motor centres and the effectors of the body. The subjective experience of these operations is that of perception, judgment, " voluntary " decision, and so on.

Another effect of the correlation psychons is the great diffusion of entering impulses, brought about through their psychonic action. The psychons are closely packed together

in these centres and the activation of one psychon thus causes
many juxtaposed psychons to react ; the disturbance, entering
at a single point, rapidly spreads over an area commensurable
with the intensity and freedom from inhibition of the entering
impulse. A highly activated set of psychons causes a large
diffusion through the correlation centres, and vice versa.
And of course, the greater the diffusion, the greater will be
the amount of psychonic energy involved and the greater
the associative consciousness of the stimulating object, or
of thought-processes concerning it.

It should also be noted that the greater the diffusion in
the correlation centres and the more intensely and multitudin-
ously the psychons in this part of the organism are activated,
the greater will be the simultaneous inhibitory effect upon the
motor centres. This effect is not to be thought of as a mere
absence of excitation ; rather it is an active influence, but
active in a negative sense, an active opposition which may
even result in a distinct diminution of the constant tonic
discharge to the musculature of the organism.

When the selection is finally made in the correlation centres,
however, the selected pattern of impulses passes along the
connector nerves to the motor centres and, entering there,
is once more combined with the pattern of (motor) self-
activities already present. Further selective processes then
occur at the motor psychons. The subjective experiences
of *feeling tone* and *emotion*, we suggest, correspond to these
operations at the psychons of the motor system, and in the
later chapter on Emotion we will show how the phasic motor
impulses (those entering the motor centres from without,
i.e., from the correlation centres) give rise to the unit emotional
reactions of Dominance, Compliance, Inducement, Submission,
and their compounds, depending upon the relationship which
the entering impulses bear to the existing (self) motor condition. When all this has occurred and the pattern of
impulses destined for the final common motor path has at
last been selected, the final pattern is dispatched on its way
over the efferent nerves to the effectors.

It is in these three regions, then, at the psychons of the
sensory, correlation, and motor centres, that consciousness
enters the unit response and, partly through the operation
of modification, inhibition, and selection, determines the
pattern of the response. Once again we emphasise the fact

that consciousness is a psychonic part-reaction of the whole unit response in any given case.   Within the unit response, however, it may have an important determinative bearing by reason of the fact that the energy manufactured at the psychons is relatively higher and more intense than any other energy taking part in the whole response pattern.   When the response engages many psychons and a large amount of psychonic energy is involved, this part of the unit response may be determinative of the whole response ; in other cases, when but few psychons take part, it may be relatively unimportant.   But only in those cases when no psychons at all are involved in the organism's activity (and these are very few indeed), can psychology leave out of consideration this part-reaction of the unit response called " *consciousness* ".

CHAPTER XIV

SENSATION

Introductory

AT the outset of our investigation of sensation it must be carefully borne in mind that when we use the term, sensation, we are really speaking not at all about the whole unit response, and not even about that subdivision of the response that comprises the activation of the sensory system of the organism. We are speaking, in fact, only about a part-reaction which itself is included within that combination of part-reactions that constitutes the sensory portion of the unit response ; and that is the activation of the psychons within the sensory system of the organism.

Thus in the present chapter we theoretically sever the connections between the interior limit of the sensory system and the rest of the organism. And we make the usual assumption that, if the organism were to be composed exclusively of this portion of its present self, the phenomena of sensation would still occur. Again, within this limited portion of the body, we shall really be concerned only with what takes place at the psychons ; generally speaking, those parts of the sensory system where the psychons are present, are within the head.

Here we come up against a difficulty which, if not introduced by behaviouristic theory, has at least been greatly emphasised therein. This difficulty consists in the prevalent attempt to describe sensation (which is a fundamentally inherent element of conscious experience) in terms of the reaction evidenced by the sensing organism. Thus, let us say that in the presence of a vibration-rate which we call the colour, red, the pupils of the eyes dilate. This, of course, is not the case ; it is taken as a simplified illustration of the point to follow. Then whenever the pupils are observed to be so dilated, the behaviourist will assert that the sensation, red (or as much of this phenomenon as can properly be excluded from the charge of verbal hallucination) is present. Such, naturally, is not the case ; not only will similar reactions result from different stimuli, and in this statement we include almost every type of symptomatic reaction that can be behavioristically observed, but also the eyes of no two persons will dilate in exactly the same way ; not even will [the eyes of a single subject respond in the same fashion on different occasions of the same kind.

This continual slight variability of the same kind of reaction results from the fact that every such reaction is but a part-reaction within an entire unit response, and unit responses, being built up of complicated combinations, are never twice the same. In other words, the reactions which the behaviourist terms " sensory responses " in his experiments, are themselves governed by the unit responses of which they are parts. Nor will the unit responses avail as indices of consciousness, because consciousness, as we have pointed out, is not a unit response but an at present inaccessible, psychonic part-reaction within the unit response.

It is true that the very strict behaviourist would deny any " sensation " at all, asserting that he did not know what is meant by this subjective term. Nevertheless, leading exponents of behaviourism, Lashley and Hunter for example, have addressed themselves to the translation of " conscious " phenomena into behaviouristic terms and many behaviouristic experiments have been conducted on questions that, to all except the behaviourists, appear to involve sensory consciousness.

Of course, in actual practice, the behaviourist, just as every other experimenter, really accepts the common, subjective experience, as evidenced by the subject's verbal report, as his criterion for the presence of consciousness. And despite some writings to the contrary, we must note that by this " sensation " of his he really means *something different from* the verbal report upon which the evidence of its presence rests. This point is clearly acknowledged in Hunter's " irreversible SP-LR relationship ", which is proposed as the criterion of the subjectivists' " consciousness".

However, it would still seem that behaviouristic theory is responsible in large part for the confusion that allows it to be supposed that sensation can be described either by

Y

descriptions of part-reactions that are not psychonic or by descriptions of total responses which, as units, are not conscious. To sum the matter up, it is the conscious experience of sensation that is the common element by an appeal to which alone sensory experiments can be conducted. If we wish to deal with this common element objectively, we shall be dealing in fact with a psychonic part-reaction of the given unit response, and only with that psychonic part-reaction that takes place within the sensory sub-division of the organism in question.

Sensation as Viewed Physiologically.

Aside from the strict behaviouristic denial of sensation as such, almost all other theories of sensation may justly be termed physiological. The ordinary list of the five senses, which was never fully comprehensive, has long since been done away with in favour of more physiological tabulations. There are a great many such physiological lists in existence, and the following may be taken as a typical example :

Skin sensations : Touch
　　　　　　　　 Warmth
　　　　　　　　 Cold
　　　　　　　　 Pain
Kinaesthetic sensations : From Joints
　　　　　　　　　　　　　　 Tendons
　　　　　　　　　　　　　　 Muscles
Taste sensations : Salt
　　　　　　　　　 Bitter
　　　　　　　　　 Sweet
　　　　　　　　　 Acid (also perhaps metallic and
　　　　　　　　　　　　 astringent)
Auditory sensation
Equilibrium sensation
Visual sensation
Olfactory sensation
Also pain sensations not cutaneous, i.e. not originating
　　in the skin
Hunger sensation
Thirst sensation

There are, of course, other types of list not physiological in character, since, in order to arrive at them, one need never have heard of an end-organ or a nerve. We append such a list for comparison with the physiological one just cited :

Auditory sensation
Visual sensation
Olfactory sensation.
Gustatory sensation
Tactile sensation
Kinaesthetic sensations : i.e., sensations of movement, either of the whole organism or of any of its parts.
Coenaesthetic sensations : Including all sensations resulting from stimuli originating within the organism, e.g. hunger, thirst, equilibrium, muscular tension, etc.

Neither of these lists would seem to be perfect from a psychological point of view, but there can be little doubt that, of the two, psychologists have chosen to follow the first in dealing with the subject of sensation. Not only is it evident from the type of lists to be found in psychological text books that the general outlook has been preponderantly physiological, but the theories of sensation that have been offered by psychology up to the present time appear to have been based almost entirely upon details of end-organ and afferent nerve function. Weber's and Hering's end-organ theories of cutaneous sensation, the audition theories of Helmholtz and Rutherford, the theories of equilibrium sensation based exclusively upon the reactions of the semi-circular canals, and even the findings of Cannon and Washburn regarding hunger sensations, are all cases in point. Such instances of " psychological " theories of sensation could be adduced in great number and in relation to each kind of listed sensation. At the moment, we only wish to point out that everything definitely advanced in this type of theory emphasizes, and seems to be based upon, the physiology of the receptors and connecting nerve systems.

Visual Theories (Physiological).

In order to make clear our objection to the physiological type of sensation theory in psychology, as well as to contrast these theories with our own proposal, it will be necessary to consider in brief detail some of the current theories of the kind under discussion. For this purpose we have selected the sense of vision, since here is a sensation complex enough to exhibit well the differences between the physiological and psychological treatments.

A preliminary difficulty in all theories of vision is the fact that physicists can give us very little satisfactory information as to the real nature of light. Light seems to be a substance, that is, it possesses inertia, which is the definition of what used to be called matter. But different light phenomena necessitate now the wave theory and now the quantum hypothesis ; and these two view-points are mutually inconsistent and contradictory. Evidently we are still far from understanding its fundamental nature.

Thus we must go forward more or less in the dark, since we are ignorant even of the real character of the stimulus for the visual sense. It has been possible, however, to divide this sensation into three categories : sensations of light, of form, and of colour. Sensations of form are supposed to be allied with other kinds of spatial perception and rely upon the triangulation introduced by binocular vision, and upon combination with other sensations and their images, such as those of touch. Thus many sensations of form are not truly sensations at all, but really percepts, and with these we will deal later on in the chapter on Thought. Sensations of colour can again be divided into three classes : those of colour tone or hue, corresponding to the wavelength of the light ; those of brightness, relating to the intensity of the light ; and those of saturation or tint, corresponding to the complexity of the light.

All the chief theories of vision are based upon the existence in the eye of certain hypothetical substances whose decomposition under the influence of entering light-rays, is conjectured to produce the necessary effect upon the end-organs of the retina, namely the rods and cones. The discovery of " visual purple ", a redly pigmented substance in the rods, whose pigmentation varies under the influence of different kinds of light, has naturally strengthened this type of theory.

We also find various functions assigned to different structures of the retina. Visual acuity, for example, is supposed to depend upon the cones. And certain nocturnal animals have been found which possess vision and in whose eyes occur only rods ; from this fact, among others, it is argued that perception of low intensities of light is connected with the rods. Without going further into the details of the general theory of vision, we can now consider several of the most famous specific theories. We shall be able to notice only what they advance in respect of colour sensations, since to go into them fully would necessitate at least a chapter in itself, and we only wish to show that they are as typically physiological as the theories now held regarding all other sensations.

In the early version of the Young-Helmholtz theory, three kinds of nerve fibres were presupposed in the retina ; this was later changed to three hypothetical substances. These, when decomposed by the wave-lengths of different kinds of light, arouse in the conjoined end-organs those impulses that produce the sensations of the three primary colours, red, green and violet. The mentioned colours were chosen as being primary because of certain facts of colour mixture and also because they remain visible at low intensities of light, after yellow and blue have both disappeared. The black-white series of sensations occurs when all the substances are equally affected in various degrees, black corresponding to the absence of excitation.

Hering, on the other hand, considered that black resulted from an active process in the eye and not from the mere absence of stimulation. His theory supposes pairs of antagonistic primary colours resulting from physiologically opposite actions within the eye ; these colours are black-white, green-red and blue-yellow. The pairs of primary colours are based upon the action of three supposed substances. Regarding these substances, Hering proposed a complicated theory of metabolism whereby, depending upon the light stimuli affecting them, they either ascended or descended a scale of potentials ; when descending to a lower potential, white, red and yellow resulted from the action of the respective substances, and when ascending, black, green and blue sensations were produced. In a state of equilibrium the result was neutral grey. The actual seat of the substances was left undecided ; it was not even said whether they were situated in the eye or in the central nervous system. Moreover, Hering himself preferred to postulate only a single visual substance having three modes of reactivity which would correspond to the operations of the three substances presupposed in the theory that bears his name.

According to Wundt's theory separate substances exist in the eye for the sensations of light and of colour. The latter substance is complexly constituted, thus offering the possibility of many different colour sensations.

One of the most recent physiological theories of colour vision is that advanced by Mrs. Ladd-Franklin. In this theory also we find the inevitable three substances, or as she prefers to call them, molecules. The first of these, which decomposes under any kind of light stimulus, is to be found only in the rods. The second, a partially differentiated substance sensitive to yellow and blue rays, resides in the poorly developed cones of the intermediate section of the retina. The third, a triply differentiated substance capable of responding to the influence of red, green and blue rays, is contained only in the cones of the central region where the colour sense is believed to be most acute. The genetic aspect of the evolution of these substances is emphasised in the view that the last and most highly differentiated of them is biologically the most highly evolved. As in almost all the other colour theories the question as to the place and manner in which the actual sensations arise, is slurred over. It seems to be supposed that they result directly from the action of the hypothetical substances upon the afferent nerves with which these substances are believed to be in contact, or at best that by this means they are directly aroused in the cerebral sensory centres. In the earlier theories the rods and cones were supposed to have a vibratory effect upon the nerve endings ; but as we have seen, of recent years it has become fashionable to substitute a photo-chemical effect produced upon the nerve endings by the hypothetical visual substances.

Naturally a vast amount of experimentation has been made upon visual sensations and many ingenious methods have been devised whereby, for example, the light can be introduced into the eye and the subject himself can see the various structures, such as blood vessels, in the walls of his own eye. It is interesting to note, in respect of these many experiments, that although the theories are almost entirely physiological in character, the experimental results upon which they are founded, are not at all physiological. By far the most work has been done either by means of verbal reports of their experiences obtained from the subjects or by the even more subjective method of introspection. For instance, not one of the famous visual substances, if we except " visual purple " (which is analogous to these substances, but is not one of them), has ever been located in the eye or its presence even hinted at, physiologically or neurologically.

We believe it will be seen that the problem of visual *sensation*, as distinct from the mechanics of the eye, has not even been approached, much less solved, by any of the theories mentioned. Yet it is the matter of sensation which, so far as concerns psychology, is the only question at issue; the morphology and histology of the eye may quite properly be left to those who have been trained and have specialised in these subjects, since presumably their special abilities in such directions are superior to those of the psychologist. The point which we cannot too greatly stress, is that the psychological problem does not arise until after the light stimulation has entered *and passed through* the eye. Strictly, what happens within the eye is scarcely within our province ; but what is our problem is how the excitation furnished by and from the optic apparatus to the visual centres of the cerebrum, becomes visual sensation. It is just at the beginning of this problem that all the foregoing colour theories leave off.

General Theories of Sensation (Physiological).

It may be well to mention briefly certain generalizations regarding sensation as a category of experience, that have been developed from the physiological outlook evidenced by the preceding visual theories, the same outlook that runs the whole gamut of sense theory from thirst to equilibrium.

Two such generalizations are embodied in Weber's and Fechner's famous Laws. We are reminded that Weber's Law refers to the stimulation of the sense receptors in general. It takes account of the fact that the stimulability of a receptor is partly determined by its previous stimulation ; and states that there must be an increase in the stimulation of the receptors, such increase bearing a particular ratio to the degree of stimulation existing previously to the increase, before sensation can arise. It will be seen that here again, as also in Fechner's logarithmic Law of the relation between stimulus and sensation, we meet the end-organ emphasis typical of the physiological view-point. To an inquirer coming upon statements of the two Laws for the first time and unaware that these psychologists in fact believed sensation to be located in the head brain, it would seem as if they supposed sensation to appertain to the receptors, since these receive the great preponderance of attention.

Johannes Müller's doctrine of specific nervous energies represents one outstanding attempt to transfer the origin of sensation qualities from sensory end organs to afferent nerves or possibly to special sensory areas in the brain. Müller supposed that each sensory nerve or each special sensory brain area possessed a specific energy which produced in consciousness the appropriate sensation qualities. This theory of Müller's was certainly a step towards an effort to formulate a real psychological theory; that is, a theory which should account for the origin of sensations in consciousness. But the theory of specific nervous energies seems to have little foundation in fact. Mere electrical excitation of a sensory nerve or of the corresponding brain centre does not produce consciousness. Neurologists have discovered that differences in stimulus qualities are probably communicated to the brain by different rates, rhythms, or volumes of afferent nerve impulses. These quantitative differences in nerve impulses seem to be originated and determined by the appropriate sensory receptor organs with which the afferent nerves connect. Once the psychons of the brain have been excited by the appropriate volume and rhythm of nerve impulses in this manner, consciousness of the appropriate sensation arises. Moreover, once the central psychon has been excited in the right way this excitation apparently leaves a trace so that the same sensations may be subsequently evoked by stimulating these same sensory centres by impulses through other nerves, or by electrical stimuli. For example, persons without retinal end organs from birth never become conscious of visual sensations, whereas persons who become blind after once experiencing visual sensations can be made to experience these sensations again as a result of recall or electrical stimulation. Müller, it seems, moved in the right direction toward a truly psychological theory of sensation consciousness ; but his neurological hypothesis was based upon insufficient data.

The Physiologists Relation to Theories of Sensation.

It would seem proper to point out in this place that our discussion of the foregoing physiological theories of sensation should not be construed as a criticism of physiology. Indeed, we have a high regard for physiologists and find it necessary to apply to them for valuable information—so long as their results are drawn from within the confines of their own field of investigation. But it seems clear enough that, in the investigation of the receptor mechanisms, physiologists have been unable to leave out of their procedure references to the psychological element of sensation, an element that, in our opinion, belongs more particularly within the field of psychology.

Nevertheless, since they have in fact used the subjective data of sensation in the construction of their theories of stimulus reception, it has happened that these same theories have been very easily taken over bodily into psychology, with the result that psychologists themselves have become prone to confuse sensation with the functioning of the sensory receptors.

There are certain general points that apply in common to this hybrid physiological-psychological view. In the first place there is the predominant position given in its theory of sensation to the structure of the special end-organs involved ; this is physiology. In the second place, another predominant position is given to the functioning of the sensory nerves, notably in the doctrine of Specific Nervous Energies ; and this is neurology. It seems to us that none of these theories are psychological theories and that none of them render either an adequate or a satisfactory account of sensation.

The Panpsychic Theory of Sensation (Psychological).

So far as we know, there are only two actually psychological theories of sensation ; they are L. T. Troland's panpsychic theory and our own psychonic theory. We shall consider Dr. Troland's theory first.

His view belongs to a category which, in our chapter on

Consciousness, we classed as vitalistic; that is, he considers the phenomena of consciousness to be of a different order than that of the phenomena of physics and of the other natural sciences. Nevertheless, he asserts that, as regards human beings, the phenomena of consciousness arise " as a result of " certain physical activities of the cerebral cortex. Since we have already given attention to the physiological theories of colour, we may take the panpsychic theory of colour vision as an example of the way in which Dr. Troland's general theory of sensation works out.

In the first place we have the question as to the impulses sent over the optic nerves from the visual receptors in the eyes, and these can vary in only two ways; they can be widely separated (few per second) or closely packed together (many per second) and their rhythm can be regular or irregular. When their rhythm is regular, we have the black-white series, ranging from black (widely spaced pulsations) to white (very closely packed pulsations).

We now meet with the three hypothetical photo-chemical substances in the retina, which, in the case of this theory, are supposed to suffer decomposition under the influence of the wave-lengths corresponding to the three primary colours of red, green and blue. When these substances are decomposing at equal or equivalent rates, the pulsations over the nerves are equally spaced; the greater the intensity of the light, the more pulsations per second, and thus the impulses preliminary to the black-white series. The frequency of the impulses accounts for the brightness of the colours.

But if the three retinal substances are breaking down unequally, the rhythm of pulsations in the nerve will become irregular. Upon the regular frequency an irregular rhythm will be superposed and the particular modulation in a given case will account for the particular hue resulting in consciousness. The matter of saturation is considered to be a measure of the departure of the modulated rhythm from regularity.

When these impulses, with the above characteristics already impressed upon them, reach the visual regions of the cerebral sensory centres, a further process takes place. There are supposed to exist here six sets of cell arrangements whose structure is such that they are " tuned ", as in the case of radio receivers, to pick up those frequencies, either regular or modulated, that correspond with the six psychologically principal colours, black, white, red, yellow, green, blue. Their action is thus individually selective, and when several of them are acting in concert, the result is one of the many colours that can be derived from a combination of the six principal ones. The black receiver is activated to the degree that the white receiver is not activated.

In addition to this, it is necessary that the incoming visual impulses, or their influence, spread beyond the visual areas proper of the sensory centres into the adjacent association areas before sensations of colour can arise. In his discussion of the conduction of the visual nerve impulses, mention is made of the fact that the impulses cross various synapses, but no stress is laid upon this fact and no function assigned to the modifying influence of the synapses upon the impulses. In fact, it would seem to be a necessary implication of the panpsychic theory of colour vision that little or no influence is so exerted, an implication, it must be said, which is certainly contradictory to neurological finding.

When all the foregoing has taken place, visual sensations of colour result, but Dr. Troland is very careful to insist that the mentioned cerebral operations are not themselves, either in whole or in part, the sensations. According to the panpsychic view, all consciousness, including of course sensory consciousness, is made up of fields of some indescribable kind of force, and such conscious force fields bear certain relationships to the fields of electrical force that compose all physical matter, including the human cerebrum.

At first glance this may seem a most obscure and complicated theory, largely perhaps because of the employment of the conception of two fields of inter-related but different forces. It is only necessary, however, to have the concept of fields of force clearly in mind in order that the panpsychic view should be seen in its actual simplicity.

As we know, the conception of a field of force has grown out of modern, mathematical physics. In the case of a wire carrying an electric current, certain influences of a magnetic nature, attributable to the current in the wire, exist in the space around the wire. The space within which these influences function is spoken of as a field of magnetic force and has specific characteristics that can be formulated mathematically. However, there are more kinds of force than the magnetic variety; all space is supposed to be filled with combinations of the fields of these various forces, and by some it is considered that the electrons and protons of matter itself are simply those points in the general physical force-field where the intersections of lines of force, or concentrations of force influences, exist. This is the electro-magnetic conception of matter which displaced the former theories based upon a hypothetical ether. The most recent researches suggest the displacement of the electro-magnetic conception in turn, but we need go no more deeply into physics than this to understand the concept of fields of force employed in the panpsychic theory of consciousness.

According to the panpsychic theory of colour vision, the physiological situation in the cerebrum, which we have been engaged in describing, might theoretically be reduced to a mathematical formulation of the field of electro-magnetic force there present. It is this field which would then bear some sort of corresponding relation to the " field of consciousness " that we call sensation of colour. It is because of the stress that Dr. Troland lays upon the non-physiological aspect of conscious sensation that we believe his theory to be a truly psychological one. Moreover, the Troland theory is based upon a modern and scholarly compilation of neurological facts and theories.

But after all is said and done, we venture to think that, apart from this unseating of physiology as the central fact in sensation, nothing very definite is put forward in the panpsychic theory of sensation. We are confronted by a metaphysical view as to the nature of consciousness that can be shown to be an almost exact reproduction of a certain tenet of doctrinal Buddhism. By the very nature of the case this view is insusceptible of proof under present conditions, nor does Dr. Troland put forward any proofs, arguments by analogy excepted. The theory thus rests for its acceptance upon the question as to how plausibly it affects the hearer, and the final decision is quite plainly due to an intellectual prejudice one way or the other. Even in this theory we find everything definite that is advanced to be either physiology or neurology. From the standpoint of a psychology exterior to its subjects, the psychological portion of the panpsychic theory is really philosophical.

To sum up, from our own point of view it seems to us that

the panpsychic theory is valuable : (1) Because it is based upon a real knowledge of neurology and does not make absurd assumptions contrary to neurological fact ; (2) because it clearly recognises that the retinal mechanisms are only the gateway to sensation, and not the sensation itself. On the other hand we believe that, as a scientific theory, the panpsychic view suffers from three defects : (1) Consciousness is treated as non-physical ; (2) purely imaginary aspects and forms of an unknown force are assumed which are arbitrarily asserted to correspond with consciousness, whereas a proper theory should correlate the known phenomena of consciousness with some measurable type of matter or energy ; (3) it puts forward no reason why some parts of the brain structure cause consciousness and others do not.

The Psychonic Theory of Sensation (Psychological).

The psychonic theory of sensation is designed to answer the strictly psychological issue : how is sensation-consciousness itself produced ? In contrast to other theories of sensation, therefore, the psychonic theory regards sensory stimuli in the environment, sensory receptor organs of the body and afferent neurons connecting these receptor organs with sensory centres of the cord and brain, as mere adjuncts to the sensation-making apparatus proper which we assume to be the psychons of the sensory centres. Stimuli, receptors, and afferent nerve trunks are essential but supplementary mechanisms, from the psychonic point of view. We regard them in this way not because these organs are intrinsically less important than the consciousness-generating tissues : but merely because we are engaged in the study of psychology and therefore must, for the sake of convenience and expediency, retain the strictly psychological point of view which lays its major emphasis upon integration-consciousness mechanisms and phenomena.

From this psychological point of view, then, we must seek to discover how the sensory receptor organs and afferent nerves are able to communicate differences in sensory stimuli from the environment to the psychonic tissues of the brain, where these differences give rise to ultimate differences in integrative activities and correspondingly create differences in sensation consciousness. The psychonic theory regards the various types of sensory receptor organs in the body as physiological instruments capable of evoking in afferent nerve fibres different rhythms, intensities, and volumes of nervous impulses. Our theory regards the afferent neurones as neurological instruments capable of propagating the disturbances thus evoked by the receptor organs and communicating them in due course to the sensory psychons. A detailed study of all the complexities of sensory receptor organ structure, afferent neurone organisation and behaviour is wholly beyond the scope of the present book. Besides, as psychologists, we are not primarily interested in such studies. We are quite content to leave them to the physiologists ; assembling our own supplementary data from the total mass of physiological findings. It is sufficient, we believe, for psychological purposes to mention one or two general aspects of receptor organ and afferent neurone behaviour.

In a previous chapter we have outlined at some length the various types of receptor organs which exist throughout the human body together with their chief structural and functional characteristics. We have further noted that the various receptors are individually adapted to different types of environmental stimuli. We cannot pretend to know as yet the exact structural mechanisms whereby many of these receptor organs are enabled to differentiate between stimuli of the same general type, as, for example, the ability of the visual receptors to respond differently to different wave lengths of light. It seems clear, however, that sensory receptors in general do respond differentially to differences of stimulation within the same mode. And it seems equally certain that sensory receptors in general are capable of communicating, to the afferent nerve fibres with which they are associated, these differences in their response to environmental stimuli.

How, then, are the afferent nerve fibres able to register differences of excitation originating in the sensory receptors ? And how are these groups of afferent neurons able to communicate the differences thus registered to the psychons of the central nervous system ? We have considered at some length, in previous chapters, the general physiological and neurological findings with regard to the laws of nervous excitation and conduction. At the present point of our discussion. it seems necessary only to emphasise a single fundamental neuronic law and its consequences. The law to which we refer is the so-called all-or-none law of nerve conduction, which states that any nerve fibre, if it is excited at all, must be excited maximally. The consequences of this law of nervous conduction rule out immediately a considerable number of allegedly psychological theories of sensation. For instance, all the older theories which maintain that differences of intensity of physical stimulation result in differences of intensity in impulses carried over the afferent nerves may be categorically denied. Again, theories of sensation which remain satisfied with real or hypothetical differences in photochemical phenomena of the visual receptors and similar end-organ phenomena in other sensory organs, must be regarded as obviously inadequate and futile from the psychological point of view. No matter what happens in the sensory end-organ, the real question which must be answered is : How are these supposed differences in end-organ behaviour translated into differences of afferent nerve conduction ? The answer which present-day neurologists give to this latter question must, we should think, be accepted by psychology as the basis for any authentic theory of sensation.

Neurologists inform us that nervous impulses over the same nerve fibre may differ, within the normal range, only with regard to rhythm and volume. That is to say that maximal impulses might be sent over a given nerve path in quick succession or at widely spaced intervals ; the rhythm impulses might differ within the limits of the stimulation thresholds of those particular neurones, in much the same way that the rhythm of electrical telegraphic currents differ in sending the dots and dashes of the Morse code. It would seem to us a very probable assumption that sensory end organs are so constructed that they are able to communicate characteristic rhythms of nervous excitation to the afferent nerves with which they are connected.

The other way in which nerve impulses may differ, that is, with respect to volume, must depend upon a number of different factors including the rhythm of nervous impulses set up in each individual nerve fibre as suggested in the preceding paragraph. A rhythm consisting of very brief intervals would naturally tend to increase the volume of excitations delivered to the psychons : while more widely spaced rhythms must be supposed to result in less total volume of excitation. These differences are doubtless so minute that present instruments are inadequate for their measurement. The most obvious source of differences in volume seems to lie in the known differences in the number of individual nerve fibres communicating with a given set of of receptor organs ; and also the known differences in the number of individual end organs located in a given area of the body. Besides these sources for volume differences in nervous excitation, we must also remind ourselves that the number of interconnections between afferent nerves of origin at the outlying synapses and in the spinal centres determines to a very great extent the total volume of sensory impulses which will be delivered at the more central psychons in sensory areas of the brain. To account, therefore, for differences in total volume of nervous excitation delivered to the central psychons we must consider rhythm of nervous impulses, number of end-organs in a given area, number of individual nerve fibres associated with the given receptor organs, and number of afferent nerve trunks combined together in the outlying and intermediate synapses of the nervous system.

In summary, then, all differences in final sensory integration activity and correspondingly in sensation consciousness must be caused by the following differences in nervous excitations delivered to the central psychons. First, differences in individual nerve fibre rhythms and differences in various combinations of these rhythms received from the nerve trunks. Second, differences in total volume of nervous excitement determined by the factors considered in the preceding paragraph. Upon these two quantitative differences in psychonic stimulation, therefore, must depend the ultimate differences in sensation, no matter what theory of sensation we choose to adopt.

There is one other datum of extreme importance which integrative psychology emphasises throughout the fields of sensation, thought, and emotion. This is the constant tonic or " self " excitation which is continuously going on, from birth to death, as a result of stimulation constantly delivered by the organism's own stimulus mechanisms. It is impossible to consider sensory integrations as taking place primarily between two separate batteries of nervous impulses both evoked by transient environmental stimuli. The primary and deciding factor in every sensory integration would seem to be, in all normal cases, the constant psychonic sensory excitement of the "sensory self"; just as the decisive factor in thought integrations must be the "mental self" and the most important factor in emotion integrations must be the "motor self". Psychology has long recognised the fact pointed out in preceding chapters that sensations, or "sensory responses", are not determined by the absolute nature of the environmental stimulus, but are determined rather by the relationship between a given environmental stimulus and the existing state of receptor organ stimulation. Weber's law, the theory of "physiological zero", "hearing the silence", and the intrinsic light of the retina are examples of recognised combinations between existing stimulations of the sensory apparatus and the presence or absence of additional sensory stimuli from the environment. To neglect this most important factor of constant or self excitation would seem impossible in any adequate theory of sensation. In the psychonic theory of integrative psychology the constant or self excitation of central psychons is regarded as the basis upon which all characteristic forms of integration, with their corresponding qualities of consciousness, are built.

General Statement of Psychonic Theory of Sensation.

In order to recapitulate and summarise our position, we may now state the psychonic theory of sensation in general terms before going on to give examples. We suggest that the psychonic energy arising at the synapses within the sensory centres of the organism constitutes sensory consciousness. Sensation consciousness is thus regarded as synonymous with integrative activity of the psychons. The differentiations existing within sensory consciousness, that is to say the different modes, intensities and qualities of sensation, are accounted for by the distinctions between the various types of sensory psychonic energy generated by the psychons in question. Psychonic energy is integrative energy; and differences in integrative energy must be caused directly by the different nervous excitations which impinge upon the psychons and are there integrated. These differences in psychonic excitation are traceable, in turn, to differences in rhythm and volume of afferent nerve excitement; which

z

differences ultimately may be traced to differences in receptor organ structure and functioning.

A much clearer idea of the general psychonic theory of sensation may be obtained by applying our general concept, in some detail, to the theory of one particular mode of sensation. The integrative theory of vision may best be selected to serve as an illustrative example since the physiological and neurological findings in the field of visual sensations and structures are more complete than the experimental findings with respect to any other sensation.

Integrative (Psychonic) Theory of Vision.

The classical theories of vision, notably the theories of Hering, Young-Helmholz, and Ladd-Franklin are really theories of differential mechanisms within the visual receptor organs. All these theories hypothecate three or more photochemical substances which are supposed to exist in the rods and cones, and which are supposed to break down or regenerate under the influence of different coloured light rays. But, as we have tried to point out in the preceeding paragraphs, it seems rather fatuous for modern psychologists to sit complacently with a full supply of these hypothetical photochemicals in their laps, fully convinced that in the unexplored virtues of these imaginary substances lies a secret formula of colour consciousness. So far as these theories are concerned their proponents have only attempted to describe the highly complicated physiological apparatus for transforming physical light stimuli into photochemical nerve stimuli. No one, we suppose, who concedes the existence of consciousness and assumes that the description of this phenomenon is psychology's proper task, would rest content with the idea that the reaction of a photochemical substance in a retinal receptor *is* the consciousness of a corresponding colour sensation.

Let us abandon, to start with, all discussion of imaginary photochemical substances, assuming only that somehow or other the visual receptors of the retina are able to function differentially in response to appropriate wave lengths of ight. Let us deal, throughout our further discussion of visual sensation, only with experimentally established facts. Two sets of facts seem to us of primary importance, namely, the existence of a so-called " intrinsic light of the retina ", and the microscopically discernible difference in structure between the retinal rods and cones.

Black-White Sensations.

In discussing visual theories few psychologists seem to have laid emphasis upon the existence of an ever-present retinal self stimulation, with its correspondingly ever-present gray sensation. Yet we have that curious, constant visual sensation known as "the intrinsic light of the retina" to serve as an ever-present background against which are perceived brightness, darkness, and colour. The "intrinsic light," or seemingly constant grey sensation, seldom comes to the attention of the average individual, since his eyes are open during most waking moments, and the usual light stimulation from outside over-whelmingly obscures the "intrinsic light". It can readily be observed, however, at any time, by shutting the eyes and protecting the lids from light stimulation. Its origin is obscure. L. T. Troland[1] supposes that the stimulation arises from "a spontaneous decomposition of the photochemical substances or, at least, an automatic activity of the retinal apparatus". Mrs. Ladd-Franklin[2] regards the intrinsic light as due to pressure (intra-ocular ?) exerted upon the retina. There is, furthermore, some evidence that the retinal cones are responsible for the constant visual sensation rather than the rods. Whatever its origin, this intrinsic light furnishes a constant flow of sensory visual impulses, with which transient visual excitations must be integrated in the formation of the more readily introspectable sensations of brightness and colour.

Rod vision has been associated particularly with brightness and darkness sensations, since the rods seem to be our retinal mechanism for twilight vision when no colours can be seen. Besides the obvious structural difference in shape between the rods and cones, there also exists some observable difference between the type of bipolar cells with which rods and cones form synaptic connection, and necessarily, therefore, some difference in the type of initial synaptic connections of rods and cones with the conducting fibres of the optic tract.[3] Here, at least, is a known rather than an hypothetical dis-

[1] L. T. Troland, Quotation from letter, 1927.
[2] Christine Ladd-Franklin, Quoted opinion from letter, 1927.
[3] Herrick, C. J., *Introduction to Neurology*, p. 228 ff.

tinction between rods and cones, which readily lends itself to correlation with the distinction in function relative to colour v. colourless vision.

Just as certain reflexes of low order may, on the motor side, facilitate or conflict with the constant tonic motor discharge without affecting the magnitude of this discharge itself, it may be supposed that afferent visual impulses of low intensity, received through the rod mechanisms of the retina, may either facilitate or impede the constant stream of intrinsic light impulses, without in the least altering the initial magnitude of the constant, intrinsic light excitation. We would suggest that the mutual facilitations of these two groups may be perceived as brightness, while mutual interferences may register in consciousness as darkness.

Such a suggestion seems to be in accord with a large number of known facts concerning the series of so-called black-white sensations. We know, for instance, that the sensation black is not only a positive experience, but that it can only occur when the eye is exposed to a surface or area less illuminated than that brightness to which the retina is at that moment adapted. Dark adaptation may, apparently, take place down to the level of the grey value of the intrinsic light sensation. Light stimulation below this threshold might well be supposed to set up afferent impulses of a frequency so low as to conflict with those producing the intrinsic light sensation ; while stimuli of an intensity greater than intrinsic light stimuli, but less than stimuli producing the grey to which the eye might at any moment be adapted would tend, similarly, to set up afferent impulses calculated to reduce the total existing excitation by way of conflict and inhibition. Such an integrative relationship of sensory antagonism, rising at the central psychons to psychonic energy, or consciousness, might constitute darkness sensation.

It may also be significant in this connection, that light so intense as to blind the eye, temporarily, also produces a marked sensation of blackness. It would seem that such overintense light, like the subliminal stimulus just considered, would tend to set up afferent impulses having an inhibitory or conflicting effect upon the intrinsic light impulse stream.

A parallel of integrative principles involved immediately suggests itself, not only with other modes of sensation, but also with the psychonic explanation of pleasantness and unpleasantness. In clinical and class work, during the last several years we have obtained reports from students and clients with respect to their colour preferences and with respect to the relative pleasantness of darkness and brightness. In general—though our results are as yet far too few for statistical presentation—we have found that there is some tendency, particularly with girls and women, to find brightness pleasant for its own sake, entirely aside from pleasant experiences which may have become associated with light. We have, as yet, found no corresponding tendency to find darkness or even total blackness sensation unpleasant. There appears, however, with both women and men, a seemingly *marked tendency to experience unpleasantness while illumination of any visual field is being reduced, and to find the brightening of a visual field pleasant.*

No exact parallel between actual brightness and darkness and actual pleasantness or unpleasantness of any given stimulus is to be expected because of the complexity and previous conditioning of the central nervous system. The only exact parallel suggested by our present discussion is the parallel between the integrative principles used to form the simplest motations of pleasantness and unpleasantness, and the integrative principles responsible for the simplest visual sensations of brightness and darkness.

Let us state the integrative theory above suggested from a different angle of approach. Let us start with the integrative psychons upon which the sensory consciousness of brightness and darkness is manufactured and see what happens there when the rods are stimulated and grey sensations result. First we observe these psychons, as it were, while the eyes are closed and covered so that no visual stimulation from the environment can occur. The psychons are in a state of very mild excitation which gives rise to the constant "intrinsic light" sensation consciousness. Let us assume that this constant mild excitation of the psychon is caused by a constant flow of afferent nerve impulses from the cones of the retina.

Let us now uncover our subject's eyes and expose them to dim light stimulation. Immediately the retinal rods, which are sensitive to twilight vision, become active. They communicate their activity over their own afferent paths to the integrating psychons. The previously existing, constant excitation of these psychons is thereupon facilitated and increased. The integrative membranes, in short, join together the intrinsic excitations from the cones, and the phasic or new excitations from the rods. This fusion, as it occurs, constitutes the sensation-consciousness of brightness.

Now let us diminish the light stimulation to which our subject's eyes are exposed. An opposite photochemical reaction takes place within the rods. Nerve impulses of a different or opposite rhythm are initiated in the afferent nerves. The new and conflicting nerve impulse rhythm reaches the integrative psychons in turn where it comes into opposition to the previously existing excitations. The intrinsic light excitations, let us remember, are not changed but remain constant on these psychons. These intrinsic psychonic impulses, facilitated as they were just prior to the arrival of the new antagonistic excitations, are now brought into psychonic conflict with the new impulses representing dimunition of light stimulus. The psychonic conflict thus produced actually constitutes the sensation consciousness of darkness according to our view. The extreme of this conflict is what we call the positive sensation of black. Thus black sensation represents a maximum psychonic conflict resulting from minimum light stimulation of the rods and constant intrinsic stimulation of the cones.

Black-white sensations, therefore, according to the integrative theory, are the product of simple alliance and antagonism relationships, on the integrative psychons, between constant or intrinsic visual sensation, and phasic or transitory sensations arising from extrinsic stimulation of the rods of the retina.

Colour Sensations.

During our previous discussions of integrative relationships within unit responses we observed that another set of integrative relationships besides simple alliance and antagonism could be shown to exist. This second set of relationships, as previously noted, consists of increases and decreases of the existing self-excitation in response to the influence of the environmental stimulus. We observed that alliance of psychonic impulses might be combined with either increase or decrease of the self impulses ; while antagonisms of psychonic impulses might similarly be coupled with increase or decrease of self activity. Thus a series of compound integrative relationships arises with four nodal points consisting of alliance and increase of self, alliance and decrease of self, antagonism and decrease of self, antagonism and increase of self.

The integrative theory of vision finds in the series of colour sensations with its four psychological nodal points, red, yellow, green and blue, an interesting parallel with the compound integrative relationships described above and previously named inducement (red), submission (yellow), compliance (green), and dominance (blue). We suggest that colour sensations arise whenever a sufficient amount of increase or decrease of the constant visual sensation or of the existing visual sensation is coupled with facilitation or conflict between this sensation and sensations arising from retinal rod stimulation as outlined in the preceding section. In short, whenever increase or decrease of constant visual sensation co-exists to a sufficient extent with facilitation or impeding of visual sensation, colour consciousness results from the compound integrative relationships thus set up.

We may suggest the fundamental relationships in these integrative principles as follows :

> BLUE : Stronger phasic impulses conflict with self-impulses ;
> GREEN : Weaker phasic impulses conflict with self-impulses ;
> YELLOW : Weaker phasic impulses facilitate self-impulses ;
> RED : Stronger phasic impulses facilitate self-impulses.

This situation may be diagrammed in a colour circle that will correspond to the unit response circle as in figure 40.

Formation of a visual colour hypothesis based upon the above suggestion is not difficult, nor is the resulting theory complicated by a necessity for the elaboration of imaginary substances or new types of mechanisms. The known facts of the matter seem to be that there exists a constant stream of afferent visual impulses, producing the intrinsic light of the retina ; that different wave lengths of stimulating light produce quantitatively different batteries of transient visual impulses, corresponding to different colour experiences ; and that the intrinsic light impulses must be integrated according to some definite set of integrative principles, with the transient colour impulses. The only theoretical part of the proposed schemata, therefore, consists of the conceptual formulation of four basic principles of unit response integration, and the subsequent application of these same principles to the sensory visual integrations which we know must occur prior to the appearance of visual sensations in consciousness.

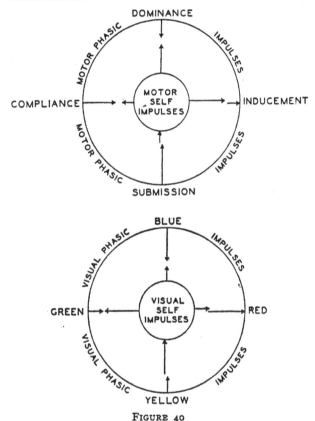

FIGURE 40

Comparative Diagrams of Emotion Circle and Colour Circle

Attention is called to the fact that the relationships between phasic impulses and self-impulses in the two circles above are precisely reversed. In the emotion circle the self-impulses are represented as stronger than the phasic impulses in dominance and inducement, and weaker than the phasic impulses in compliance and submission. In the colour circle, however, the visual self-impulses which are concerned in the blue and red integrations, supposedly corresponding to dominance and inducement, are represented as weaker than the phasic impulses; while the opposite relationship obtains in green and yellow integrations, which correspond with compliance and submission. For fuller explanation of this reversal of relationship see *Psychonic Theory of Vision* as discussed in the present chapter; and also the last section of Chapter VII above.

Blue-Dominance.

If we apply the dominant principle of integration to the sensory manufacture of blue consciousness, we have first to observe that the wave-lengths of blue light are shorter than those of any other primary colour stimulus. Thus we may assume that a more intense stimulation of retinal cones results, with each cone energising close to the maximum number of individual nerve fibres with which it is directly connected. The dominant factor in a final sensory integration evidently would be the transient stimulus, rather than the constant, intrinsic light ; thus reversing the roles played, on the motor side, by constant tonic discharge and transient antagonistic stimulus. This is a purely logical rather than factual assumption, and is based only upon the supposition that, in emotions, it is the self (or constant motor discharge) that is acting upon the environmental stimulus, while on the sensory side it is the environment that is acting upon the self (constant afferent excitations). If this be the fact, it is easy to see how the most intense visual stimulus within the nodal intensity series, or octave, would be best qualified to overwhelm, or dominate, the entire existing flow of intrinsic light impulses. Blue light seems to be the shortest wave length of the spectral series so far as its relationship to the retina goes, since still shorter wave lengths begin the colour circle all over again by mingling red, the longest wavelength colour, with blue sensation to produce violet.

Moreover, just as there exists a circular mechanism composed of proprioceptive muscular reflexes by which the constant tonic motor discharge can be increased or decreased in effecting integrative relationships with phasic motor impulses, so we find in the retina itself a mechanism by which the constant stream of intrinsic light impulses might be altered at the very inception of a transient light stimulus. All end organs of the retina transmit their impulses across an initial set of synapses in the external molecular layer of the retina, to neurons of the second order whose cell bodies lie in the internal layer. Some of these second order neurones spread the impulse laterally, while others conduct directly to a third set of synapses with the so-called " ganglion cells " of the retina. It is apparent that the laterally conducting cells of the second order may, when excited, affect all the afferent fibres leading into the optic tract ; and some of the fibres thus affected must be carrying continuously the intrinsic light impulses. Thus it would seem that there is a possibility of summation or inhibition of the intrinsic light stream, at the very beginning of the conduction of each transient colour impulse toward the brain. That is to say, each light stimulus may increase or decrease the total intrinsic light excitation at the same time that the transient impulses proceed as a separate unit toward the central synapses where, eventually, they must form their typical, or definitive relationship with the intrinsic light stream.

If then, a blue light stimulus, with its short wave lengths, causes an initial reduction by way of inhibition in the intrinsic light volume, and later forms a dominant junction with the unit mass of intrinsic light impulses, compelling the latter to follow the " blue " path toward further integrations at higher brain levels, we might logically characterise the sensory event thus described as visual domination of the organism by an intense blue light stimulus. For the sensation blue, thus analysed, would consist of diminution of the visual self (constant grey sensation), by an intense or dominant light stimulus, with the dominant stimulus overcoming and directing the self at their integrative juncture.

When the final juncture occurred between blue stimulus impulses and intrinsic light impulses, some facilitation would, of course, inevitably result. This would contribute to the blue sensation whatever brightness it possessed. Yet it is to be observed that the dominant form of integration seems to involve some mutual interference and possible diminution of the absolute value of one or both component impulse groups, prior to their final unification. Thus, it would not be expected, if the suggested analysis of blue sensation is correct, that blue would possess a maximum brightness. Such logical expectation is, in fact, in accord with experimental findings. Blue is not, under any conditions, the point of maximum brightness in the spectrum.

Yellow-Submission.

Yellow, on the other hand, contains the spectral area of greatest brightness to the light-adapted eye. Following our above suggested schemata, we might suppose that the sensation yellow is formed by an integration in which the yellow visual impulses submit to the visual self, or constant, intrinsic light stream. Yellow light, of course, is composed of much longer wave-lengths than is blue light. Yellow light, in fact, is to be found within the long-wave half of the spectrum, and it seems, therefore, to follow that the ensuing excitation of retinal cones is less intense. If we may assume, then, that these feebler impulsions are of requisite volume initially to increase rather than to diminish the intrinsic light stream, by way of the circular nerve fibres of the retina or some other appropriate synaptic mechanism, the suggestion follows that the yellow impulses may be of proper relative volume to yield to and may be directed by the constant visual impulses at their definitive juncture. In such a relationship no mutual interference or conflict of impulses could occur at any stage, and a maximum of mutual facilitation should result. According to the brightness theory suggested above, this maximally complete alliance relationship at the integrating psychons should produce the maximum brightness of the spectrum; which, in fact, it does.

When the intensity of illumination of the spectrum is increased, without change in the wave-lengths of any component light, the hues of the long-wave half of the spectrum change to yellow, and then to gray; while the colour sensations produced by the short-wave half of the spectrum assume a bluish tint, and finally shift into black-white sensations. (Green as an exception to this rule will be noted at a later point in the present discussion). All colours, when thus transformed into yellow and blue, possess great brightness but very low chroma. On the other hand, if the intensity of light be similarly diminished, spectral colours change to red, green, and violet, all very dark and of varying, though low saturation. These facts seem closely in accord with our fundamental premise, namely that *intensity of stimulation of the cones is the differential stimulus factor upon which integrative manufacture of colour sensations is based*, rather than specific effects of different wave-lengths of light upon different photo-chemical substances.

Also, these phenomena seem to offer evidence that the " blue-yellow " zone of the retina may be colour-blind to red and green light merely because a sparse allocation of cones, such as that existing in the blue-yellow zone, is not capable of generating sufficient volume of nerve impulses to integrate definitely with the intrinsic light stream except when the few cones simultaneously stimulated are energized to the maximum of two nodal points, one capable of dominating the intrinsic light energy and the other submitting to it. For, as we have seen, if any retinal cone is stimulated with maximum intensity, whatever the wave-length of the light used, it gives blue sensation, and finally simply brightness; while any cone can be made to produce yellow sensation by supplementing the low intensity of long-wave stimuli up to the point where they naturally submit to, and completely blend with the intrinsic light.

The marked access of brightness and diminution of chroma, also, as the intensity of stimulation is increased, seems in close accord with the idea that brightness is the awareness of simple facilitation of the intrinsic light sensation. After this constant visual stream had been initially increased or diminished to its extreme limits, only facilitation could occur upon juncture with a specific light stimulus, and the integrative relationship which has been suggested as the basis of colour consciousness would be expected to disappear, just as colour sensation does, in fact, disappear, at sufficiently high and low intensities of stimulation.

Green-Compliance

The application of compliance, as an integrative principle, to an attempted postulation of the manufacturing formula for green sensation is made easy by the close connection of this formula with the submission formula for yellow. Spectral green light is composed of wave-lengths next in series to the wave-lengths of spectral yellow, the green waves being slightly shorter than the yellow. It will be remembered that we supposed yellow light to be of such a stimulation intensity that it increased, initially, the afferent intrinsic light stream, which then became of just sufficient volume to draw the yellow impulses into its own course at the junctional synapses. We may now suppose that the green stimuli, being of next greater intensity to the yellow, result in a volume of nerve impulses which increase the intrinsic light excitation initially, just as do the yellow impulses. But we must suppose further that the green impulses, being greater in volume than the yellow, turn out to be approximately equal at the junctional synapses, to the initially enlarged intrinsic light stream and so form a mutually independent juncture with the latter, rather than forming the submissive juncture entered into by the yellow impulses. The green excitations would then pursue their own course, which would nevertheless be harmonized, at common psychons, with the path of the intrinsic light stream, producing mutual facilitation within these conjunctive centres.

Such an integrative picture of green sensation might be expected to yield an amount of facilitation nearly as great as that produced by the submissive type of juncture hypothecated as a basis for yellow sensation. The intrinsic light stream would be increased, and it would be, to a large extent, synchronized with the green stimulus impulses, though not quite as completely as the yellow excitations which, in submissive relationship, must merge themselves completely in the intrinsic light stream. If then, brightness sensation is psychonic facilitation, spectral green should prove to be, as in fact it is, nearly as bright as spectral yellow.

According to the integrative formula suggested, the lower the initial value of the intrinsic light volume, the greater should be the increment of facilitation produced by green light as compared to the increment of facilitation caused by yellow light. For whereas the simple, initial addition to the intrinsic visual stream, which both yellow and green impulses have been supposed to produce, would not be interfered with by an unusually low intrinsic volume prior to stimulation, no matter how low this prior volume might be, the yellow impulses might find a submissive juncture with too low a total volume of intrinsic impulses partially impossible to effect. The green type of co-operative integration, on the other hand, might just as readily be made with low total volumes of intrinsic excitation, as with greater volumes of these same impulses. That is to say, only part of a battery of yellow impulses might be able to submit to a very small intrinsic light stream ; whereas all green impulses, no matter how voluminous should find no greater difficulty in co-operative juncture with a small intrinsic stream than with a large.

This theoretical result harmonizes very well, apparently, with the so-called Purkinje phenomenon, in which it has been found that the maximum brightness of the spectrum shifts from yellow to green when the eye is dark adapted and the intensity of spectral illumination is decreased. According to the above suggested schemata, the yellow, submissive type of juncture should begin to fail when the intrinsic light stream prior to stimulation is low, and the intensity of yellow stimulus is thereafter reduced below the point where its initial increase of the intrinsic stream compensates for this low preliminary volume sufficiently to permit total submission of yellow impulses to the intrinsic stream.

The fact that green does not change hue, as the intensity of illumination is increased, until it finally passes into completely colourless sensation, also seems easy to account for on the integrative principles suggested. A co-operative relationship of integration, once established, should not be altered by simultaneous increase of both factors integrated, except to increase the total amount of facilitation (brightness). If increase of intensity of green wave-length stimulus reached the blue intensity before all chroma was lost in brightness, then initial diminution of the intrinsic light stream might be expected to replace the initial increase supposed to result from normal green stimulation ; and in such case we might expect that green would turn to blue, before giving way to simple brightness. But it seems in accord with the known relationships between the number of discriminable hues and the wave-length intervals of this portion of the spectrum to conclude that this would not be likely to occur.

Red-Inducement

The light waves which act as adequate stimulus to the red sensation are the longest in the spectrum. We might assume, therefore, that the resulting intensity of stimulation had reached a low point in the spectral series, corresponding to the high point of intensity of blue stimulation, and productive, therefore, of the same initial inhibitory effect upon the intrinsic light stream that we have assumed to be exercised by blue stimuli. With intrinsic impulse volume thus reduced, the red impulses might force their way into the intrinsic light stream path. This type of juncture, with low volumes of impulses entering the eventual facilitating relationship, could not be expected to result in maximal brightness according to the integrative theory under discussion as, in fact, it does not.

Inducive integration, however, like dominant integration, might be expected to be very positive and definite in the establishment of its relationships, since the stimulus impulses constitute active agents, comparatively greater in volume than the intrinsic light stream, which they join under their own power, as it were. Perhaps this assumption might serve to account for the known fact that the spectral blue and spectral red are the most saturated hues of the spectrum.

Complementary Colours

Finally, it may be noted that complementary colours may very readily be described by means of the integrative theory proposed. If two diametrically opposite types of integration are attempted, simultaneously, with the same stream of intrinsic light impulses, by two opposite types of stimulus impulse volumes, it would certainly seem that the equal and opposite influences upon the intrinsic light impulses must cancel one another out, leaving the double volume of stimulus impulses to form a simple, uncharacteristic juncture with the intrinsic light stream. Such juncture would, of course, result in marked facilitation, but would permit no colour sensation to result. Exactly opposite types of integration, therefore, would produce brightness sensation, but no colour, which is the effect arrived at by all pairs of true complementary colours. The same effect might be anticipated, under this theory, whenever the intensity of a colour stimulus fell below that of the intrinsic light stimulation. As a matter of fact, it has been discovered in practical colour photography that the intrinsic light of the retina has a tendency to obscure colours at low intensities of illumination.

Now one of the difficulties that has beset the path of colour theorists who have postulated one photo-chemical substance for blue-yellow, and another photo-chemical substance for green-red, has been the fact that pure spectral green and red, though forming convenient and logical starting points in the colour rectangle, for various reasons, do not constitute truly complementary colours. In fact, their simultaneous presence on the retina produces yellow. This seeming whimsicality of primary colours led Hering finally to choose blue-red (really in the purple series) and blue-green as his photo-chemical primaries. These colours are complementary, surely enough, but are of little use in satisfying the various other requirements of colour vision theory. Mrs. Ladd-Franklin finally cut the Gordian knot, so far as photo-chemical theories go, by boldly manufacturing, in imagination, a sort of egg-cell-like differentiation of yellow substance into daughter substances of green and red, with the supposition that both the offspring had to join the male parent, blue substance, if the grandparent substance, black-white, were to be reassembled. On the other hand, according to this ingenious theory, green and red substances released simultaneously, would unite (chemically ?) again forming yellow substance. This yellow substance must then, we suppose, stimulate the retinal nerve endings in its distinctive way, setting up afferent impulses appropriate to the final sensation, yellow. We should then have the same basic problem to solve that we had in the first place ; i.e. what impulse relationships constitute the sensation yellow ? And we might answer that question in the manner suggested above, or in some similar manner.

If, however, we do not choose to avail ourselves of the ample and convenient supply of imaginary photo-chemicals just mentioned, for the purpose of mixing our colours in the retina, we have an equally logical, and perhaps a somewhat more realistic method available under the integrative principles above proposed. For it may be noted that while the principles of dominant and submissive integrations are exactly opposite, one to the other, the integrative principles of compliance and inducement are not, in their entirety, opposed. It is true that compliance is based upon a relative decrease in the compliant element while inducement calls for an increase in the inducive element, and, so far, the principles are opposites.

But, in compliance relationship, the stimulus accomplishes its harmonization with the sensory self merely by remaining in its own path, and this cannot be said to be opposed completely to the integrative procedure of entering the path of the intrinsic impulses. The opposite of entering the path of the intrinsic impulses would be to compel these impulses to enter the path of the stimulus, which is the second part of the domination principle.

We note, then, that the inducement principle finds an opposite for its first phase (increase of stimulus) in compliance integration (decrease of stimulus) and that it finds an opposite for its second phase (entering intrinsic impulse path) in domination integration (compelling intrinsic impulses to enter path of stimulus). A mixture of all three integrative principles, inducement, compliance and dominance would be required to cancel one another out and produce simple facilitation ; just as we know, in fact, that a mixture of all three colours corresponding to these three principles, red, green, and blue is required to abolish colour sensation and to leave only, brightness. Mixture of inducement and compliance alone (red and green) would result, most probably, in no relative change in stimulus volume, since the opposite first phases of these two integrative principles might be expected to cancel one another.

But the second part of inducement (entering the intrinsic path) might be expected to become the controlling factor, since it is the only positive one, in its conflict with the second part of compliance (merely remaining in *statu quo*). A yellow (submissive relationship) combination of impulses should result rather than a red relationship, since the stimulus had failed initially to be relatively increased, and the red stimuli, without such increase, being originally weaker than the yellow, might prove to hold the same proportionate relationship to the intrinsic stream that yellow impulses would hold after initial relative decrease. The entire phenomenon, in short, is one of relative proportion between stimulus impulse volume, and intrinsic light volume ; and the relative proportion productive of yellow sensation may just as readily result from combination of red and green integrative principles as from the adequate yellow light stimulus itself. Thus we might explain the behaviour of red and green in producing yellow, without recourse to any supplementary mechanisms whatever, over and above the integrative principles first postulated. Such a simplification and unification of visual theory seems, at least, worth attempting.

The above discussion of the mingling and inter-action between the four integrative principles proposed suggests that a graded series of integrative relationships probably exists, in which the " primaries " merely represent nodal points, where distinct and clear-cut shifts of integrative principle can be detected. Such a continuous series of integrative relationships would be exactly in accord with the continuous colour series of the spectrum, on the one hand, and with the continuous series of distinguishable emotional tones, on the motor side. " Primary emotions " and " primary colours," thus defined, should escape the stigma of artificiality with which physical scientists, statisticians, and others are apt to condemn any definite formulation of admittedly diverse phenomena into a small number of supposedly basic elements.

The scope of this chapter is not sufficient to discuss at requisite length the phenomena of positive and negative after-images or complementary colours, and simultaneous induction of identical or complementary colours. Suffice it to mention, in passing, that the data of neurology offer a rich assortment of diverse rules of behaviour of nerve impulses at the synapses, in terms of which it should be comparatively simple to account for these colour phenomena, once we concede that the manufacture of colour sensations is an integrative affair. After discharge, for instance, might account for positive after-images ; but we also have, very possibly, the phenomena of "immediate induction," and irradiation and central spread of reflexes to utilize. For contrast colour effects we might examine the applicability of "successive induction," "rhythmic alternation," "post inhibitory rebound," "electrical reversal," or some adaptation of "postural reversal" to sensory integrations.

With photo-chemical theories of vision we always have a difficult time trying to stretch a very few, imaginatively endowed, retinal substances to cover a multitude of colour phenomena. With an integrative theory of vision, our chief difficulty lies in selecting intelligently the pertinent principles of nerve-impulse behaviour from a great mass of painstakingly prepared material furnished us by the physiologists. After such a tentative selection, moreover, our experimental task, as psychologists, in testing the accuracy of our selection, must be kept in very close alliance with the sound and dependable laboratory results of the neurologists, if we hope to demonstrate the reliability of our psycho-neural theories as physical facts.

The integrative theory of vision suggested in this chapter does not in the least pretend to have effected a complete alliance with neurological data or terminology ; it is presented only as a first approach toward such a desirable union. The specific nerve impulse mechanisms of the four conceptual principles herein formulated have yet to be selected and tested out both by psychological and physiological procedures.

The Psychonic Theory of Sensations Other than the Visual

In considering the senses other than the visual, which we believe are properly to be described only upon the same principles of psychonic integration already employed, it is necessary to allude once more to the fact that in every case the receptors concerned in the first step of the process of sensory stimulation, are *constantly* subject to stimulation. Sometimes, as in the case of equilibrium sensation and the receptors in the walls of the semi-circular canals, this constant stimulation is of the same self-type as are the impulses resulting from the "intrinsic light" of the retina. In cases like that of the cutaneous touch sensation receptors the constant stimulation is probably to be referred to causes exterior to the organism in question, atmospheric pressure, pressure from garments, air currents, etc.; but in these cases, too, such constant stimulation will bear the same relation to the varying phasic stimuli as is otherwise borne, in some of the senses, by the stimulation of the self-originated impulses. We may add that at present evidence appears to be accumulating in favour of the view that all sensory receptors without exception are subject in some degree to self-stimulation by the organism.

Consequently there must take place the same general type of integration between the phasic stimuli and the constant stimuli that we have already described in the case of visual sensation. Facilitation and conflict will undoubtedly be important elements in the resulting psychonic processes. On the other hand the possible complication and variation of the integrative processes will be governed to a large extent by the structure of the respective receptors that receive the stimuli proper to the various senses. The eye is the most complicated receptor organ in the human body; from this degree of complexity we descend through a series of gradations, through the auditory, olfactory, gustatory apparatus, etc., to the simple end-organ structures in the skin and muscles. It is worthy of note that the so-called distance receptors of sight, smell, and hearing, for example, are the most highly developed in the organism, while those receptors concerned with the transmission of stimuli connected with the conditions and changes within the body itself, are the simplest. This fact may turn out to be of the utmost significance for psychology, but we shall have no opportunity of discussing it in the present book. We wish to point out, however, that the relative powers of discrimination within the various senses depend upon these varying complexities of their respective end-organs for the reason that the more complicated the receptor apparatus is, the more varied will be the types of integration taking place at the psychons between the impulses transmitted from these end-organs.

FIGURE 41

Suggested Sensation Integration Relationships Illustrating Psychonic Theory

SENSATIONS	END-ORGANS	PSYCHONIC INTEGRATION RELATIONSHIPS
Visual :		
brightness-darkness	rods	facilitation and conflict with self impulses
colours	cones	facilitation-conflict plus increase-decrease of self impulses
form	rods and cones	PERCEPT type correlation responses (see next chapter on thought processes)
Auditory :		
tone-noise	auditory cells of Corti	facilitation and conflict with self impulses
pitch	auditory cells of Corti	facilitation-conflict plus increase-decrease of self impulses
Olfactory :		
spicy	olfactory vesicles	facilitation and conflict
flowery	in upper nasal	plus increase-decrease of
fruity	passages	self impulses
resinous		
foul		
scorched		
Gustatory :		
salt	taste buds	facilitation-conflict plus
bitter		increase-decrease of sel
sweet		impulses
acid		
Kinaesthetic :		
back and forth movements of joints	Pacinian corpuscles	facilitation and conflict with self impulses
stretching and relaxation of tendons	Organs of Golgi and Pacinian corpuscles	facilitation and conflict with self impulses
contraction of muscles	Nerve endings in muscle spindles	facilitation of self impulses
Cutaneous :		
pressure	Meissner's and Merkel's corpuscles	facilitation of self impulses
warmth	Ruffini's corpuscles	facilitation with self impulses
coolness	Krause's end bulbs	conflict with self impulses
pain	free nerve endings	conflict with self impulses
Non-cutaneous :		
pain	free nerve endings in smooth muscles of viscera	conflict with self impulses
hunger	receptors in stomach walls	conflict with self impulses
thirst	receptors in mouth and throat	conflict with self impulses
Equilibrium :		
balance-unbalance	receptors in semi-circular canals	increase and decrease of self impulses

The Function of Sensation in the Unit Response

We must now add a word about the function of sensation in the unit response. Our unit responses actually commence with sensation ; in some cases the sensation initiates a process that passes through the stages of thought and feeling to action, and sometimes, as in the cases of the lower reflexes, sensation seems to pass directly into a motor response. There are also the more complicated situations in which sensation is transformed into thought and in this guise continues to be stored up for various periods before finally issuing as implicit (glandular, etc.), or overt (muscular) behaviour.

All this the psychonic theory takes into account in its inclusion of different combinations of part-reactions in different unit responses. The impulses which, as they cross the sensory psychons, give rise to sensation do not thereafter vanish ; these impulses constitute energy units that must, of course, produce subsequent effects somewhere in the organism. The type situation is found when they pass through the correlation centres and thence become stimuli for the motor centres, there arousing further impulse patterns which finally result in glandular activity or muscular contractions. In certain cases this entire arc is not brought into play ; a switch-over connection may be made, for example in the spinal cord, whereby the afferent impulses pass directly into the motor system, before ascending to the higher correlation centres in the cerebrum ; such a situation exists in the case of the knee-jerk and other low-order reflexes. On the other hand, the sensory impulses, after entering the correlation centres, may circle about there for long periods until eventually they reach those parts of this system where the correlation end-process takes place and results in stimuli for the motor system. It would seem that in this fashion in the correlation centres these impulses may be, as it were, stored up in the form of potential energy for later release. It will thus be seen that the psychonic theory offers a factual explanation for the various roles that sensation has been held to perform in subjective psychology.

From the view-point of the present writers the controversies that have raged around the sensationalist and empiricist positions seem to be largely battles of words, rather than of real meanings. We have attempted to emphasize throughout this book that the only real occurrence in psychology is the unit response. This response, in most cases at least, *is initiated* through the sensory centres that give rise to sensation at the sensory psychons ; since science has been historically interested in tracing out cause and effect relationships, the initiatory place of sensation in the total response has been especially open to emphasis. Nevertheless, it is equally possible to centre one's attention upon the mental or the emotional sub-divisions of the whole process, and certain schools, although fewer of them, have adopted such positions.

To us, however, it seems that the tripartite division of the unit response into sensation, thought, and emotion, while a convenient assumption and one based indeed upon the factual constitution of the human organism, is an artificial one from the ultimate point of view. We do not agree with the implications of Gestalt psychology that such division is meaningless ; on the contrary we believe that this three-fold division can, and should, be made, and that the distinctive processes taking place within these divisions, and even subsidiary processes within each division, can, and should, be separately investigated. But our final position is that, during the progress of such investigations, it must never be lost sight of that each separate process is in fact a part of the whole unit response, that no one of the three major divisions should be given a predominant place or emphasized at the expense of the others ; and finally, that each part-process possesses its actual significance and importance only in proportion to the relation it bears to the fundamental unit response in question.

CHAPTER XV

THOUGHT-PROCESSES

Introductory

THE general opinion of mankind has usually considered thought-processes to be of a very mysterious nature. Here were activities which took place without any overt movement, apparently without physical accompaniment of any kind; they were unheard, unseen, imperceptible. Yet by means of these mental activities men were enabled to perceive the significance of situations, to devise ways and means of meeting them to their own advantage, and in general to wield a tremendous power over even the animate part of nature. Evidently thought was not only invisible but also powerful. The inevitable conclusion was that thought was immaterial; and the next association was to the effect that it was " spiritual," not of the same order as those crass objects that can be touched and felt and grossly moved. Even nowadays, when souls have vanished from psychology and consciousness has taken their place, there is scarcely a psychologist to be discovered who does not confound consciousness with thought and the mysteries of consciousness with the unplumbed depths of mental functioning.

For our part we consider the general situation as perfectly definite. There are three kinds of consciousness, sensory, mental and emotional, and it is a fallacy to imagine that one kind of consciousness is more like consciousness, or more characteristically conscious, than another kind. From an objective point of view consciousness is a particular kind of energy; although this energy may possess differentiation within its entire range, nevertheless it is all of the same fundamental energy type. Between sensory, correlation and motor psychonic energies there is far less distinction than there is similarity.

With sensation, i.e. with the energy arising at the sensory psychons, we have already dealt, and we shall consider in the next chapter the psychonic energy at the motor psychons, which is emotion. In this chapter we shall be concerned with that psychonic energy which occurs at the psychons of the correlation centres, and it is our position that objectively this particular kind of psychonic energy is thought. Thus it will be seen that we do not consider thought to be some sort of immaterial mystery, much less a "spiritual" one; on the contrary, it is a specific form of physical energy, and, as such, its nature and its functioning are to be investigated and described.

Contemporary Theories of the Nature of Thought

We must acknowledge at once that our position is probably both novel and unorthodox. For the reader interested in psychology it is therefore necessary to be acquainted with the most prominent contemporary theories on this subject and for our own purposes it is necessary that we give these theories in brief outline and show wherein we believe their respective weaknesses to lie. Within the compass allowable we shall accordingly explain what we understand to be the introspectionist, the behaviourist, the Gestalt and the "Middle Grounder" positions and shall briefly add what can be a criticism of each only in the most general terms.

The Introspectionist Position

Introspectionism has been dealt many a hard blow since the days of the controversy over "imageless thought," but it is by no means dead. On the contrary it is steadily drawing to its standard many who revolt against the extremities to which behaviourism has carried the objectivist position. Although ourselves of the objectivist persuasion, we can well understand the estrangement that many psychologists feel when confronted by a view which would make psychology little more than a physiological investigation. Such converts to introspectionism have naturally modified the introspectionist position until it might better perhaps be indicated by the term, subjectivism; but since introspection remains one of the chief tools of investigation of this school, no doubt the earlier name serves as well as any.

Dr. Bernard Hart, in his *Psychology of Insanity*,[1] has

[1] 3rd Edition, 1916, p. 9, Cambridge University Press.

summed up the subjectivist view-point very concisely as follows : " The psychological conception is based on the view that mental processes can be directly studied without any reference to the accompanying changes which are presumed to take place in the brain. . . ." The crux of this statement lies in the words, " mental processes can be directly studied." Such a direct study of Thought, as it were *in vacuo*, can be carried forward by two means only ; either one can think about Thought, or one can introspect upon it. Thinking about Thought results in a description of Thought in terms of itself, a logical fallacy so obvious that it occurs in no other science than psychology. It is exactly as if a botanist should attempt to enlighten us regarding the apple, exclusively in terms derived from the apple. Thus he would tell us that the apple has an apple-stem and that its apple-skin is ordinarily of the usual apple-colour ; and when we reminded him that these points were precisely those upon which we expected his elucidation, he would shrug his shoulders and reply that the botanical conception was based on the view that apples could be directly studied without any reference to the chemical, biological, or geological phenomena involved.

Similarly, to attempt a description of Thought in terms of Memory, Percepts, Concepts, and so on, which themselves are all thought-terms, is simply to systematize a series of subjective words whose actual significance thereafter remains as vague and as subject to private interpretation as it did before. We have no objection to the psychological employment of terms like Concept, but in our opinion the first task of a psychological *science* is to define all such terms so accurately and moreover objectively that no one can mistake their meaning when subsequently used. We do not believe either that everybody is in agreement about the subjective meanings of subjective words or that such a lack can be supplied by the simple process of offering definitions based upon further subjective words, e.g. the definition of Concept in terms of Percepts. This kind of subjectivist procedure does not appear to be a scientific one at all ; it consists only in an ever-widening series of logical errors.

Having defined his terms in the way just described, the subjectivist then proceeds to investigate these " mental processes " by the technique of introspection. We have already pointed out that introspection can prove both sides of the same question ; as a matter of public record this achievement is already to its credit. The plain fact seems to be that with the utmost sincerity, skill and integrity on the part of the introspector, this technique is unalterably influenced by the subjective prejudice of him who uses it. We suggest that a physicist would soon abandon a spectroscope that displayed the remarkable property of producing evidence in support of whatever physicist happened to be using it.

In our opinion a science that is not objective is not a science. One may have as much subjective experience as one wishes, but when it becomes a question of using this experience for scientific discussion and for the establishment of common psychological fact, it must be reduced to purely objective terms. Subjective prejudice and private interpretation are so nearly the same as subjectivity itself, that under present conditions and with such techniques as are presently available, the destruction of one is the destruction of the other. Such destruction is at the very foundation of all scientific procedure, for science aspires, within its strictly defined range, to establish truths that remain commonly valid despite personal opinion to the contrary.

The present volume is not the place to enter into a prolonged discussion of the various further objections that may properly be urged against the subjectivist attitude in psychology. And indeed we believe that the two objections just outlined are quite sufficient, when thoroughly understood, to show that this position must be definitely abandoned.

The Behaviourist Position

So definitely have the behaviourists abandoned the subjectivist position that they have abandoned both thought and consciousness along with it. The subject of consciousness appears to be utterly beyond the speculative abilities of this school and the behaviourists present the appearance of finally denying in exasperation the existence of a factor so incompatible with their view-point.

The position of the behaviourist regarding Thought seems to have been dictated by his exaggerated interest in the muscular reactions of the body, the same interest which is probably responsible for his apparent acceptance of the discredited Lange theory of emotion. Thus he proposes, first, that there is no such phenomenon as conscious thought, second, that such thought as does exist is a matter of words, and third, that words are really muscular contractions of the throat and vocal chords, together with any further immediately associated musculature. Thought, in short, is a series of vocal or sub-vocal speech habits and the facts of imagery which, like those of consciousness, will not fit into the scheme at all, are accordingly denied any existence.

We must confess that to us this position seems hastily constructed for the purpose of getting on with the more interesting task, at least for the behaviourist, of investigating overt behaviour. We can see no reason whatsoever for identifying Thought with muscular contractions rather than with the motor nerve activation that causes the contraction or with any other part of the purely verbal process. Furthermore it seems to us that there exist many complexities in the phenomena of thought-processes that have very little to do with words or with speech habits and that these complexities have obviously played an important part in the construction of behaviouristic theory. Even in that realm of Thought where verbal labels do indeed exist, it does not seem possible that a muscular explanation can ever be satisfactorily made ; for example, the names of many symbols used in the infinitesimal calculus and in the mathematics of quantum physics are so long that their muscular pronunciation, even if purely " implicit," would consume a period a thousand times as long as it takes to think them. We cannot appreciate that the behaviourists have offered an adequate explanation of Thought even in its verbal aspects, much less as regards those much more intricate details which constitute the real psychological problem involved.

In order properly to present their position, however, we must add that behaviourism admits the possibility of certain substitutes for the speech habits of the throat and associated muscles. Thus, due to conditioning, various manual and visceral habits may become connected with verbal habits and on occasion serve as substitutes for them or as links in a given thought-process. (The emphasis, as before, is on muscular contractions and is open to the preceding objections.) A whole thought-process, as in the solution of a problem set to a subject, may thus be of a segmental character, first verbal, then visceral, then verbal again, next manual, and at last, in the final formulation of the answer, once more verbal. In this fashion the behaviourist reaches his conclusion that Thought is perhaps after all not simply a series of speech habits, but that when a man thinks he does so "with his whole body"; i.e. that all the principal segments of his musculature may be involved and he thus thinks "as a whole."

This conclusion is so typical of the Gestalt school that, although we believe the behaviourist announced it before the Gestaltist did so, we shall defer our criticism of it until the succeeding section.

The View-point of Gestalt Psychology

So far as we know this school has not definitely formulated its position in regard to the general subject of thought; however, it has been made clear that it views all problems from a certain defined direction, and since by far its most important investigations have been made in the field of perception, we believe its view-point as to Thought may be explained without much possibility of injustice.

"Gestalt" is a German word for which no exact English equivalent exists; its most appropriate translation appears to be the term, "configuration." As is suggested by its name this school places much importance upon the general form or configuration of any subject with which it is dealing. Thus, in perception, the configuration of the whole object is what gives significance to its various parts and when an experimental subject is confronted with a particular situation, it is the configuration of the whole situation to which he is alleged to react.

The great and overwhelming emphasis in Gestalt psychology is thus upon "the whole." In this view a percept is not built up of sensory parts; on the contrary, each sensory part is dominated and even intimately conditioned by the whole percept of which it is a portion, its existence as a part is dependent upon the existence of the whole and in the absence of the whole there is no part. All this is equivalent to asserting that there can be no auditory sensation, i.e. no experience of sound, unless such sound is part of a perception; and in this case the properties of the sound itself are most fundamentally determined, not by the air vibrations or even by the sensory mechanisms, but by the whole percept which contains it. In supporting such a view the Gestaltist, we believe, would be forced to contend that no sound has ever been humanly experienced that was not, at the same time, part of a perception. There is, of course, not the remotest objective evidence for this or similar contentions. That a percept loses its distinctive character *as a percept* when it is analyzed into parts, no one will deny in the face of the many Gestalt arguments and experiments showing this to be true. It is even true that a part, considered separately, is a different thing from the same part when it is related to a larger whole. But in this instance the statement of the case itself asserts the difference ; it amounts to no more than saying that different conditions are different conditions. The difference already exists by definition ; it is not due to some magic existing in wholeness or configuration.

In the same way the Gestaltist maintains that the individual views external situations as unanalyzed wholes. The famous Gestalt experiments in which mammals and fishes have been conditioned to differences between two objects (thus to a relation inherent in the total situation rather than to the objects themselves) has been held to discredit the behaviouristic-type experiments in which it has been supposed that the animals were conditioned to particular objects. To us it appears that this sort of reasoning involves a serious non-sequitur. To establish that an animal can be conditioned to a relation, most assuredly does not prove that it cannot also be conditioned to an object *per se*. For ourselves we definitely do not believe that it will be possible to prove such a negative, in view of the hundreds of experiments which have very clearly established the validity of the behaviouristic theory in certain cases. The Gestalt hypothesis declares that in the case of a coloured object the significant element is the perception of the relation between object and background, but the experiment in which chicks were conditioned to red kernels against many differently coloured backgrounds goes far to disprove the universal application of the hypothesis. The only thing actually proven by the widely cited Gestalt experiments is that the animals in question can *also* be conditioned to a relationship ; what is not in any way proven is that they cannot be conditioned to a simple object, or to an isolated sensation such as the colour red.

That the Gestalt school has succeeded in showing the importance, in certain circumstances, of wholes, we are entirely prepared to admit ; what we object to is the insistence upon the exclusive importance of this view. Their position would seem to be that no separate investigation of the eye is allowable since the eye is a part of the face and can only be properly investigated in relation thereto. On the contrary we believe that the eye can be separately investigated without any assumption as to what it is a part of and that the knowledge acquired by such an investigation may be equally as important as knowledge of the eye in relation to the face as a whole; under certain conditions it may be vastly more important. This does not mean that the eye is not a part of the face; but it does mean that for particular, but nevertheless important, purposes that fact is practically without significance.

The Gestalt view, however, carries the significance of wholes everywhere. And we believe we do not misrepresent it when we assert its position to be that thinking is an activity of the whole organism. Even modern text-books not of the Gestalt school, e.g. that of Perrin and Klein, maintain that thought-processes cannot be limited to the cerebrum with the receptors and effectors excluded. And we have seen that the behaviourists also, from their own point of view, believe that the whole body is, or may be, involved in thought-processes.

We must seriously object to any such contention. From our view-point a man does not think with his whole body any more than he eats or breathes with his whole body. In western countries at least the effectors in the legs and feet take no part in the feeding processes, nor does the sexual apparatus, nor do the ears, nor do a hundred other parts of the organism, although, of course, from a strict point of view they are all affected in non-significant ways. This is not by any means the first time that psychologists have been interested in the significance of wholes and relations, but at such recurrent periods it seems inevitable that attempts should be made to stretch this significance beyond all limits and make it cover everything.

Perception is an integrative process. The opposite of integration is analysis. Accordingly, when an integration is analyzed, it is no longer an integration. This obvious consideration seems to be the burden of the Gestalt contention. But from this it does not at all follow that any objection can be raised against the description of an integration by means of describing its parts *and* the way in which they are combined.

In fact such a means is the only one whereby an integration can be described.

As to Thought in general we cannot avoid feeling that the Gestalt conclusion is hastily drawn from the newly perceived importance of wholes. We believe that the importance of this factor finds its correct application not to the phenomena of Thought as such, but to the phenomenon of the unit response. The fact is that no man ever thinks, in the sense of being solely occupied in thinking. He is always engaged in a unit response which also includes at least both sensing and feeling, but this does not mean that the *Thought* portion of the unit response involves more than the correlation centres. The present confusion consists very simply in the confusion of a part-reaction with the whole unit response. Thought-processes, just as sensory or emotional processes, are part-reactions *within* a given unit response. To us it seems that it is only as part-reactions that they can correctly be dealt with. It is both proper and necessary to consider thought-processes, in the first place, separately from the different, although simultaneously occurring, part-reactions of the organism ; in the last section of this chapter we shall consider the place they occupy in relation to the unit responses of which they are parts.

In concluding this section we cannot refrain from pointing out that, with all its emphasis upon relations, we can as yet find no detailed mention in the Gestalt literature of the particular relationship which is the most important of all for psychology. This is the relationship existing between the individual and the external world, which, for psychology, is represented by the relation between the stimulation coming into the organism from without and the constant self-stimulation of the organism itself. Upon the resulting integrations between these two fundamental factors is based the entire psychology of human beings and animals as we know them. That phasic impulses do come into the organism cannot be doubted ; nor can it be doubted that they come into an already operating organism, into one that is already the site of much similar impulse-activity. The plain fact is that such phasic and self-impulses *must* combine with each other in some fashion ; and we believe that the four fundamental principles of integration which we apply to sensory, correlation and motor phenomena successively, form the actual neurological basis of these inevitable combinations.

The View-point of the " Middle Grounders "

By far the greatest number of contemporary psychologists adhere to none of the special schools already mentioned. They represent the so-called conservative element in psychology and to them Professor Woodworth of Columbia University has applied the term, " Middle Grounders." At different times they make use of the view-points and procedures of all the different schools and attack whatever problems they are dealing with, by the means that appear most applicable. On one occasion they will use the subjective technique of introspection, on another they will temporarily adopt the methods, and thus become involved in the assumptions, of behaviourism. They also continue to make use of various older views that have come down from the structuralist and functionalist schools of the past ; as regards Thought, we still find such statements as that Thought is primarily a process employed in getting out of difficulty, or the variant rendering that Thought is mental trial and error. A great profusion of labels of this character is applied to Thought in psychological text-books, such as perceptual thought, creative thought, stereotyped thought, and so on ; labels that are ultimately derived from the results flowing from the activation of thought-processes, but which go only a very little way toward describing the processes themselves.

This generalized outlook and willingness to make use of various, even contradictory, methods on the part of the Middle Grounders, presents an outward appearance of great tolerance and breadth of view. We cannot but feel, nevertheless, that there is a certain hollowness presently to be perceived in this appearance. For example, when one engages in an introspective experiment or bases one's contentions upon the subjectivist view, the corresponding objections will be raised. These objections are not met at all by reason of the fact that next week one carries through a behaviouristic experiment upon another problem ; on the contrary not only do the former objections still apply with undiminished force to the first procedure, but furthermore a whole host of new objections is raised against the second procedure. By successively applying the view-points of contending schools the only result is that one becomes subject to all the objections that may apply to all these schools. And the point is that these objections are not of such a nature that they can cancel each other out. To be alternately a subjectivist, a behaviourist and a Gestaltist, has no further meaning than that anything to be said against any one of these schools applies to a portion at least of one's own work.

The defence is that there is much that is correct in the views of all schools ; what is wrong is the extreme to which their positions are carried. Therefore one should use their views, but in moderation. In some instances we are in hearty agreement with this proposition, but in most cases we find it very difficult to be so. Thus the Gestalt concept of the whole is important for psychology ; but its importance is in an entirely different direction than that proposed in the Gestalt application, it does not consist in a modification of that application. And as to introspection, it does not appear to us that if a tool is proven untrustworthy by its inherent nature, such untrustworthiness is eliminated by using the tool on an occasion other than that on which its unreliability was established. Indeed its employment in simple problems is more dangerous than in complex ones, since in this case the falsity introduced by its use will be much less apparent.

In general we would say that what is correct in the positions of the various special schools of contemporary psychology is not to be incorporated by the simple eclectic process of adding together particular points chosen from among the several views represented. That there is a portion of truth in all these views we believe to be correct ; but it is necessary that such portions be combined from a new standpoint that will unify them and thus give them a *new* meaning almost completely lacking in their original formulation. Thus, while on many points we find ourselves in complete agreement with the Middle Grounders in psychology, we do not feel that we can by any means adopt their general view-point.

" Mental Association "

A vast amount of work of the subjective kind has been done in investigating what is called " mental association " or " associative thought." Free and controlled association tests were very popular not so long ago, the sort of exercise in which the subject responds to a list of words with the first verbal response that " occurs " to him ; and free association is still used as an important part of the psychoanalytic technique.

As far back as the times of Aristotle psychologists were

busy devising lists of the subjective " laws of association " ; this occupation has accompanied psychology through most of its modern course, e.g. in the English associationist school of the nineteenth century, and even in the period following 1900 such laws were still being codified. A typical list of the laws, or conditions, governing association was as follows :

> exercise :
> > frequency
> > recency
> > intensity
> effect (i.e. success or failure)
> similarity
> contiguity
> combination (or conditioned reflex)
> congruity

Now to us it appears that the above laws, and all others like them, are not laws referring to the intellect or to Thought, but that they really refer to stimulus conditions that themselves are *antecedent* to the true thought-processes. The situation seems clearly comparable to that which we previously discovered in the matter of sensation, where the determinable factors of the sensory stimuli themselves, or alternatively the effect of such stimulation upon the various receptor mechanisms, was supposed adequately to account for the phenomena of sensation. We have already argued that such a view is fallacious, that a description of light waves or of retinal processes, all of which occur antecedently to the arousal of the conscious event of sensation in the cerebral sensory centres, is neither an account nor an explanation of the sensation itself.

In exactly the same way we believe that a formulation of the environmental conditions leading to the occurrence of thought-processes offers neither an account nor an explanation of the thought-processes themselves. In the matter of congruity, similarity, contiguity, and so on, these qualities refer in the first place to the exterior situation of the organism, in fact to the external stimuli to which it is subjected ; such qualities are then introjected, referred to the *resulting* interior processes, and it supposed that we now have an adequate account of the interior processes themselves. How can this possibly be true ? The interior processes remain as much shrouded in mystery as ever, for by describing qualitatively the external stimulus *conditions* leading to Thought and by referring these descriptions inward, we are still left with no more than a formulation of conditions, we have no description at all of what the processes may be that take place under these conditions. To describe retinal rod and cone stimulation is not to explain the succeeding fact of conscious vision ; to formulate causative conditions such as congruity or combination is not to describe the thought-processes that result from such conditions. It is not possible to allot space for detailed examples of all the associative categories that have been suggested as furnishing these so-called laws of Thought, but in our belief all laws of " mental association " without exception will be found to suffer from the criticism just offered.

The Objective View-point as to Thought

The psychonic theory of Thought is not derived from subjective experience nor is it based upon introspective data ; it is founded entirely upon the objective view-point. The objective data upon which it is built consist of our present neurological knowledge of what occurs in the connector or correlation centres, for, as previously explained, we believe that the psychonic energy arising in these centres objectively constitutes Thought.

When nerve impulses pass out of the sensory centres, they enter the correlation centres of the cerebrum and are there combined or integrated with other correlation impulses already present in these centres. The psychonic theory of thought-processes states that when such impulses now integrate at the correlation psychons, they arouse at these definite points that special kind of psychonic energy to which, borrowing the general subjective term, we give the name of Thought.

In thus dealing with only one of the three major subdivisions of the nervous organization of the body the situation is comparable to that considered in the previous chapter on Sensation ; only now we must theoretically sever the connections on the one side between the sensory centres and the correlation centres and on the other between the correlation centres and the motor centres. The general flow of impulses will be inward from the sensory centres and outward to the motor centres, and of course the *incoming impulses from the sensory centres* will in this case constitute the entering, phasic stimuli for the correlation system. For our present purposes we are left with only the correlation centres themselves to deal with, and within these our special interest will lie in the question as to what happens at the included psychons.

From the direction of subjectivity *we believe Thought to consist essentially in a consciousness of relationship*, but not in a consciousness of some abstract, formalized Relationship in general ; rather we believe Thought to be the consciousness of certain definite and distinct relationships that exist neurologically (not psychically) in the cerebrum. Just as sensation is the consciousness of the effect of external, phasic stimulation upon the already existing constant, or self, stimulation of the organism, so Thought is the consciousness of a given relationship existing between certain impulses or patterns of impulses in the correlation centres. These relationships are brought about at the correlation psychons and, of course, the resulting consciousness is the psychonic energy there arising.

The Six Types of Relationship Underlying Thought

Upon reflection it is evident at once that there is no single, simple type of relationship involved here. Out of the large number of relationships actually existing, it is possible, however, to discover six general types under which all the many cases may be included. They are :

(1) relationships between different groups of sensory impulses.

(2) relationships between groups of sensory and correlation impulses.

(3) relationships between groups of sensory and motor impulses.

(4) relationships between different groups of correlation impulses.

(5) relationships between groups of correlation and motor impulses.

(6) relationships between different groups of motor impulses.

We may represent these several relationships in the following chart by the correspondingly numbered lines, if it be carefully remembered that the lines only indicate, in a simple diagrammatic fashion, the pathways within which those integrations take place that result in a consciousness of relationship :

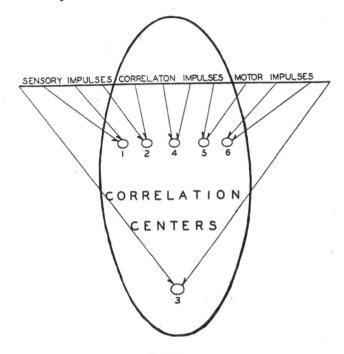

Chart showing the Types of Integration Relationship Underlying Thought Processes

The large oval on the above diagram is intended to represent schematically the total correlation areas of the cerebrum. All six types of integration relationships constituting thought as discussed in the text must occur within this area. The horizontal line near the top of the oval indicates the points of origin of sensory, correlation and motor impulses which come into relationship with one another in the correlation area. The six small ovals represent correlation centres in which these impulses integrate, §3 indicating the typical thought process from the functional point of view.

It is difficult to see how there can be any further relationships than those just listed, since objectively there exist no further impulse-groups between which a relation can occur in the correlation centres. We shall next consider separately these six types of relationship in serial order.

(1) *Relationships Between Different Groups of Sensory Impulses*

The first integration of a non-sensory character that takes place between the impulses caused by the stimuli continually entering the body from outside, may be said to occur between those impulses that have already passed through the sensory centres and then enter the correlation centres. Thus, impulses that have passed through the auditory, olfactory, visual and/or other sensory centres may, almost immediately upon entering the correlation centres, form a joint integration. Such an occurrence gives rise to perception, and any integration of this character is called a PERCEPT.

Let us take an example illustrating this very common type of mental process. We will suppose that a man has just pushed open with his hand a freshly painted gate. The first result, drawing his attention to the object, is a sticky sensation originating from the touch receptors in his fingers and hand. There is also a kinaesthetic sensation of the " opposition " type from the receptors in the muscles of the hand and arm, permitting a judgment of the relative softness or hardness of the object. Then, as he looks at the gate, the man receives through his eyes a complex visual impression, embracing colour sensations, the visual pattern of the whole gate and its various parts including the general form of the gate, the forms of its parts, their juxtaposition, and so on. In addition there will be olfactory sensations, caused by the volatile elements in the paint, which affect the receptors in his nose. Thus far we have only sensations, occurring in the various sensory centres and described in our previous chapter ; they are separate and easily distinguishable. It is when the impulses issue from the various sensory centres and are combined in the correlation centres that the consciousness of the gate *as an object* arises. The different sensations are then referred to a common exterior source, the gate, which in experience exists, not as touch sensations plus visual sensations plus olfactory sensations, but as a simultaneous combination or integration of these.

It is by this process, namely perception, that all objects as such are built up in experience, both inanimate objects and animate ones, even including those objects that we call our own bodies. Subjectively they have no existence except as various combinations of sensations ; once these component sensory elements are taken away, nothing, no object, remains

—a fact long since pointed out by " idealistic " philosophers like Berkeley who wished from this to draw the (incorrect) conclusion that therefore no objects existed. It may be worth while, however, in passing to mention that no such things as the actually *perceived* objects exist ; the intervening processes of receptor stimulation, sensory activity and correlation function are much too lengthy, indirect and complicated to permit of the percept having anything more than a rough approximation to an accurate representation of the object perceived. There is, in fact, just close enough an approximation to allow an adequate motor response to be made to the object ; we may suppose that the main purpose of perception, as developed biologically, was to serve this practical end and even now perception has little other value, as modern physics has demonstrated in its own astonishing but more accurate description of those same objects to which our percepts refer.

It is possible to emphasize the statement that percepts are combinations of sensations in two different ways, viz. combinations of *sensations*, or *combinations* of sensations. The latter way is correct, for the essence of a percept is relationship ; what makes a given percept is the specific manner of combination of different sensory impulses, the way, in short, in which they are integrated at the correlation psychons. From the objective point of view the psychonic energy in such integrations is perception.

Since sensations may be divided into two general kinds, namely those referring to objects or events outside the body and those whose function it is to report interior bodily conditions, and since both kinds of sensory centres discharge their impulses into the correlation centres, there to be combined, there results a class of percepts that can easily be distinguished from those perceptions that build up the objects of the external world.

This second class of percepts as such seems to have received little definite attention from psychology, but we believe them to be equally as important as the perceptions of external objects. The integrations, in the correlation centres, of the impulses issuing from the kinaesthetic and equilibrium sensory centres, for example, produces the perception of balance, and the general integration of all the interior sense-impulses present at a given moment, produces the awareness of one's body as a body. Among this kind of integrations there is one which, because of its subjective interpretation, is of very great importance. This is the so-called awareness of striving, the " feeling of conation," as it has been called. " Conation " is a term frequently used by psychologists to designate the striving or effortful feeling now to be considered. We believe this feeling to be a perception based upon an integration of impulses from bodily sensation centres ; the prime element in it seems to be the " resistance sensations " from the receptors embedded in the muscles, but to this are added integrations of balance and other interior-sensation impulses.

This perception acquires its undue importance because in the past it has provided a basis for many imposing speculations concerning the so-called human Will. That the phenomenon is perception is clearly shown by the fact that, when the " resistance sensation " is present alone, no question of Will arises ; it is when the " resistance sensation " is integrated with other internal sensations and the " feeling of conation " results, that large claims about Will-power commence to be made. Naturally there is little basis for the self-congratulations that theorists have deduced from so slender a premise. What actually exists is not a Will, but a conative perception, and although this awareness is not subsequent to the integration of which we have been speaking, neither is it antecedent thereto. In fact, objectively this awareness *is* the integration, and the elements of which that integration is composed are certainly antecedent to the integration itself.

Nowadays almost all psychologists have abandoned any mention of Will. And even the purposivists, for whom Purpose seems to be subjectively considered as a sort of pale shadow of the Will, are prepared to admit that Purpose is not something added to the response either subsequently or antecedently, but is simply a label to be attached for convenience to a special kind of response. However, as we shall hope to show in one of the following sections, Purpose is an Attitude, a phenomenon quite different from the conative perception that used to be called Will.

In spite of all this there is a distinct class of persons, not psychologists, who in their subjective experience seem naturally to attach so great an unconscious significance to the conative perception, that they come to *identify themselves* with this part-element of their consciousness. They feel that *they are* this perception, and if asked seriously to say what is their most intimate self, it is to this that, after reflection, they will point. Thus for them the conative perception constitutes self-consciousness.

We shall have something further to say, both about Will and about the other two varieties of self-consciousness in the later sections on the several kinds of relationship consciousness that arise in the correlation centres.

(2) *Relationships Between Groups of Sensory and Correlation Impulses*

The incoming impulses from the sensory centres, either in sensory groups or as already integrated into percepts in the outlying correlation centres, cannot long avoid meeting and therefore combining with groups of typical correlation impulses already passing in various directions through the correlation centres. The latter impulse groups, i.e. those which, whatever their original source, are at any given moment in possession, as it were, of the correlation centres, correspond to concepts, abstractions, and so on, and constitute what is popularly considered as the typical thought-processes. Needless to say, our own position regarding thought-processes includes much more than this single category within the term, Thought; in fact, those correlation groups consisting of concepts, and so on, are but one of the six general types of mental function, and will be dealt with in detail under sub-heading (4) of the present discussion. In this section it is only necessary to point out that the relationship involved here is between such groups of correlation impulses and the entering sensory groups.

Objectively, then, we have the integration of these two types of impulse-groups at the correlation psychons; and subjectively, the awareness of the relationships involved in such impulse integrations constitutes *intellectual meaning*. The term intellectual meaning is, perhaps, a redundant expression, for from our point of view all meaning is intellectual, since it occurs in the correlation centres and is one of the essential subdivisions of Thought. Meaning, however, has three clearly defined aspects; they are practical meaning, purely mental meaning and emotional meaning. The relationship now considered is that of practical meaning.

In illustration let us say that a group of entering sensory impulses corresponds to the perception of a horse ; let us further say that these percept impulses now meet with correlation impulses corresponding to the concept of horses in general. How this extraordinarily apposite meeting comes to take place will be considered later ; here it is only a question of what happens *when* it takes place. As will also be shown later, the concept, horse, includes much more than the percept, horse ; to take but one instance, it includes the ride-ability of horses. Accordingly, when the integrative relationship is established between the percept group and the concept group impulses, the two fuse and instead of " horses are ride-able " we have " this perceived horse is ride-able." The quality of being-able-to-be-ridden, not involved in the original percept, now becomes definitely attributed to the object represented by that percept and a certain practical significance or meaning arises.

Illustrations like the above are, of course, subjective, and we cannot too often caution the reader against the view that our theory is based upon such subjective interpretations of experience. It is true that the problems of Thought, like those of sensation and emotion, arise from subjective experience ; it is that which is to be explained and accounted for. But our position must continue to remain the same, that the only scientific account that can be rendered must be in the objective terms of neurology and physics and must carefully avoid the fallacious procedure of explaining subjectivity in terms of itself. Thus our illustration must not be confused with our explanation ; what actually happens when practical meaning enters subjective experience is an integration at the correlation psychons between groups of sensory and correlation impulses.

(3) *Relationships Between Groups of Sensory and Motor Impulses*

This is actually the typical relationship produced by the correlation system, since the correlation centres are interposed between the sensory and motor centres and serve the prime function of a selective connection between them. Nevertheless, as we have seen, this typical relationship is only one of a number of relationships, or integration processes, that may take place within the correlation centres.

The subjective name for this particular kind of relationship is ATTITUDE, i.e. the emotional relation to outside stimulation. As has been explained, external stimulation subsequently results (already within the correlation centres) in perception ; but this successive process is so rapid as usually to pass unnoticed in subjective experience, with the result that Attitude, as used subjectively, generally refers to the emotional relation to outside objects or events. As previously mentioned, affective consciousness (feeling and emotion) occurs at the psychons of the motor system and sensation at the psychons of the sensory system ; the connection between these psychons takes place through the psychons of the correlation system, and here the consciousness that is based upon their joint relationship, must arise.

It is necessary to keep clearly in mind that in the present section we are not speaking of affective consciousness itself ; pleasantness and unpleasantness, Dominance, Compliance, Inducement, Submission and their multifarious compounds are not now in question, but only the *relation* between the various sensations and these also various affective states. Such relations we have summed up as Attitudes.

There are various Attitudes, of which we will mention the three most important, at any rate the most important in the history of psychology. The first is the Purposive Attitude, the Attitude in which it is proposed to do something about the given sensory stimulation. This Attitude, it seems to us, has been vastly over-exaggerated in certain schools of psychology, where it is supposed to be at the very core of human, and even of animal, psychology. To us this appears to be far from the case ; this Attitude is simply a part-reaction within the whole response-arc, and the consciousness of purpose only arises *as a result of* the psychonic integrations that simultaneously occur at the correlation psychons between the sensory and motor ones involved. Purpose itself seems to be nothing except a consciousness of the relationship existing between the phasically activated parts of the sensory and motor systems, and this relationship actually exists within the correlation system through which the other two systems are connected.

A sort of special case of purpose is Will, the Conative Attitude. As we have made plain in an earlier section, we believe what is usually referred to by the term, Conation, is the Conative Perception. But due to the fact that Conation has been so deeply involved in the controversies that have raged about the question of the Will, the issue has been thoroughly confused and it would seem that some psychologists have really been referring, in such discussions, to a Conative Attitude rather than to the Conative Perception. Thus it will be necessary to discuss Conation briefly under the present section also.

To be sure, Will departed from psychology shortly after, if not at the same time with the soul ; and we can scarcely avoid suspecting that the frenzied attempts to over-emphasize Purpose are but belated efforts to resuscitate Will, with a perhaps unconscious implication of eventually re-introducing the soul itself. It may be that we do an injustice to the " purposive " schools of psychology, but whether intentionally or not, such seems to us to be the direction of their efforts. Having thus made it plain that we can see nothing to be particularly emphasized about this kind of Will, we may now say that we see no objection to applying the label of Will to an especially clear-cut or definite example of the Purposive Attitude ; provided, of course, that it be borne in mind that what we mean by Will is a special case of a particular kind of relationship (the purposive), occurring in the correlation centres.

That relationship which is the opposite of the Purposive Attitude may also occur ; and this will be the Indifferent Attitude. In the first case we may suppose that the sensory impulses pass through the correlation centres to the motor centres, as it were, compactly ; their pattern is definitely maintained during their journey and when it is productive of more or less immediate motor effect, the result will be as if a low-order reflex had been lifted to the higher levels of the cerebrum—a very different view of purpose than that ordinarily held. On the other hand, Indifference will result if the sensory impulses pass to the motor centres not compactly but on a broad front as we might say, and have no immediate effect of muscle activation. In the latter case the motor centres will, of course, be activated and there will be an emotional reaction, but there will be no necessary contraction of muscles, or overt behaviour ; the impulses will be absorbed in the general activity of the motor centres without their own special pattern reaching any final motor pathway. The relation of such a motor effect to the sensory impulses will, in the correlation centres, constitute the Indifferent Attitude And in a similar fashion any Attitude will consist of the psychonic energy engaged in the general integration brought about by the correlation centres between sensory and motor activity.

(4) *Relationships Between Different Groups of Correlation Impulses*

Naturally it is possible for certain groups of impulses, themselves of correlation-centre type, to form integrations with each other. Subjectively, the best known phenomena of this kind consist in the combination of percepts into CONCEPTS. Thus from many perceptions of the objects called horses, there arises the Concept of the horse in general It is very obvious that the attributes of this Concept are not made up of a successive addition of the attributes of the percepts from which it has evolved ; for instance, we may have had perceptions of a thousand horses, but when we are conscious of the Concept, the horse in general, the object we then refer to does not possess four thousand legs. It possesses the generalized legs of all the horses we have perceived, and this generalization is a combination, or integration, of many percepts. A Concept, then, is the subjective name given to the psychonic energy that occurs at those correlation centres where groups of impulses coming from other correlation centres, are integrated with each other.

Neurologically the human nervous system achieves its utmost refinement and complexity in the correlation system of the cerebrum ; in addition to those simplest integrations of correlation impulses which we have called Concepts, it is possible for these conceptual integrations themselves to form further mutual integrations with each other. Thus we find generalizations based upon elements which are also generalizations but of narrower scope. The narrower scope generalizations are Concepts ; the wider generalizations built upon them are the typical components of ABSTRACT THOUGHT, although the Concepts are also, on a lower level, abstract in nature, since their bases are less complex integrations of the same general type.

Subjectively, Abstract Thought may take many different forms. The abstract idea of Justice, divorced from any practical application or connection with concrete objects (percepts) and situations, is an example of this kind ; the idea of Truth is another. And of course the processes of higher mathematics exhibit numerous and high degrees of mental abstraction. Basing ourselves upon the neurology of the cerebrum, we would say that Abstract Thought is the psychonic energy arising at the psychons where integration takes place between those groups of already integrated correlation impulses which themselves constitute Concepts.

There exists also a slightly different kind of relationship, still of this general type, wherein two or more groups of correlation impulses may be integrated in a third correlation centre. Thus Concepts may not only be related to an Abstraction as its component parts, but there may also be an awareness of a relation, e.g. similarity, between a particular Concept and the Abstraction of which it is an integral part. Such an awareness may arise as the result of an integration taking place through another arc of correlation centres than the one already engaged in the integration of the given Abstraction itself. The sort of comparison process thus possible, may also occur between Concept and Concept, Abstraction and Abstraction, or between any other two or more groups of correlation impulses. And here we have the basis for Mental Introspection, whose counterpart, Emotional Introspection, will be mentioned in a following section. A similar instance of integrative relationship between groups of correlation impulses forms the basis for the consciousness of Mental Meaning.

Furthermore, when the definite comparisons and formulations that may make the process introspective, are absent, we may find that vague type of consciousness which consists of an indefinite combination-awareness of several mental part-processes going forward at a given moment. There is a large class of persons who seem to identify themselves sometimes with this particular part-reaction of their unit responses, and for them the psychonic energy involved at these psychons will constitute self-consciousness.

(5) *Relationships Between Groups of Correlation and Motor Impulses*

Corresponding to the type (2) thought-processes, namely those which neurologically are the basis for practical meaning, we find on the motor side of the cerebrum the integration between groups of correlation and motor impulses which underlie Emotional Meaning. It will be recalled that we believe that the psychonic energy arising in the motor centres is experienced subjectively as emotion. Neurologically it is true that, although the general course of the cerebral nerve impulses is from the correlation to the motor centres, there are certain return entrances through which groups of motor centre impulses may pass back again into the correlation system. Such a circumstance will cause the meeting, and inevitable integration of correlation and motor impulses, and sub-jectively the resulting experience will be one of the attribution of emotional significance, or Meaning, to the intellectual experiences represented by the correlation impulses. Obviously this occurrence constitutes a combination motor and correlation phenomenon, but since both the subjective emphasis is upon the significance involved and objectively the event actually occurs in the correlation centres, the pheno-menon is properly to be included among the thought-processes.

(6) *Relationships Between Different Groups of Motor Impulses*

The occurrences now to be considered, on the motor side of the correlation system, correspond to what takes place on its sensory side during perception. Subjectively, they comprise the relations felt to exist between different, and distinguishable, emotional elements. Objectively, they consist of the psychonic energy arising in the correlation arc which connects two different motor centres or groups of motor centres, with each other ; such arcs or some of them pass through the correlation system and thus the consciousness that arises is mental rather than emotional.

Let us consider the situation when one is asked, for example, how much envy there is in one's dislike of a certain man, or how much self-interest there is in his alleged love for a particular woman. We can predict, of course, that the public answer will be made up of a series of self-justifying rational-izations, as plausible as the person interrogated can devise. But let us also suppose that this person has a certain self-respect and sincerity toward himself which demands that he be clear in his own mind as to the true answer to these questions, no matter how much he may seek to deceive his questioner. How will he proceed to determine the matter ? Although there are better means, he will probably attempt to weigh the constituents of his whole emotional state directly against each other and thus to determine whether there is any of the subjective state he calls " envy " involved, and if so, to what degree. The ensuing judgment will scarcely be very accurate, yet in a vague way it may indicate that there is indeed an element of " envy " present, although whether this element is slight or large we should hesitate to say upon such a basis. The man himself will doubtless say with great conviction that it is slight.

Here we have what is evidently a typical introspection upon emotional states. The introspection itself is plainly a thought-process, a mental occurrence that can only take place if there is some mental connection between the emotional elements judged. Objectively considered, these emotional elements arise in the motor centres ; there are correlation-centre connections between various motor-centre groups and we propose that the impulses passing through such correlation connector centres between motor groups give rise to psychonic energy which is the introspective consciousness here mentioned.

There is, however, another point to be mentioned before we leave the discussion of this particular type of relationship-consciousness. There appears to exist a large class of persons for whom this special kind of consciousness constitutes what in a previous section we have called self-consciousness. We have not been using this term, self-consciousness, in its colloquial sense, i.e. we have not been using it in the sense in which it means one's opinion regarding the opinion of others toward oneself and in which it is sometimes equivalent to bashfulness. We use self-consciousness here to mean that this large class of persons are accustomed to identify themselves with their consciousness of just the type of inter-emotional relation that we have been discussing. In other words, they feel that *they are* the relationships of this type that consecutively arise in them.

Perhaps the question here involved will become clearer if we take another example. We will postulate a man who walks out through the fields on a spring morning. His general affective state is one of Dominance, but there are many minor elements also present ; there is the pleasantness of the view and the fresh smell of the spring air, there is the unpleasantness of crossing a boggy corner of the meadow and the Compliance he makes with the obstacle formed by the brook at its edge. At any moment there are at least several of these elements of emotional consciousness present, and the general, combined effect of all of them is what he thinks of as himself. That is, this general effect is what he thinks of as himself in retrospect ; if he introspects upon these emotional combinations *as they occur*, they then become the objects of introspection and the man can no longer identify himself with them but must now identify himself with the introspective process. In this case the awareness of the relationships we are discussing, changes from self-consciousness to introspective consciousness. It is only as he looks back upon the past that he feels such (unintrospected) awareness of relationships to have been what he then was.

The general combination of motor impulses underlying this phenomenon takes place, of course, through those correlation centres which connect the motor centres involved as the elements of his emotional consciousness. And the psychonic energy in such correlation centres is the vague and unformulated awareness of the relationships which we are considering in this section. We must carefully point out, however, that we do not maintain that everyone has a feeling of self-identification with this same type of relationship-consciousness; nor do we assert that there is any fundamental justification for such an identification, when it does occur, either in this case or in the other two cases already discussed where the identification was made with sensory or with correlation processes. We merely wish to point out that in a large number of cases self-identification with these types of part-reaction is a fact ; when the present type of self-identification takes place, the identification is actually made with the psychonic energy arising in the correlation centres that serve as connectors between different groups of motor centres.

Thus there will be two quite distinct kinds of mental consciousness associated with the psychonic energy considered in this section. When weighing and comparison takes place, this psychonic energy will be subjectively called Emotional Introspection ; when comparison and similar activities are absent, it will be called Self-consciousness by a particular group of persons.

2C

Summary of Type-relationships

In general terms we have now briefly described the six type-relationships that compose Thought. In subjective experience Thought comprises the awareness of one or more kinds of the relationships described; for an objective psychology the psychonic energy at the correlation psychons where the above impulse-group integrations occur, constitutes Thought.

There is still, however, an important point to be made. We see no reason to suppose that the integration activities involved in Thought must always take place in the same correlation centres; indeed what evidence there is upon correlation functions[1] seems to suggest that the typical functions of this system are not localized, in the higher animals and man, in any particular cortical or sub-cortical areas, but that any of the correlation centres may evince any of the correlation functions.

This would seem especially true of the kind of integration activity we have been discussing. Since the process is simply one of integration between groups of impulses passing through the correlation centres, such groups will be combined wherever they chance to meet, one likelihood being that integrations between groups of sensory impulses and between groups of motor impulses will usually, but not necessarily always, occur in the neighbourhoods of the sensory and motor centres respectively.

There seems also to be one other likelihood, concerning which we hesitate to speculate, since the evidence for it rests upon purely subjective grounds. We refer to the apparent appositeness, mentioned earlier, with which, for example, the impulses representing the Percept, horse, come into contact with those representing the Concept, horse. It may be that such occurrences are in fact only chance happenings which receive an attention in subjective experience from no other cause than that they are in fact apposite, those times when such appropriate meetings do not occur, although far more numerous, remaining unnoticed. Most people, however, would probably believe otherwise, and it may indeed be that

[1]See especially K. S. Lashley's experiments at John Hopkins on the learning function in white rats, *Psychobiol.*, 1917, I; *Arch. Neur. and Psychiat.*, 1924, 12; *J. Comp. Psychol.*, 1926, 6; and others.

something of the nature of specific gravity or of an electromagnetic attraction between *pattern*-similarities of impulse groups, at least leads these groups into regions where their chances of mutual integration are enormously increased.

But in respect of Thought in general we may look upon the correlation centres as a relatively large area, anywhere within which the integration-relationships here discussed, may take place. Within the correlation system different centres or arcs of centres may serve a similar purpose at different times ; what remains constant is not the function of special correlation centres but the six kinds of possible integrative connections that can be made at any correlation centre, and thus the six types of relationship-consciousness that compose Thought.

The Four Primary Integration Types

We have said that Thought is the awareness of relationship, and we have been describing the various possible elements between which these relationships can occur ; but we have not said as yet of what types the relationships themselves may be.

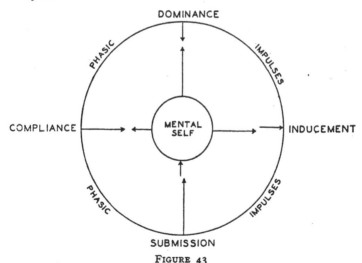

FIGURE 43
Elementary Types of Thought Integrations

It will be remembered that, with regard to the sensory system, some degree of constant stimulation is delivered by the organism itself to certain, and perhaps to all, of the receptors. In the case of the motor system, the self-originated, constant tonic discharge to the musculature of the body fills this role of self-stimulation. In respect of the correlation system there is no known mechanism to fulfil this function, but the obvious fact that phasic stimuli must, in this case too, always affect an already operating system of centres, creates the same situation.

The general situation with regard to integration processes as such is the same in the correlation centres as it is in the sensory and motor systems. When we consider simply the integrations themselves, leaving out of account for the moment whatever the special elements may be between which the integrations take place, we find once more that all the types of possible integration may be plotted on the circumference of a circle. Such a circle will possess the four nodal points of distinction which, in treating of emotion, will be called Dominance, Compliance, Inducement and Submission ; this will be so because, within the correlation system also the same distinctions between incoming and existing impulses will have to be made as elsewhere. That is, the impulses integrated in these centres may be divided not only into the six classes already described in the preceding sections but also into the two even more fundamental classes of incoming (phasic) stimuli and constant (self) stimuli.

It is further to be remembered that when, as we are now doing, we speak of the correlation centres as a separately distinguishable system within the body as a whole, the phasic stimuli for this system will consist of those impulses which enter the correlation centres for the first time, having already passed through the sensory centres. Thus the afferent nerve impulses constitute phasic stimuli for the sensory centres, within which they then undergo a series of selective integrations ; it is the impulse-patterns or groups that result from these processes, which then, and only then, become in turn phasic stimuli for the correlation centres. But there are already probably millions of impulse-groups passing through the correlation centres when such new, phasic impulses make their incursion into the correlation system. The newly entering impulse-groups must combine in some fashion with those already present when they arrive. And there are, as usual, the four primary ways in which they may do so ; they may be in alliance or harmony with the existing impulse-

patterns and either stronger or weaker in effect ; or they may
be in conflict and again either stronger or weaker.

If we may speak of the sum total of the impulse-patterns
existing at any given moment in the correlation centres as
the Mental Self, then from the view-point of the Mental Self
the integrations resulting from the just mentioned relations
will be of the respective types of Submission, Inducement,
Compliance, and Dominance. And between the four so-called
nodal points in the integration circle where these relations find
their maximum expression there will occur all the possible
mutual modifications and combinations of these primary type
integrations with each other.

It may be somewhat confusing at first glance to keep clearly
in mind the difference between the six types of integration-
relationship that we have earlier listed in accordance with the
nature of the elements, i.e. impulse groups, integrated, and the
four types of integration-relationship just listed in accordance
with the nature of the integration itself. Such a distinction,
however, is not at all difficult to make when it is understood
that with regard to the first six kinds of elements taking part
in the integration, any of the latter four kinds of integration,
or their compounds, may occur. Furthermore, within the
correlation system proper it is to be remembered that the
impulse integrations corresponding to percepts, concepts, or
to any of the other types listed earlier, may, in a given instance,
represent either the phasic or the pre-existing elements in the
next succeeding integration in which they take part.

Dominance-Type Thought-Processes

In considering the simple, primary integrative types of
Dominance, Compliance, Submission and Inducement, we must
remember that these elementary or nodal integrations almost
never occur simply or singly in actual experience of either the
sensory, emotional or intellectual variety. In real life there is
to be found no simple, unmixed dominance emotion, nor is
there a correspondingly unmixed dominance thought-process.
The dominant thought-process is, however, fairly easy to
isolate by analysis from the more involved compound
intellectual responses in which it occurs.

The nature of this dominant thought experience is to be
distinguished when any new material, derived through sensory

channels is forced to give way or to conform to the existing ideas or mental content which we have called the Mental Self. This simple, dominant aspect of the thought-process always treats its subject-matter as antagonistic and inferior to the mental content already existing, or to the thought experience already going forward when the new material seeks entry.

Two of the most easily recognizable examples of the dominance-type thought-process, one normal and the other abnormal, may be called Analysis and Prejudice. In Analysis the new material is broken down into simpler and more familiar elements that can take part in the subsequent processes of grasping and comprehending ; such an event may be very useful biologically and thus seems to serve a normal function from the objective view-point. Prejudice, on the other hand is intellectual dominance carried to abnormal lengths ; the fanatic whose opinion can never be altered, no matter what new evidence may arise bearing upon his position, is not suffering from "logic-tight" compartments in his "mind" ; the impulses representing the new evidence enter the correlation system but they are not magically kept separated from the impulse groups representing the pre-existing prejudice, they are swamped and inhibited by the prejudice impulses. It is noteworthy that the arguments against a particular fanaticism can never be fairly stated by the fanatic, as should be the case were they present in a separate compartment of his "mind" ; on the contrary, they always reappear in distorted and mutilated form, if indeed they have not been so far destroyed as to become unrecognizable. In Prejudice of this kind we have an exaggerated instance of intellectual Dominance ; it is pernicious both sociologically and biologically, and we have little hesitancy in naming it abnormal.

Compliance-Type Thought-Processes

According to our formula the experience of intellectual Compliance consists of giving way to, or complying with, new mental material that is antagonistic to and stronger than the Mental Self. Just as emotional Compliance must precede emotional Dominance in the normal sequence, so intellectual Compliance should precede intellectual Dominance in the healthfully functioning thought-processes. It is obvious that any new fact (sensory datum) must be given way to intellectually and allowed to pass freely through the correlation centres before it can either be memorized or indeed comprehended.

Such a subjective experience is easily recognizable when we consciously " give way to facts ". In this experience we go through the intellectual process of recognizing that a new mental fact which we already knew to be contrary to our Mental Self, is actually stronger than the Mental Self, whereas we previously believed it to be weaker. For example, one may believe that all red-haired people have terrible tempers. A red-haired subject comes to the psychological clinic and after a great deal of careful analysis and study the psychologist can discover no trace of what is usually called " temper ". For a long time the psychologist attempts to compel this new datum to fit into his previous conclusions, but at last he gives up the attempt and his Mental Self admits the new conclusion that some red-haired people do not have uncontrollable tempers. The core of this experience is mental Compliance.

In grasping and comprehension mental Compliance plays as essential a role as that of mental Dominance, a role moreover which in the usual case is prior to that of the latter.

Submission-Type Thought-Processes

The experience of intellectual Submission would seem to be easily recognizable in the frequently recurring control of our ideas or thoughts by apparently spontaneous association with such new ideas or sensory data as " intrigue our interest ". In the experience of so-called " creative imagination ", both voluntary and involuntary, this intellectual submission-type of integration would seem to play a very important part. The incoming impulses seem to attract to themselves other impulses representing an extended train of imagery, thoughts and ideas previously existing in the Mental Self. Of course there is a simultaneous changing and interpretation of the new thoughts in accordance with the previously existing ones of the Mental Self, and such a process is not Submission and should not be confused with it. But the free and pleasant yielding of our own ideas to the control of a new thought or concept seems clearly to constitute intellectual Submission.

The conversation of women gives evidence of a very clear-cut example of this intellectual Submission. Mention of a hat or of a new style of dress calls forth, apparently, an almost exactly similar stream of ideas and thoughts from all the other women present. In general, women's ideas are apt not to be controlled by any ordered or organized plan of the Mental Self. They seem to follow casually and in more or less unorganized sequence the intellectual attraction or Inducement of any new thought or idea suggested. This is intellectual Submission on the part of the Mental Self. It is characterized integratively by an attitude of alliance with the new mental material, which is regarded as stronger than the ideas and concepts already existing in the Mental Self.

In our present society examples of intellectual Submission on a large scale abound on every side. They are to be found every day in the acceptance of false and illogical ideas by vast multitudes of people as a result of reading such ideas in newspapers or magazines or hearing the new material from the lips of people whom they regard as authorities. Advertising in peace time and propaganda during war rely upon the submissive intellectual tendency of those addressed. Especially in the latter case the degree of intellectual impertinence displayed by the paid propagandist is exceeded only by that of the gullibility with which every implication in his " atrocity " stories is swallowed by the " patriots " who employ him.

Inducement-type Thought-processes

In this type of intellectual response the Mental Self is regarded as allied with but superior to the new ideas of sensory data. The process of Interpretation of the new ideas is characterized predominantly by mental Inducement. The new idea is not analyzed out dominantly for the purpose of grasping or comprehension, but rather it is drawn successively into various previously existing thought-patterns of the Mental Self, with which it is regarded as being closely allied. In the process of Interpretation the new correlation impulses may be induced into a combination with previous impulse roups that completely overwhelm and absorb the entering groups, so that the new idea becomes almost unrecognizable to anyone except the subject who does the interpreting. In such a process of Interpretation there is also a simultaneous, but lesser, Submission activity with respect to the previously existing thought-elements of the Mental Self.

Compound Unit Responses of the Intellect: Grasping

Just as in the sensory and motor centres what actually occurs is not the simple, primary integrations but the more complicated compound unit response type of integration, so in the correlation system also the latter, more involved phenomenon is the usual occurrence. Perhaps the most usual and typical mental response is that of Knowing, which in turn is made up of two compound unit responses of the intellect that we may call Grasping and Comprehending.

Grasping is an intellectual response corresponding precisely in integrative type with the compound emotional response of Desire. Mental Grasping is composed of active intellectual Dominance and simultaneous passive intellectual Compliance. The existing correlation impulse groups comply with the entering, phasic impulses (representing the new idea that is to be grasped) to the extent that the entering impulses are allowed to maintain their own individual patterns ; at the same time the new impulses are forced into arrangements or combinations with the previously existing impulse groups in such a way that the latter maintain their original structure unimpaired.

In subjective terms, the mental grasper passively complies with a new fact or sensory datum which seems antagonistic to the existing Mental Self by permitting the new fact, despite its antagonism, to remain intact in the intellectual centres that are performing the integration. Simultaneously the new fact is actively dominated by analyzing it into terms of the previous mental content and by forcing an arrangement of these terms compatible with the existing organization of the Mental Self. Finally the new material is memorized, in order that it be available at any later time for intellectual manipulation.

Curiosity seems to represent the compound mental response of Grasping tinged with the concomitant emotional response of Desire.

Comprehension

This compound unit response of the intellect corresponds with the compound emotional response of Satisfaction. Here we find active intellectual Compliance coupled with passive Dominance of an intellectual kind. After we have grasped a new datum or idea mentally, we normally strive to comprehend it. The outstanding integrative element in this process is an active Compliance with the new thought or fact. The Mental

Self is actively readjusted to allow room, as it were, for the new fact or idea unaltered. Simultaneously, however, we resist intellectually the passage of this new datum into the Mental Self sufficiently to make it conform to the present nature and pattern of the Mental Self. This combination of active Compliance and passive Dominance results in a mental assimilation of the meaning of the new material in the same way that the nutritive values of food are assimulated by the blood during the process of digestion which is accompanied by the emotional compound unit response of Satisfaction. And in fact Comprehension carries an inevitable emotional consequence of Satisfaction just as mental Grasping is connected with an affective Desire.

Intellectual Complex Unit Response of Knowing

When the intellectual compound unit response of Grasping gradually blends into and combines with the compound unit response of Comprehension, the result is the complex unit response of Knowing. This corresponds precisely with the emotional complex unit response of Appetite which combines Desire and Satisfaction in the same way.

As an example of the knowing process in operation, let us take the case of an orthodox physicist confronted for the first time with Einstein's General Relativity Theory. He decides that here is something important for the science of physics. Initially he must make the new theory fit into the background of general physical problems and outlook, and he accomplishes this result by forcing the theory into place, rather than the background; to this extent the existing Mental Self actively dominates the new data. But his second process is quite different, for he must now allow the new theory to modify the very background into which it is absorbed and his attempt is to realize in definite terms just how the general theory of physics is to be modified by Relativity. Far from expecting that the general outlook shall remain unchanged, his whole effort is in the direction of an harmonious blending of the two elements into a new and fuller knowledge.

Thus, from the view-point of the Mental Self, we can write down the whole Knowing process as (1) Grasping : = passive Compliance, active Dominance; + (2) Comprehension : = active Compliance, passive Dominance. The formula is then pC aD + aC pD.

In this connection it is interesting to note that many of the people we meet in daily life can, with little effort, be classified as Graspers or as Comprehenders. The Graspers are those who never get beyond the first stage of the Knowing process; superficially they appear to have taken in your remarks and indeed they have fully grasped them, but they never succeed in achieving a complete comprehension. The Comprehenders, on the other hand, do not omit the first process of Grasping, for that is essential to Knowing; but they also go beyond the grasping stage, they intellectually welcome the new information and, by welcoming it, succeed in incorporating it intimately with themselves.

Compound Unit Responses : " Creative " Imagination

Just as Passion is a totally different compound response from Desire, so Imagination represents a totally different type of intellectual integrative combination from mental Grasping.

Intellectual Imagination represents an active Submission of the previously existing thoughts of the mental Self to the control of a new idea or sensory datum, and also a passive Inducement of the new mental material into allied combinations with previous thoughts and ideas. In short, Imagination is a compound of the intellectual unit responses of active Submission and passive Inducement, thus pI aS.

In the first place " creative " imagination is a *thought* process that must be distinguished quite definitely from " sensory imagination," which consists merely in the reinstatement of sensations or " sensory images " as they were formerly called. On the other hand, we must also distinguish creative imagination from the total process of mental creation of which imagination forms an important part. " Creative " imagination, as suggested above during our discussion of mental submission, is a thought process which consists, for the most part, of placing the previously existing Mental Self under the temporary control of a new Percept, Idea, or Concept.

The new or phasic mental material is permitted momentarily to draw to itself, as it were, allied and associated thought contents already existing in the mind, and to rearrange these contents according to a new pattern dictated by the new mental Idea or Concept. According to the popular phrase, the new and inducive idea " takes a firm grip on the imagination " of the subject.

At the same time, the Mental Self strives in a more or less passive way, to attract and hold the new Concept in its focus of attention. The mind, one might say, eagerly presents its existing materials to the uses and control of the new Idea for the purpose of making the new Idea as vivid as possible. The Mental Self, in short, passively induces the new Idea to control and manipulate existing mental content, and insures its retention in the correlation centres by voluntarily holding forth mental materials for the new Idea to work upon. The Mental Self, therefore, at the same time actively submits to, and passively induces the continued presence of, the new Idea. This simultaneous combination of the two thought processes constitutes a compound mental response which we call Imagination, designated as " creative " Imagination in contrast to the simple, mnemonic, sensory-image process.

It is quite easy to differentiate, by objective observation of other people's mental behaviour, compound unit responses of Imagination from compound unit responses of Grasping or Comprehension. Certain types of person habitually react to new mental material with Imagination rather than with mental grasping or comprehending, and the obvious result is a set of Thoughts or Ideas which bear little resemblance to original fact, and which also manifest a certain peculiar absence of logical coherency. " Just a flight of the imagination " we say, meaning that the Imagination process took place with little or no admixture of Grasping or Comprehension of the new material. In the final, verbal response, the stimulus material comes forth highly coloured and sometimes wholly concealed beneath an unrecognizable mass of Ideas and Concepts which the stimulus has drawn to itself from the previous content of the Mental Self. The resulting verbal statements of the imaginative person have no objective validity for the very reason that the mental material which they contain has been drawn forth from the subject's own Mental Self. And the imaginative statements have little logical coherency because the material has been drawn together and assembled about the stimulus Idea, not by Compliance-Dominance reactions (logic) but by Inducement-Submission responses which depend upon chance alliances between the new Idea and certain parts of the previously existing Mental

Self. The mental response of Imagination, in short, forms a precise counterpart of the emotional response of Passion. When a rich young man responds with uncontrolled erotic passion to a beautiful dancer, let us say, without waiting to react, first, with Desire for adequate and suitable means for forming a love union with the girl, or with satisfaction toward the present parental supply of money, such Passion response is bound to be impractical, ineffective and futile. It is just the same way that a mental response of Imagination lacks all correspondence with objective fact when Imagination takes place immediately without previous Grasping or Comprehension of the stimulus Idea.

Children, at certain stages of their mental growth, are normally addicted to " creative " Imagination responses, without previous mental Grasping or Comprehension of new Percepts and Ideas. This uncontrolled Imagination results, of course, in untrue statements, " fairy " stories and other imaginative reports of things that never happened. This normal stage of development of the child mind might properly be described as " mental adolescence." This occurs, of course, long before physical adolescence since the mind is now thought to be nearly mature at the age of fourteen or sixteen.

" Artistic " individuals, " geniuses " of various types, " aesthetes " and " impressionistic " persons, especially women, represent adult personality types wherein Imagination response is developed at the expense of mental Grasping or Comprehension. In " creative artists " Imagination is adequately balanced by and combined with the appetitive type mental processes, with constructive results in the artist's own special field. In other fields of endeavour, however, a typical artist is likely to manifest an over-balance of Imagination activity, at the expense of mental Grasping and Comprehension, with proverbially impractical results.

Explanation

This process may be regarded as the complement of Imagination, in just the same way that the compound emotional response of Captivation is the complement of Passion, both being composed of the identical primary elements, Inducement and Submission. Explanation is a compound of *active* Inducement and *passive* Submission, thus containing the converse phases of both primaries to those composing Imagination. While the Mental Self strives, in Imagination, to surrender its innermost treasure to the attraction of the stimulus Idea, the same self attempts, during the response of Explanation, to draw forth for the stimulus those parts or materials which can be made to blend most harmoniously with Thoughts and Concepts already present in the Mental Self.

The word " Explanation " is used to designate this type of compound mental reaction, not because it is a completely satisfactory term, but because it is a very broad term in popular usage, reasonably free from conflicting psychological meanings. To be sure, it becomes necessary to note certain possible confusions in its use as here proposed. The word " explanation " may carry with it, to some minds, the suggestion of verbal responses, or actually spoken words uttered for the purpose of explaining something to somebody. " Explanation," as we use the term, includes only the thought process or mental part-reaction which must always precede coherent verbal exposition, but which is not by any means always succeeded by spoken words or even by subliminal " twitchings of the larynx." In fact, the compound thought process which we propose to call Explanation, may finally expend its neural energy, and complete the unit response of which it is a part by gross physical actions of very different sorts.

Suppose, for example, that a timid person is awakened from deep sleep by sounds like footsteps just below his bedroom window. He peers anxiously through the darkness, but can see only a vague shadow moving on the lawn below. His mind first begins to Imagine, and then to Explain, both of these responses occurring without any preliminary Grasping or Comprehending of the stimulus. He imagines a human form below his window, and explains the stimulus as a burglar. But these mental reactions are not followed by any sound whatsoever from his larynx ; in fact, the mental responses of Imagination and Explanation which have taken place both produce a strong motor effect of inhibition upon all his bodily movements. The poor fellow scarcely breathes lest the imagined intruder shoot with the revolver which is part of the mental " explanation " already completed.

Suddenly, however, the well-known cry of a courting cat breaks the silence of night. The anxious householder cannot actually see the object on the lawn below any more clearly than before. But new mental responses of Imagination and Explanation are set up, with very different Thoughts resulting, and with great differences, also, in the final bodily reactions of the subject. Still quietly, and without a single spoken word, he reaches carefully behind him for his shoes, finds one, and hurls it fiercely at the shadow on the lawn. A new type of feline screech attests the accuracy of his markmanship ; two cats leap out into a patch of light from the window ; the house-holder's mental responses change from Imagination-Explanation to Grasping-Comprehension ; and verbal expressions highly derogatory to his midnight visitors follow tempestuously.

This illustration serves to bring out the point that spoken words are no more necessary or essential results of the thought process of Explanation than of C—D types of mental response to an identical stimulus. Nor do we believe it likely that the Imagination and Explanation responses above described took place, mentally, in the form of words ; the entire thought process was too quick for that. The mentally created burglar probably entered our subject's consciousness in the form of a visual rather than an auditory image, or, more likely still, he was an Idea. In short, the troubled householder's Explanation of his vague Percept did not take the form of " saying to himself " : " There is a burglar ! " but rather of *thinking the Idea* " burglar," or a broader Idea, " danger," of which " burglar " might be a part. Words, we believe, have no peculiarly significant connection with the compound mental response of Explanation.

There are very many forms of Explanation response which play important parts in every-day human behaviour ; in fact, the marked tendency to *explain* unfamiliar phenomena before *comprehending* them constitutes one of the most frequent and widespread sources of intellectual error in human thinking. One of the best-recognized instances of such importunate Explanation response is the reaction called " rationalization." A girl sees an attractive boy on the beach, hurries into her most abbreviated swimming suit, and strolls slowly along the shore with seeming insouciance. The condition of the tide calls to her attention the fact that it will not be time to swim for several hours to come, and she responds to this Thought by mentally Explaining that she put on her swimming suit early to get a sun bath. The girl " rationalizes " her own conduct, in short, by substituting the more pleasant Explanation reaction for the more difficult and unpleasant response of comprehension. We say that she " is not honest with herself " ; and we really mean that Comprehending her own motives and emotions is an unpleasant type of thought process from which she shrinks, reacting, instead, with the more agreeable Imagination-Explanation sequence of mental activities. Because there are very many occasions when all of us lack the courage to Grasp and Comprehend the real facts about ourselves, yet find ourselves compelled by the force of the stimulus situation to respond to it mentally in some fashion or other, we very generally fall into the bad intellectual habit of rationalizing, or Explaining our own behaviour in such a way as to preclude both ourselves and other people from Grasping and Comprehending it. In certain types of psychopathic cases, large and important complexes, and even secondary personalities may be built up as a result of such exaggerated and perverted use of Explanation response.

Examples of strong and well-developed Explanation activity may be found in the mental behaviour of scientific researchers, certain types of applied mathematician, economists, criminal investigators, special article writers, political economists, and others. We may note that Explanation response, when it occurs in the thought processes of these types of efficient worker, habitually predicates itself upon preceding mental reactions of Grasping and Comprehension.

The Complex Response of Realization

We have already noted, in the examples given above, that Explanation naturally follows Imagination, just as Captivation, on the emotional side, normally overlaps and succeeds Passion. During the compound mental response of Imagination, the new, or stimulus Idea is in control, and the submission of the Mental Self is active, its Inducement passive. As Imagination gives way to Explanation, the Mental Self begins to assume the controlling role by more and more actively inducing suitable mental elements in the stimulus Percept or Idea to blend into and unite with previously existing parts of the Mental Self. The Self's Inducement, then, changes from passive to active, and its Submission changes from active to passive, thus causing Imagination response to change gradually into Explanation reaction. In the instance of the imaginary-explanatory cat affair, discussed in the preceding section, it would be very difficult to tell just where Imagination left off and Explanation began. But as soon as both these mental reactions had occurred in their natural sequence and blending, one into the other, the householder suddenly *realized* that the intruders on his lawn were love-making cats. Without essentially altering the ordinary word meaning, therefore, it seems justifiable to use the term Realization to describe that complex, but very common mental process which combines Imagination and Explanation in successive but overlapping sequence. The unit response formula for Realization would then be : Mental pIaS + aIpS = R (R being the symbol for Realization).

Realization means, literally, making something real to the subject. This seems to be a fair subjective description of the consciousness which results from the successive combination of the mental responses of Imagination and Explanation. Common experience informs us that we may both *grasp* and *comprehend* a mental stimulus without regarding it as *real* to our Mental Selves. But when Imagination has supplied the stimulus with an adequate context from our own minds, and Explanation has united the new thoughts with our old ones, the new Idea or knowledge becomes truly real to us ; that is to say, the complex mental process whereby the mental stimulus assumes intellectual reality may properly be termed Realization, from both subjective and objective points of view. When we have mentally grasped and comprehended a fact, we *know* it ; when we have treated it imaginatively and explained it, we *realize* it, having united it in complete alliance with the Mental Self.

Intellectual " Creative " Responses : Origination

The simultaneous combination of Grasping (pC aD) and Imagination (pI aS) result in the originating of new thoughts, ideas and concepts in just the same way that the combination of Desire (pC aD) and Passion (pI aS) result in the emotional unit response of Origination. In the intellectual combination of responses resulting in intellectual Origination response the acquisition of mental material is made for the sake of the Imagination of new ideas, just as emotional Desire is controlled by Passion, so that Desire is felt on behalf of the statue or other object to be produced rather than for the self.

Transformation

Comprehension (aC pD) may combine simultaneously with Explanation (aI pS) to make the intellectual response of Transformation. This corresponds to the emotional combination of Satisfaction (aC pD) and Captivation (aI pS) which makes emotional Transformation response. In the intellectual reaction, Comprehension of the new mental material is undertaken for the purpose of Explanation in terms of the individual's own ideas and concepts and mental imagery, when the two combine to transform the new mental material into new meanings. In the same way Satisfaction of the child's needs is sought for the purpose of captivating him and controlling his behaviour so that he will be transformed into new personality or physical developments.

Mental " Functions "

We have now considered the six classes of integrative relationship that may take place within the correlation system and also the most important or typical intellectual unit responses that may occur there. From the point of view of an objective psychology based upon the neurological integrative phenomena occurring in the human body, the foregoing discussions constitute a description of the chief elements to be considered under the head of the Thought-processes. There remain, however, further mental processes, sometimes called " functions " after their designation by the older functionalist school in psychology which believed that the science should be investigated from the direction of these supposed specialized functions.

Among such " functions " we have already considered the processes of Association (which we believe is not a thought-process at all), Perception, Conception and Abstraction. In the chapter on Learning we have explained the objective activities involved in Learning, Retention and Recall, the latter two being the activities which are comprised in the " function " of Memory. With regard to these it is only necessary to add that the conscious activities that go by these names correspond, for an objective psychology, to the energy manufactured at the psychons engaged. There remain several other mental " functions," however, to which a brief space must be allotted.

Imagery

If Imagination is a mental process it may well be asked what part images play in it, for, verbally at least, they seem to have an intimate connection. We must now consider what an image is.

In the first place, when afferent nerve impulses, coming from the various receptors, cross the psychons in the central sensory centres, sensation arises. Similar impulses in the sensory centres may, however, be centrally initiated in recall processes rather than enter from the receptor nerves, and in this case the resulting consciousness at the sensory psychons is not sensation but sensory imagery. It is subjectively sharply differentiated from sensation by reason of the fact that sensory imagery is not projected outward (except in the phenomenon of eidetic imagery) and its qualities attributed to external objects as in sensation ; the cause of imagery is recognized as being within the body rather than outside it.

The same sort of process may be carried further and result in mental imagery. When groups of impulses from the sensory centres, such impulses having originated in the usual way from the organism's receptors, integrate in the correlation centres the result is a Perception ; and when, in recall, similar impulse-groups similarly integrate, the corresponding image arises. This sort of process can take place not only in regard to Percepts but also as regards Concepts, Abstractions, Introspections and Attitudes, although in these cases it is not customary to speak of the repeated integrations as images. All of these elements, however, may take part in various kinds of Imagination under the same guise as the sensory images ; it is at this point that Memory enters into Imagination.

Concentration

A more characteristic mental " function " is Concentration. In Concentration we may suppose that the involved impulse-groups effect activities in a relatively small number of correlation centres ; many such impulse-groups will converge upon a limited number of centres. The result will be a high degree of psychonic energy-intensity arising in a strictly localized area, with the characteristic intensity-effect of Concentration in subjective experience.

Attention

A special case of Concentration is Attention. There is almost always a " focus of attention " in mental activity ; it is unstable and constantly in motion, as it were, and at some times there is a " higher degree of attention " than at other times. The focus of Attention at any given moment will be in those centres where most impulse-groups are being integrated and where, consequently, the greatest amount of psychonic energy is being generated. Thus Attention may be focussed within the sensory or motor systems as well as in the correlation system at different times ; Attention itself is only the subjective name given to the phenomenon that occurs when a preponderant amount of psychonic energy is present in one locality rather than another within the organism. Attention may " wander " and even disappear entirely when it happens that there is no especial concentration of psychonic energy at any particular locality.

It will be impossible in the present chapter to give further space to the many other functionalist designations which, in any event, are nowadays receiving much less prominence in psychology than formerly. We will merely propose that where the named " functions " do not refer to the general psychonic conditions of the organism, as in the case of Attention, their detailed explanation is to be found in various combinations of the primary integrative activities of the correlation centres.

The General Psychonic Theory of Thought-processes

When nerve impulses pass out of the sensory centres, they enter the correlation centres of the cerebrum. The psychonic theory of Thought states that when these impulses, now within the correlation centres, cross the correlation psychons, they arouse at those definite points that special kind of psychonic energy that, in subjective experience, is Thought.

Integration has an extremely important place in all Thought-processes ; and integration takes place at the psychons. The various kinds of Thought that we have distinguished depend primarily upon the different types of integration to be found within the correlation centres.

Thought, in the psychonic theory, is subjectively defined as the awareness of relationship ; not of relationship in general, but of the relationships that can occur between the six principal combinations of correlation impulses. Such relationships, or integrations, can be of four primary kinds, corresponding to those that, in the motor centres, go by the names of Dominance, Compliance, Inducement and Submission. These may be combined in various proportions, giving compound integrations ; and the whole extended range of the various combinations that can occur, results in the well-recognized complexity and subtlety of Thought-processes. From the objective point of view our position is that Thought as such *is* the psychonic energy thus arising at the correlation centres of the organism.

The Function of Thought in the Unit Response

We have already made it plain that Thought is a part-reaction within the whole unit response. What then is its relation to, and its function within, this whole of which it is a subordinate part ?

The primary function of Thought is identical with the primary function of the correlation system within which it arises. That is, it serves as the *connection* between the sensory and motor systems ; moreover, its most important attribute is that it forms a *selective* connection between these. The fact of selection is based upon the essentially integrative character of the correlation system and its integrative character is based again upon its physical structure. It is not merely a series of connecting nerves, however complex ; it is a vast accumulation of synapses, containing millions of psychons within its limits.

Thus it comes about that the impulses entering the correlation system from the sensory centres, are not simply transferred across to the motor centres. These impulse-groups are combined with other entering groups and also with those which they find already passing through the correlation centres upon their own arrival. The result is a selective process that permits some of these impulses to reach the motor centres only in greatly modified form ; others are passed through with less interference, and still others wiped out entirely. Then there is a fourth kind of occurrence in which the entering impulses are caught in a sort of whirlpool motion and continue to circle within the correlation centres for a long period before eventually making their exit into the motor system in some later integration.

Certain phenomena, involving a sudden release of energy when no adequate stimuli have been recently presented, occur especially in pathological cases. In some of these instances we may suppose that a group of impulses has been circling about in certain correlation centres ; in other instances this may take place in the motor centres, but in either case the effect is as if a considerable amount of potential energy had been stored up. Such energy can be released by adequate stimuli entering through the sensory centres ; the adequacy of the entering stimuli will be determined by their ability, when combined with the already circling impulse-groups, to effect an exit into the motor centres and through them to the efferent nerves. But in the case where no such new (stimulus) impulses enter, the same result may occur by reason of a lowering of the motor system threshhold for the circling impulse-groups. Such a lowering of threshhold may consist in nothing more than the temporary diminishment of the number of other correlation impulses seeking entry into the motor centres, or it may be due to many other factors of synaptic conduction entirely unrelated to the immediate effect of the sensory centres upon the correlation centres. In these terms, then, we have an explanation of the puzzling phenomena offered by such sudden and apparently uncaused energy releases.

In conclusion we may point out that the tremendous number of psychons present in the correlation centres of the organism give a fully adequate basis for all the subtleties and complexities that make up the sum total of our Thought-processes. It cannot be too greatly emphasized that the underlying principle of all Thought is *integration* and that Thought thus furnishes a very definite basis for the identification of mental processes with the phenomena of psychonic energy.

CHAPTER XVI

EMOTION

PART I: FEELINGS AND EMOTIONS

Introductory

We come now to a consideration of emotion, the last of the three chief divisions of conscious experience. There seems certainly to be something distinctive about feelings and emotional responses that sets them off from both sensations and purely mental activities and that has led to the attempt to deal with them separately in psychology. And if it is legitimate for the psychologist to place sensory and mental phenomena in different categories and to render a separate, preliminary account of them before combining such accounts in a final description of the whole organism in action, the latter of course constituting the only finally adequate account, then emotional processes also must have their separate preliminary treatment. In the actual phenomena of the fully operating organism there are not two, but three, distinct and distinguishable, fundamental elements; these are sensation, thought and emotion, and the last is just as distinctive in quality of consciousness as the others.

Although emotion seems to be perhaps more subtle than thought, even if it does not reach the complexities of the more involved introspective thought-processes, yet it appears not to have been considered so. In fact, while thought seems to have been considered more mysterious than it really is, emotion has suffered a contrary fate and has been dealt with in a much simpler manner than is adequate. Our first task will be to see how psychology has hitherto envisaged the essential nature of the emotional element in experience.

Previous Theories of the Nature of Emotion

During the modern epoch psychologists, almost without exception, have put forth the greatest exertions to force emotional phenomena into the patterns of some part or other of the sensory system. They appear to have held a compulsive belief that, come what might, this *must* be the solution ; and the most delicate experiments of the physiologists have been necessary in order finally to explode the most ingenious of the resulting theories.

By far the best known of such theories, the grandfather, as it were, of them all, was the famous James-Lange theory of emotion. Lange believed that he had traced the origin of emotion to the afferent impulses from the visceral musculature ; it was James who added that the sensations caused by such sensory impulses *were* the emotions. This position could be, and was, summed up in the following illustration : when you suddenly meet a bear while walking through the woods and precipitately take to your heels, you do not run because you are afraid, but you are afraid because you run. Such a statement held all the intriguing qualities of an apt and startling *bon mot* ; psychology was so thoroughly hypnotized by it that for the succeeding twenty or thirty years it has been quite unable to look anywhere outside the elements involved in this epigram for a solution of the problem. Even Dr. Watson, opposed as he is to Jamesian theories, has adopted a manual, verbal and visceral classification of reaction-systems, the last apparently corresponding to what is left of emotion under behaviouristic treatment.

In the chapter on Consciousness, in treating the nerve trunk conduction theory of consciousness, we have already mentioned the work of Sherrington on the transection of the vasomotor nerves in the dog, Goltz' work on emotional patterns and Cannon's investigations of bodily and visceral changes during emotional states, the three most important researches bearing upon the above theory. There have been other researches of a like nature, the underlying principle being to prevent the afferent impulses from the viscera from reaching the cerebral centres, either by cutting the nerve trunks through which they are conducted or by destroying those cerebral regions where they enter, the common assumption being that no sensation arises until the impulses have passed into the cerebral centres. The existence of emotion was judged in these experiments on the usual behaviouristic grounds, i.e. by the presence or absence of overt behaviour of the characteristic muscular variety. It was found that, although none of the afferent impulses from the viscera could enter the cerebrum, the animals experimented upon evinced the symptomatic reactions of emotion under proper stimulation of other kinds ; and it must now be admitted that emotion cannot be based upon such visceral sensations. This result has obviously done away not only with the James-Lange emotional theory but with all the many modifications and varieties of this parent-theory which have sprung up since. Emotion does not consist of particular visceral sensations or of sums or patterns of such sensations.

Another attribute of modern theories of emotion, almost as characteristic as the inclusion of the sensory element already noticed, is that they all seem to involve the motor mechanisms of the body. They have attempted to explain emotion in terms of sensation, but usually in terms of sensations originating from the motor system of the organism itself. The visceral sensations of the James-Lange and other theories arise, of course, from the contraction of the smooth, or unstriped, muscles of the viscera. Others who have dealt with emotion but have not specifically stated that they consider it to consist of sensations, nevertheless have also associated it with the motor side of response. Thus MacDougall has made emotions correspond to instincts, which are patterns of motor reactions ; he has proposed a list of thirteen instincts and a comparable list of thirteen emotions.

Naturally the behaviouristic position has also emphasized the motor mechanisms in dealing with emotion. We cannot avoid suspecting that behaviourism at bottom really denies the existence of emotion as such, in the same way that it denies consciousness and thought. The behaviourist seems to admit only that certain ways of behaving have previously been given names of emotions, for what he regards as descriptions of emotions are in fact descriptions of muscular behaviour. These behaviours fall into two classes ; first, there are the implicit visceral behaviours already mentioned above and second, there are Watson's three " unlearned " types of overt behaviour which he calls the " primary " emotions of fear, rage, and love. The latter, of course, are predominantly reactions of the skeletal muscular system. Both these classes of phenomena are obviously motor ; and the behaviourist's description of emotion in both cases thus falls into the category of the description of motor phenomena.

Of particular interest to us are the latest conclusions of

physiological research, as embodied in W. B. Cannon's report[1] of experiments designed to locate the neurological centres of emotional excitement. It is well known that the cerebral centres oppose the spinal column mechanisms in the activation of the organism, the impulses from the cerebrum checking those that originate at the base of the brain and the top of the spinal column, and vice versa. The latter are concerned primarily with the automatic functioning of the organism, the unconscious processes of digestion, blood circulation, and so on, and through these centers also the motor impulses pass out to the effectors.

Experiments have already established that in decerebrate animals (those in whom the cerebrum has either been removed or destroyed by accident or operation), the rage behaviours occur with less control than in the normal case. Cannon and his assistants used decorticated animals and found these behaviours still more greatly exaggerated. Thus it became evident that the centre for this type of behaviour does not lie in the cortex. Dr. Bard, one of Cannon's assistants, next applied himself to the task of successively cutting away the nearby structures and attempting to find the exact centre for this kind of behaviour. It was found that this centre lies in the posterior half of the diencephalon. The final conclusion was that the neurological centre for rage lies near the base of the diencephalon, probably in the sub-thalamus. The size of this dominating motor-emotional area, in the cat, is less than a fourth of a cubic centimetre.

The fear, joy, and grief behaviours also disappear after the removal of this centre by operation and it is to be supposed that this particular motor centre is concerned with the origination of those nerve impulses which secondarily cause the effectors of the organism to exhibit the behaviours generally termed emotional. Pathological human phenomena, in cases where these same structures have suffered lesion, are entirely in accord with such neurological conclusions.

In concluding his report Dr. Cannon remarks that the withdrawal of cortical dominance (by operation or otherwise) causes the emotional type of response to become prominent. Since cognitive consciousness is generally associated with the cortical neurons, it becomes evident that emotional conscious-

[1] *Feelings and Emotions : The Wittenberg Symposium,* by 34 Psychologists, 1928, Worcester, Mass. ; pp. 257-269.

ness must be associated with the sub-cortical centres. The theories of the peripheral source of emotional consciousness, from sensations following changes taking place either in the effectors or in the viscera, are not supported by the facts, whereas the ascertained facts point definitely to the sub-cortical source of such consciousness.

The fact that emotional consciousness has been connected, by careful neurological experiment, with motor centres of the between-brain, is of great significance from the psychonic point of view. Its significance, in fact, is so great that we urge the reader to obtain the reference cited and study it with care, since it is impossible to give anything like a full report of it here.

Motation

Let us look at the situation from the psychonic point of view. We have earlier adduced what appear to us to be proofs of the intimate connection between conscious and psychonic phenomena. There are subjectively three easily distinguishable kinds of consciousness, sensation, thought, and emotion ; and there are also three distinguishable types of psychon in the sensory, correlation and motor centres of the human body. Therefore, if the psychonic theory is correct in describing consciousness objectively as psychonic energy, some kind of consciousness *must* arise at the motor psychons, due to the psychonic energy there present. We can see no reason at all for supposing that consciousness of a sensory kind is related to the energies in such different arcs, removed as they are both by structure and function from the sensory apparatus of the body. Similar objections exist against equating these energies with consciousness of the correlative or mental type.

On the other hand, there is no other locality within the organism where we may look for that psychonic energy upon which consciousness of the emotional variety, still to be accounted for, can be based. Cannon's experiments, and others along similar lines, prove conclusively that the most intense and " primitive " emotional phenomena occur in that motor area of the brain through which *all* the outgoing motor currents of the central nervous system are forced to flow, and within which centres, therefore, these motor excitations undergo the most concentrated integration. In view, moreover, of the neurological experiments cited above the conclusion appears to us to be inevitable that the psychonic energy arising within the motor centres, objectively *is* emotion.

The subjective, conscious aspect of this energy includes feelings and emotions, both of which have sometimes been included under the single term, affect. Due to the fact, however, that this word is both a noun and a verb and also that its various derivatives are commonly used in so different a sense than the foregoing, we think it best to employ the term, Motation, for that general kind of affective consciousness which includes both feelings and emotions. We must now deal with these two respective kinds of experience.

Feeling

Since we have decided that Motation consists of the psychonic phenomena at the psychons of the motor centres, we must now theoretically sever the connections between the correlation and motor systems and in the present chapter consider only what takes place in the latter. This is comparable to our treatment of the sensory and correlation systems in the chapters on Sensation and Thought.

Having done this, we can see at once that the phasic stimuli for the motor system will consist of correlation system end-results, i.e. they will consist of those impulse-groups or patterns which come through the correlation centres adjacent to the motor system and enter the latter for the first time.

At the same time such impulses will not represent the total energization of the motor centres. From before birth until death the musculature of the body has to be *continuously* toned up in order to resist the constant environmental forces of gravity pull, atmospheric pressure, and so on ; and this is accomplished by a mechanism which all the time keeps dispatching to the skeletal muscles what is known as the constant tonic discharge. This tonic discharge is a constant stream of efferent nerve impulses, sent out from the motor centres in the cerebrum and cerebellum to the muscles in question. Such impulses constitute a striking case of the self-activation of the motor system, as opposed to the fluctuating phasic stimulation ultimately derived from the passing and temporary events in the organism's environment.

Here then we find two quite differently originated kinds of impulses passing through the motor centres. By reason of the fact that these centres, just as the sensory and correlation ones, contain large numbers of integrating mechanisms, called synapses, integration *must* take place between these two varieties of impulses ; it takes place at the synapses, the specially energized portions of which are psychons. Thus the motor psychonic energy, like the sensory and correlation psychonic energies, is ultimately based upon integrative processes.

There are two fundamental ways in which the phasic and self motor impulses can stand in relation to each other during integration ; they can be allied or in harmony with each other, or they can be in conflict with each other. It is neurologically established that, when the entering, phasic impulses combine in a simple fashion with the self-impulses both these relations can occur without any perceptible altering of the volume of the existing self-impulses or constant tonic discharge.

We propose that integrations of this character correspond to the Feelings, sometimes called affective tones, of Pleasantness and Unpleasantness respectively. These two are the only Feelings proper, and of course they can also result from the total or combined effect of the many, more definite integrations, underlying emotions, that may be proceeding in the motor centres at the same time, depending upon whether such total or combined effect be one of alliance or conflict.

Both sensory and mental processes may be either pleasant or unpleasant. Thus when a group of impulses representing a sensation crosses through the correlation centres and produces a slight effect of alliance with the motor self-impulses upon entering the motor system, this sensation will be subjectively called a pleasant one, and vice versa. (Of course, at the same time an attitude will arise in the correlation arc through which this impulse-group has passed ; but in the cases where the impulse-intensity is so low as to result merely in pleasantness or the reverse, the activation of such a correlation arc may be so slight as to pass unnoticed subjectively, in the usual case). The same situation will hold for thought-processes, such as percepts, concepts, introspections, etc. ; these impulses, too, may achieve subsequent low-order integrations with the constant motor impulses, and thus be experienced as pleasant or unpleasant.

This kind of integration mechanism also accounts satisfactorily for the fact that the same colour sensation, for example, the same scene, or the same idea may on one occasion be pleasant and on another quite the reverse, since the impulses representing the sensory or other element in the integration, constitute only one factor ; the pattern of the motor self-impulses may in the second instance be quite different than in the first, making the integration itself of opposite type. And similarly, the total pattern of phasic impulses in the second instance, although it may include an identical former element, e.g. red sensation, may nevertheless include many perceptual, conceptual or other elements different than in the previous instance ; thus the total phasic pattern will be different and even though the motor self-impulse pattern be similar, the integration that produces the Feeling may be different.

We may make an interesting point here regarding the unpleasantness almost always associated with pain, the association that has caused so much confused reference to both sensation and feeling in the psychological discussion of pain. We have stoutly maintained that pain is a strictly sensory phenomenon and that it is not in itself either feeling or anything like feeling, but we acknowledge of course that there must be some unusually close relationship existing between the sensation, pain, and the feeling, unpleasantness. In this connection it seems to us significant that the existing evidence tends toward the localization of the sensory pain centres in the lower portion of the cerebrum and in close proximity to the thalamic motor centres, whence issues a part, at least, of the constant tonic discharge. No other specialized sensory centres have been located in so convenient a proximity to the motor system. Thus if we may suppose that, when the pain centres are energized by afferent impulses, these impulses may, and usually do, pass directly over to the motor centres without entering any correlation centres at all, and if we may further suppose that these impulses are usually of such a nature as to be in conflict with the constant tonic discharge mechanism of the thalamus, a supposition not at all difficult to make in view of the known inhibitory effect of severe pain stimuli upon this tonic mechanism ; if we may make these two suppositions, then the intimate subjective association between pain and unpleasantness becomes clear at once. It also becomes clear why pain is almost simultaneously felt to be unpleasant, apparently without the intervention of even the most brief mental process, since indeed no correlation centre activity would be involved. Furthermore, where extremely low intensities of pain impulses are concerned, there would be no bar either to an imperceptible or even to a partially allied effect of these impulses at the thalamic centres, such as might be supposed to underlie the subjective phenomena that occur when just distinguishable pain sensations are occasionally felt as indifferent or as very slightly pleasant. The corresponding connection between severe pain and fear will be considered later on in the following section on Emotions. Moreover, the psychonic theory of unpleasantness explains why any sensory or emotional experience, when it becomes over intense, becomes simultaneously unpleasant. Such over intensity of excitation in any cerebral centre must quickly overflow the normally integrated central paths, causing conflict and interference with the normal integrations in the crucial motor centres. This integrative motor conflict *is*, *ipso facto*, unpleasantness, according to the psychonic theory.

Primary Emotions

The idea of primary, or elementary emotions is a symptom of the usual scientific attempt to reduce whatever is dealt with, to its simplest terms. Just as the physicist seeks, in the physical world, to discover one, or at most some two elements which, when modified or combined in special ways will give all the items of physics and chemistry, so the psychologist, in the field of emotions, has sought to determine the smallest possible list of emotions, that in combination with each other will yield all the varied emotions experienced.

Among such previous lists those of the instinctivists have held an important place. We have alluded to MacDougall's list of emotions, corresponding to his list of instincts ; William James proposed different emotional categories and very many other lists can be found in the works of various psychologists. It is noteworthy that, while some of these lists bear resemblances to each other, none of them, so far as we know, are the same ; and the objective evidence adduced in support of them is so slight as to be negligible, being for the most part not objective but introspective.

In the case of the behaviouristic " primaries " of fear, rage, and love, the charge of subjectivism would be vigorously disputed, since the behaviourists pride themselves upon their objectivity.   Yet, as we have already seen, their overwhelming interest in motor reactions has led them to attempt to put everything, even thought and emotion, into terms of bodily (by which they really mean muscular) response.   We believe such responses to be both important and interesting, but we cannot avoid feeling that it is only another subjective prejudice to try to make them cover all the phenomena of psychology. The recent term, " Emotionality," appears to be but a more refined way of expressing the same fundamentally behaviouristic explanation of emotional phenomena.

The Primary Integration-types of the Motor System

But in common with these psychologists, whom we have criticised not because we feel no admiration for their accomplishments but rather because we cannot agree with their particular conclusions on this matter, we too believe that there exist certain primary, or elementary, emotions.   We believe this to be the case, not because we think it necessary on *a priori* grounds, but simply because the objective, integrative mechanisms wherein emotion arises, are found to be of such a nature that they produce certain fundamental integrations, such integrations being subject to further mutual and more complex combinations, in which they play the parts of elements.

We have seen that, objectively, emotion is the psychonic energy arising within the motor centres ; such energies arise because of the prime integrative function of the synapse, of which the psychon is a part, and these integrations fall naturally into four primary or fundamental classes.

How then may these fundamental integrations be described ? An integration involves a relationship between two or more elements, and we have noticed before, in the general case of the unit response, that the simplest relationships between the whole organism and its environment are those that we have called Dominance, Compliance, Inducement, and Submission.

Dominance integration means that the organism's self or tonic activity is in conflict with, but superior to, the phasic influences of environment.

Compliance integration refers to the situation where the self is weaker than environmental influences and in conflict with them.

Inducement integration represents the situation where the

self activity and environmental influences are in alliance with one another, with the self in a position of superiority.

Submission integration describes a state of alliance between self and environmental activities wherein the self activities are weaker than environmental influences.

Thus the organism plays the role of dominating, complying with, inducing or submitting to the environmental situation.

Great care has been given to the selection of the terms Dominance, Compliance, Inducement and Submission, for we believe that psychology suffers greatly from the use of a literary, introspective, and generally subjective terminology that is a distinct hindrance rather than an aid in the undertaking of genuinely scientific problems. In particular is this true in the field of emotion, where the names themselves of the various emotions are subject to the widest range of private interpretation ; and we are in the most complete agreement with the behaviouristic attempt to nail these words down and give them a strictly specific definition, although we feel that the behaviourists have not gone deeply enough into the interior functioning of the organism to complete their endeavour successfully. All modern languages without exception suffer from an inherent subjectivity which seriously impairs their value as media of scientific communication and we do not by any means believe that the four terms we have chosen as labels for the four fundamental types of possible relationship between the organism and its environment, meet the ideal requirements ; we urge them only because we feel that, within the usual limits of at present unavoidable subjective error, they best represent the actual, objective relationships involved.

We have seen how these same four primary types of relationship or integration have appeared again and again throughout the whole range of the human responses and reactions with which psychology must deal. In the phenomena of thought-processes, as well as in those of sensation, we once more discovered these integrations to be of fundamental importance ; and it appears evident that, so far as the underlying principles of their functioning are concerned, the main organic systems of the body, and especially the chief subdivisions of the central nervous system, are functional replicas, on a more restricted scale, of the whole organism. In the cases of these smaller subdivisions the large organism-environment situation is represented, on the one hand, by the patterns of constant, self-impulses proper to the given subdivision or by the existing state of stimulation present in it at a given moment, and on the other hand, by the patterns of entering phasic impulses that constitute the stimuli for that particular subdivision.

With regard to the third main subdivision of the central nervous system, namely the motor system, this situation holds very clearly. The constant, self-stimuli are due to the phenomenon of constant tonic motor discharge and the phasic stimuli consist of the impulse-groups entering the motor centres from the adjacent correlation centres. It is perfectly obvious that these two classes of impulses must be integrated at the motor synapses, whose principal function is such integration, and it is likewise obvious that during these integrations the two classes of impulses taking part can stand in four, and only four, type-relationships to each other. The self-impulse groups can be in conflict with and stronger or weaker than the phasic impulse groups ; or they can be in alliance with and stronger or weaker than the phasic impulse groups. In all these cases, since we are now discussing emotions rather than feelings, we are dealing with phasic impulse-groups integrating more complexly than those which, without altering the existing volume of the self-impulses, cause merely pleasantness or unpleasantness. The fact is well established neurologically that when these more intense phasic impulses enter the motor system, they cause an actual decrease in the amount of tonic discharge or self-impulses ; if they are weaker than the existing self-impulses, an actual increase in the volume of self-impulses takes place. The preliminary motor balance of the self-impulses within the motor centres at a given moment we may call the Motor Self ; this will correspond to the similar Sensory and Mental Selves of the other two main subdivisions.

As previously explained the resulting integrations will represent nodal or polar points in the entire integration circle. Any intermediate proportion of relative strength or weakness between the two elements in conflict or alliance with each other may as easily occur at this fundamental integration-level, but the points where the type-relationships between them reach their maxima will be taken for convenience as the " primary " points of the circle. The psychonic energy arising during any motor integration will be experienced subjectively as a particular emotion, and following both convenience and the already established psychological tradition we propose to label as the Primary Emotions those that represent subjectively the integrations of these four nodal kinds. The situation may be charted by means of the same sort of integration circle used elsewhere in this book in similar cases.

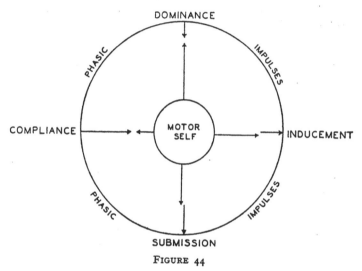

FIGURE 44

Elementary Types of Emotion Integrations

Dominance

In cases where the self-impulses are in conflict with the phasic impulses and stronger than they are, the latter will be forced, upon entering the motor system, to avoid the channels already being followed by the more powerful self-impulses. Since there is conflict and even although the phasic impulses are, on the whole, the weaker element, an increase in the self-impulses is necessary to overcome the phasic antagonists. Such increase has been shown actually to occur by means of various integrative reinforcement mechanisms.[1] Subjectively this situation will be experienced as the Primary Emotion of Dominance.

[1] W. M. Marston, *Emotions of Normal People*, p. 87, ff.

Compliance

When the phasic impulses are in conflict with the self-impulses but more powerful in total effect, the latter will be forced out of their own channels and made to comply with the entering impulse patterns by taking up a direction through the motor centres which leaves the phasic impulses free to follow their own path unobstructed. In this case also the volume of the self-impulses will be decreased. (Sherrington[1] has shown that no integrative reinforcement mechanisms exits in connection with anti-tonic reflexes). Hence there will arise the Primary Emotion of Compliance.

Inducement

It may as easily happen that the phasic impulses are in alliance with the self-impulses; and then the resulting integration between them will be of an harmonious kind. Both will be already predetermined to follow very similar courses through the motor centres, but we may assign the more influential role to whichever of the two impulse-classes is the more powerful. When the self-impulses are the stronger, the phasic impulses, already disposed to follow the existing self-patterns, will be rapidly drawn or induced into those patterns. In this process of induction, other integrative reinforcement mechanisms will be brought into play, and thus the self-impulses themselves will be increased in volume as a result of the integration. Here we will find the Primary Emotion of Inducement.

Submission

In a similar case, but where the phasic impulses compose the stronger element, an harmonious combination will take place in which the self-impulses may be said to submit themselves to the course-tendency of the entering impulse-groups. Here, as in compliance, we shall find a decrease in the self activities taking place during the process of submission to the phasic impulses. The resulting subjective experience is the Primary emotion of Submission.

It is to be noted that in the resulting overt behaviour of the organism there appear two varieties of each response, not represented in the emotion-circle chart. A dominant response

[1] W. M. Marston, *Emotions of Normal People*, p. 87, ff.

may be active, as when a situation or object is dominated by active exertions on the part of the organism ; or it may be passive, as when the same things are dominated by the resistance or immobility of the organism. An example of active Dominance would be the case of a policeman effecting the arrest of a fleeing gangster. An appelate Court might express passive Dominance toward the gangster, after he has been convicted, by denying his appeals for a re-trial. The same situation holds for the other three Primary Emotions (and in fact for Compound and Complex Emotions as well), so that we may write active Dominance aD, passive Dominance pD, active Inducement aI, passive Submission pS, and so on.

What distinguishes objectively between active and passive emotions is obviously whether or not the impulses forming the corresponding integrations achieve an outlet to the efferent nerves leading to the muscles of such a kind that active contractions result. It is not the *sensations* returning from these muscles which give the active or passive experience of the emotions, for these sensations have to do with the initiatory phase, not of the response we are now considering, but of the next succeeding one. What makes a given emotion subjectively active or passive is the psychonic energy arising at the *entrances* of the efferent nerve arcs where they begin in the motor centres.

The primary emotions may, of course, exist momentarily in pure form on infrequent occasions ; the integrations underlying them will take place almost instantaneously and be gone. During the time span of actual situations discriminated in real life the motor situation will be extremely complex ; not only will varying integrations succeed each other so rapidly that, as single units, they will probably pass undiscerned, but also various different type integrations will take place in different motor centres at the same time. A knowledge of the primary emotions therefore is principally important as a guide to the manner in which the compound and complex emotions are built up.

Compound Emotions

While there are probably not as many motor centres as correlation centres, there are nevertheless a large number of them, and it is not only possible, but almost inevitable, that at any given moment many somewhat independent integrations should be taking place within the motor system at different points. Due once again to the synaptic structure of the motor centres, such different integrative processes may be connected with each other through still another motor centre arc. If the separate integrative processes thus connected represent Primary Emotions, then the energy arising in the connecting arc (which it must be remembered is a motor and not a correlation one) will represent a combination of the Primary Emotion energies and will correspond to a Compound Emotion. Many such combinations of the Primary Emotions may occur.

It also seems highly probable that two or more primary integrations may occur simultaneously in the same motor centre, combining at once into a single, compound integration.

Desire

This is an especially important Compound Emotion, since it serves as the mainspring of the majority of Complex human emotions and very greatly influences the lives of all normal human beings. It occurs as a combination of active Dominance and passive Compliance and thus includes in itself emotional elements associated with both these Primary Emotions. Moreover, Desire may vary in its composition through a comparatively small range, and thus in a given Desire either the dominant or the compliant element may slightly over-balance its complement.

The simplest of all Desires is that which is experienced in relation to food. Desire for food must not, of course, be confused with the Hunger Sensation. The sensory impulses representing Hunger, after passing through the correlation centres, constitute only the phasic impulses involved in this desire. During the initiatory phases of Hunger, the receptors in the stomach become successively more and more activated, with the result of more and more intense impulses in the hunger sensory centres. The resulting impulses subsequently entering the motor centres from this source thus become stronger and stronger until they possess at the height of each hunger pang greater strength than the self-impulses there present. The existing condition of the motor system, and subsequently the whole train of existing unit responses, is therefore seriously interfered with. The result is passive compliance with the hunger pangs and an active dominance toward food to make strong Desire, and that this Desire is concerned with food is due to the function of the correlation centres which form the connection between the Hunger sensory centres and the Desire-activated emotional centres in this response, and which link the present sensory experience of hunger with memory traces of past satisfactions by means of food.

The nature of the Desire for food is such that the organism is forced to comply with the food by seeking it to the exclusion of all else or, if it be already present in the environment, by paying exclusive attention to eating it. At the same time the ultimate purpose of the response is that the organism shall dominate the food completely by eating and digesting it, i.e. by forcing the food to change its own nature and become part of the organism. The fact that the ultimate result is dominant in character makes the dominant-type relationship the controlling factor in Desire compound rather than Compliance. Thus the formula for this response is pC aD. This characteristic situation is first of all mirrored on a small scale in the motor centres, where the simultaneous mixture of the relationships involved in both Compliance and Dominance, when brought about by the entrance of a single kind of phasic Impulses (in this case the original Hunger sensations), gives that special emotional craving that we ordinarily call Desire.

Due to the role that is played by the correlation centres in the whole unit response, whereby Sensations, Percepts, Concepts, and so on, may become connected with Emotions, Desire may be associated not only with food but with innumerable other things, with clothes, jewelry, yachts, houses, etc., and even in abnormal instances, as we shall see later, with other persons.

Satisfaction

This is a Compound Emotion also involving the Dominance and Compliance relationships, but in this case the Compliance is active and Dominance passive, so that we may write: Satisfaction equals aCpD. Let us take, in illustration, the same example of food. When the food has once been eaten and begins to undergo the process of digestion, a noticeable change comes over the behaviour of the organism. The anxious seeking, the hurried feeding movements of the hungry person are gradually replaced by relaxation, ease, and complacency, nor, even if he attempted to do so, could this transition be avoided by the eater. The digestive process results in the stimulation of a great number of afferent nerves within the body, and sends many and powerful impulses through the sensory centres. From the standpoint of the. sensory system these impulses, since they originate within the body itself, are a form of self-stimulation, but when this same energy reaches the motor centres, it constitutes for them a group of powerful phasic impulses. Therefore, so far as concerns the motor centres and thus the emotions, the then existing motor self-impulses are forced to comply with the impulses originating from the digesting food. Nevertheless, the food is still being dominated and assimilated within the body, and in this the motor centres play a part, so that there is also engaged an element, though relatively a passive one, of Dominance. The peculiar subjective experience of this compound motor process is what we call Satisfaction.

Passion and Captivation

Passion is a Compound Emotion of the erotic type, another Compound Emotion of this kind being Captivation. In the old literary days of psychology Passion and Captivation were not distinguished. In fact, not only were these two aspects of erotic experience confused, but both emotions were described by the totally eroneous term " sexual emotion."

The adjective, sexual, refers to a difference between two types of organism, male and female. The term, sexual emotion, could therefore only be properly applied to an emotion which has its origin in sex differences. Love, or erotic emotion, is quite the opposite in this particular. Both types of erotic emotion, Passion and Captivation, seem to be of identical subjective quality in persons of both sexes. There is no reason to presuppose that the Passion felt by a woman is in any way different from the Passion experienced by men, or that the Captivation emotion of a woman is a different sort than the Captivation experienced by a man. The very fact that the erotic excitement experienced by both sexes has been given the same name, " sexual emotion," tends to show that the emotional excitement experienced, is thought of as identical in men and women. If, then, Passion and Captivation, like Desire and Satisfaction, are emotions felt by both sexes, they cannot properly be termed " sexual emotion."

Eros, the Greek god of love excitement, was worshipped

by the ancients. The term, erotic, is derived from his name. Therefore we shall use the term, erotic emotion, in our discussion rather than the more ordinary, but erroneous, term, sexual emotion.

All through literature, ancient and modern, we find descriptions of love pursuit and love capture. In many the woman is considered as the person pursued and the man as the lover pursuing. It has been assumed that when woman runs away from man, she feels the more passive sort of erotic excitement, while man feels the active, capturing excitement. A few writers of greater insight, like G. B. Shaw, have observed that woman, though she runs away, is really the captress, while man, for the very reason that he is led on by her fleeing charms, is the captured lover. This analysis represents the true psychology of the situation. Erotic capture is not made by dominant destruction of an opponent's resistance ; it is accomplished by irresistible attraction. Woman's proverbial love tactics of running away from man are merely designed to enhance her charms and make them irresistible to the extent that her lover will leave all other pursuits and follow her alone. Love is an attraction. The fleeing woman should be thought of as a magnet and her pursuing lover as a bit of soft iron attracted irresistibly by the woman's superior magnetic power.

Experimental and clinical studies have shown, as a matter of fact, that man's erotic emotions contain a prevailing element of Passion, while the erotic excitement of women is largely of the Captivation variety.[1] Passion is the self-surrendering aspect of erotic emotion. Captivation is the active, attracting aspect.

Passion is a Compound Emotion involving the relationships underlying both Inducement and Submission. Let us suppose, for example, that a man sees a beautiful dancer. He feels irresistibly excited and stirred up by this woman's grace and physical beauty. At one and the same time he wishes to give himself to this beautiful woman utterly, to throw himself at her feet and beg her to use him as she will, while simultaneously he feels a wish to seize her, to possess her, and to make her subject to his will. The first set of impulses are all submissive ; the second group are inducive. The

---

[1] W. M. Marston, " The Bodily Symptoms of Elementary Emotions," *Psyche*, no. 38, p. 70.

excited male wishes both to submit to and to induce the dancer. This simultaneous mixture of Submission and Inducement gives that special excitement which we call erotic emotion.

The control which beautiful women have always exercised over men has brought them kingdoms and vast fortunes. This control is based upon Captivation, which contains a prevailing element of active inducement. The emotion aroused in men who have thus yielded themselves to woman's erotic charm is Passion containing a predominant element of active Submission.

As has been previously explained, the female body possesses, with reference to the motor system, two types of stimulable genital organs, the internal and the external, while the male body possesses only the external type. Thus the possible motor impulse-groups with reference to these organs will differ in the cases of woman and man. Here is the real basis for the alleged distinction between the sexes in regard to erotic emotion. It is not that the emotions themselves differ. Erotic emotions, like all others, depend upon the activation of the central motor psychons that are the same for both sexes, but the genital organs of the two sexes are such that in one sex one of the erotic emotions will occur most frequently and in the opposite sex the other. Not subjective prejudices but the objective fact of organic structure determines that woman should be the leader in the love relationship ; her body is adapted by nature toward this end, while the male body is so designed as to submit to woman throughout the love experience.[1]

The Compound Emotion of Passion is to be thought of as predominantly a male emotion. It is the emotion of the soft iron irresistibly attracted to the magnet. Passion has been described again and again as a mad wish to surrender oneself to the control of a lover. The controlling emotional ingredient of Passion is the wish to submit completely to the lover's control. The longing of Passion is the longing to be subjected—to have the beloved accept the homage and services of oneself as a love slave. Passion springs from the predominant emotion of active Submission, which over-rides and controls passive Inducement in the Passion mixture. So far as the present writers know, the emotional nature of Passion has

[1] W. M. Marston, *Emotons of Normal People*, p. 317.

never been clearly emphasized in literature, and as a result of psychology's failure to point the way, both character studies and plots depicting the emotion of Passion have nearly always confused this emotion badly with the active phase of erotic emotion, namely Captivation. The heroine has at one time been shown leading her man on, teasing him with every love device known to the daughters of Eve and altogether bewildering him with the power of her love charms. At another moment this same woman may be shown as yielding herself completely to the dictates of the man, throwing herself literally or figuratively at his feet and accepting his superior love leadership in the consummation of their union. This literary error has not only spoiled many a good story but has seemingly thrown considerable confusion into many psychological discussions of the erotic emotions. Psychology has been written largely by men, who are perhaps unconsciously reluctant to concede woman's supremacy even in the matters of love.

It is only too true that women have always laughed up their sleeves at the love hokum retailed to the world by male authors who made their heroes superior to their heroines in fictional love affairs. During the Victorian age especially, love stories depicted the heroine as a clinging vine, a yielding violet and a sweet, obedient housewife carrying out her lord's commands. The fact that women who were betrayed into following this formula in everyday life frequently lost their husbands to other women who did not, necessitated the hastily trumped-up idea that this was one of the regrettable " ways of the world " ; it was one of those instances wherein the submissive woman's ideals of love somehow failed of fulfilment in a still unredeemed world. Of course the trouble was not with the world but with the typical Victorian incompetence for understanding the world as it is. The dancer, the show girl, the flirt, in fact the natural female captivatress who continued to flirt with her husband after her marriage as well as before, got her man and held him, because this is the way nature happens to have designed it.

Woman possesses the superior love power, the irresistible erotic attraction of the magnet. When she cuts off this magnetic power and tries to make herself into a bit of soft iron to be attracted by what little love magnetism the male possesses, she enters upon a disheartening experience. For one thing, men do not take any great interest in exercising magnetic love or Captivation. They soon tire of it. When any woman becomes a clinging vine and tries to submit to a man, she forthwith loses her grip on him and it is inevitable sooner or later that he should yield to the power of some other woman who continues to exercise her Captivation.

The emphasis upon Passion as a predominantly male emotion should not be construed to the effect that women do not also experience this emotion. They do, of course. Woman's Passion is probably much more profound and controlling in her life than is man's. Yet the woman successful in love affairs quickly passes from the passionate phase of erotic experience to the captivating aspect of the same love relationship. Woman's Passion occurs at the beginning of her love affair; it may persist throughout the affair, but it quickly becomes subordinate to Captivation.

As an illustration : when a young girl gets a " crush " on an older girl, her teacher, or some handsome young man, she experiences pure Passion. For the time being she does not dream of controlling in any way the object of her adoration ; it is beyond her thought that the beautiful senior or handsome college youth should yield to her or return her affection. If the object of her " crush " is some college boy, she perhaps makes herself thoroughly obnoxious to him by appearing in his path on every occasion. The boy's reaction of disgust and annoyance is a complete demonstration of the result of a feminine use of Passion as a love technique in affairs between the sexes.

The adolescent girl experiences these passionate emotions because her body has just developed into the beginning of its love capabilities. She has grown, in short, into the first stage of erotic emotion. A year or two later we find her quickly following her "crushes" with equally violent captivation attacks upon the objects of her admiration. She makes a conscious effort to control the affections of other girls for whom she feels an initial passion. She begins to subjugate young men by means of her personal charms. If she feel Passion in relation to a given young man, she immediately makes a special and ingenious feminine campaign to capture and control his attention. Girls at this stage have passed to the second and culminating love growth. They are now capable of both Passion and Captivation. True to their feminine nature, they quickly follow each attack of Passion with a greater and more prolonged period of Captivation.

With male lovers the Passion comes first in sequence just as with women, but this phase is greatly prolonged. The courtship, the long effort to succeed for the woman's sake, the process of striving to win her love favour is the man's typical part in the relationship, interspersed with brief climaxes of Captivation when the woman comes to his arms. Even in this embrace the predominance of captivation power is still retained by the woman, whose passive, magnetic role holds the balance of captivation power, while the man continues to show a predominance of Passion. It is only at the very last moment of the love-sequence that the man experiences the predominance of Captivation momentarily.

All these facts are simple expressions of the psychological laws governing these two emotions ; we have discussed them from the clinical view-point at such length because it is here that the greatest misconceptions are most widely spread and because we wish to show that in spite of current errors the behaviouristic evidence concurs in the view which the objective data of motor activation make necessary.

Indeed there can be no avoidance of the conclusion that as regards the love-type integrations (see next section) Passion and Captivation are as easily to be distinguished as are Desire and Satisfaction. In Passion the phasic impulses combine with the self-impulses in an integration containing simultaneously the elements of Inducement and Submission, but the Inducement is passive and the Submission active or predominant ; thus Passion equals pIaS. In Captivation the situation is reversed, although the elements remain the same, so that Captivation equals active Inducement, passive Submission, aIpS.

The self-impulses of the organism, originating from automatic stimuli within its own genital system, combine with appropriate phasic motor impulses caused by environmental stimulation of the genital receptors. In man the self portion of this combination of motor activities is of relatively low intensity but its supply remains fairly continuous. Woman's body has so developed as to genital structure that at times it is capable of a love relationship and at other times it is not ; the intrinsic stimulations of genital structures are periodic in function. The result is that this part of the stimulation of the motor centres varies in intensity in woman, at some times being much more intense than at others ; during the more intense periods, this stimulation is probably more powerful in woman than it ever is naturally in man.   From this it must result that, when men and women are left unmolested by spurious advice of the Victorian kind, the woman will be the periodic seeker of the love relationship while the man will be continuously receptive and prepared to respond with passion whenever his constant genital self-impulses are reinforced by the external stimulation due to the woman's presence.   Inducemnet naturally plays the important part in the woman's role and Submission in the man's ; thus Captivation, in which Inducement is predominant, will be the characteristic female erotic emotion and Passion, in which Submission is predominant, will be the usual male one.

Other Compound Emotions

Of course there are many other Compound Emotions besides the four we have briefly discussed in this chapter. In fact there will be as many of these as there are possible gradations of mixture of the four Primary Emotions.   Rather than attempting to give inadequate descriptions of a large number of such Compound Emotions, we have thought it best to use the available space in order to go fully into what are perhaps the four most practically important ones.[1]   It is more important that the principles underlying these relationships should become clear to the student of integrative psychology than that detailed accounts of a great number of named emotions should be discussed.

Complex Emotions

It is plain that the integrations representing Compound Emotions are of a kind that may be, in turn, still further compounded.   In other words, if two or more compound motor integrations are occurring at the same time at different places within the motor centres, they may be connected through still another motor centre arc, or complexly combined within the same motor centre.   Some of the resulting combinations of

[1] For discussions of other compound emotions with examples, see *Emotions of Normal People* and *The Art of Sound Pictures*. (by W. B. Pitkin and W. M. Marston).

integrative motor processes occur so frequently in experience and are of so striking a nature that they have long since received names drawn from the subjective experience of them ; such combinations of less complicated emotions we propose to call Complex Emotions. A Complex Emotion may contain as its constituent parts a Primary Emotion and a Compound Emotion, two Compound Emotions, a Compound and another Complex Emotion, and so on. As will be seen, the prime integrative function of any synaptic system here too, in the case of the motor centres, leads to great complexity.

Appetite

We have seen that Desire is a Compound Emotion described by the formula pCaD ; Satisfaction similarly is aCpD. In the usual case, e.g. in feeding, these two Compound Emotions follow each other in the sequence Desire-Satisfaction. This may be written pCaD +aCpD, and such a process, considered as a whole we propose to term Appetite, written A. Appetite will therefore be a Complex Emotion, and care must be taken not to confuse it with the Hunger Sensation, as is sometimes done. Desire will be the active aspect of Appetite and Satisfaction the passive aspect ; we may then write pCaD =aA ; aCpD =pA ; aA +pA =A.

Love

This also is a Complex Emotion, built up in a fashion similar to that of Appetite. Passion, pIaS, is the passive aspect of love ; Captivation, aIpS, is the active aspect. Thus pIaS =pL and aIpS =aL ; and pL +aL =L. As we have seen, in the situation where the love relation achieves completion, Passion, in the cases of both man and woman, precedes Captivation, but eventually is replaced, though only momentarily in man, by Captivation. It is the entire process, considered as a whole, which is properly to be called Love.

In these complex emotions the factor determining whether they are to be considered active or passive is the role played by the Motor Self. In Desire, for example, which is pCaD, the element in which the Motor Self predominates is D, and in this combination it is active. Thus Desire =aA. Similarly the Motor Self again predominates in D in the case of Satisfaction, which is aCpD ; and Satisfaction =pA. In the love-type emotions Inducement is the element in which the Motor Self predominates, and so we have Passion (pIaS) ⟶pL and Captivation (aIpS) =aL. The case is similar with whatever other complex emotions we chance to be dealing.

Creation

Reference to the earlier chapter on Drives will remind the reader that Creation responses are of two categories, termed Origination and Transformation. The corresponding part-reactions of the motor system involved in these responses, that is, the emotional components of the responses, consist of the same type-integrations but now on a smaller scale, since they occur entirely within the motor centres. Such part-reactions give the Complex Emotions of Origination and Transformation, which together constitute the Complex Emotion of Creation. Origination is a combination of the Compound Emotions of Desire and Passion ; thus pCaDpIaS or, as it might also be written more concisely aApL =O.

Likewise Transformation is a combination of the Compound Emotions of Satisfaction and Captivation ; aCpDaIpS, or pAaL =T. Origination emotion arises during such a response as the making of a baby by a mother, or the creation of a statue or painting by an artist, the originator being the active force in the process ; and so O =aCr, or active Creation. On the other hand the creative process of educating or moulding the developing responses of a growing child present the case of Transformation emotion on the part of the mother, who is a creative transformer ; and here the chief activity must be put forward by the child. The instructor, or transformer, may guide and instruct in the necessary principles, but it must be the student or child who furnishes the crucial energy by actively following the instructions or absorbing into himself the proferred information. Therefore Transformation is the passive aspect of Creation emotion and T =pCr ; aCr +pCr =Cr.

It is not our intention to go into these complexities too deeply in the present chapter. What it is important to note is that the same general principles of integration, only on a more involved scale, underlie the Complex Emotions as form a basis for the simpler Primary and Compound Emotions. In the section on Abnormal Emotions, to follow, several further examples of Complex Emotions of this type will be given and these should make the governing principles sufficiently clear.

CHAPTER XVII

EMOTION

PART II: INTEGRATIVE THEORY OF ABNORMAL EMOTION: AND THE PLACE OF EMOTION IN UNIT RESPONSE

Appetitive-type and Love-type Motor Responses

BEFORE entering upon a discussion of Abnormal Emotions it will be necessary to point out a very convenient distinction holding in general between two classes of all the preceding emotions considered. If reference be made once more to the integration-circle diagrammed earlier in this chapter and a line be drawn from a point midway between Dominance and Submission to another point midway between Compliance and Inducement, all the reactions represented above this line will be of the appetitive type and all lying below, of the love type.

The appetitive type, of which Dominance and Compliance are the chief and simplest examples, are connected with all the self-seeking activities necessary to the maintenance of the individual's bodily existence and personal welfare. In the natural course of events they are, or should be, principally directed toward *things*.

The love type reactions, examples of which are Inducement and Submission, are of an entirely different kind. The chief aim of such responses is not the welfare of the subject but of the object; and they are naturally directed by the individual toward *persons* rather than things.

Just as in the unit response situations the appetitive responses involve conflict between persons and things or persons and persons, while the love responses involve harmony and alliance, so in that smaller replica which is the motor centre within a single organism, the appetitive part-reactions involve conflict between the motor phasic and self-impulses and the love-type reactions involve alliance.

433   2F

The fact that in some cases each of these two general types of response is natural and in some cases not, brings us to a consideration of Abnormal Emotions.

Abnormal Emotions

In introducing the term, abnormal, we tread indeed upon dangerous ground. We feel no hesitation in saying that there are few words in our subjective language that are more widely misused, both colloquially and scientifically, than the two terms, normal and abnormal. Since it is not possible that these words should now be dropped from psychology, we have no recourse except to inquire into the matter of their incorrect employment and to endeavour to put forward what we believe to be their correct use.

The most obnoxious instance of the misuse of the term abnormal, and one which is very prevalent, consists in its application to those persons, things, or customs which the speaker happens to dislike. Thus we find our straight-laced moralists bandying about words like abnormal and perverted, and applying them to those who, from any sort of an objective view-point, are obviously more healthy than their accusers. On all sides we find similar, if less flagrant, abuses of these adjectives, whereas it is plain that to employ such words simply in accordance with subjective prejudice is no more than a malicious impudence.

It is a cause for congratulation that among responsible psychologists the foregoing misuse is noticeably absent. Nevertheless, we cannot but feel that the current use of " abnormal " in psychology is a mistaken one. At present the idea of abnormality seems to be hopelessly confused with the entirely different idea of a departure from the average ; what is average is supposed to be normal and what is not average is supposed to be abnormal, although objectively it is quite possible that the average may be the most abnormal of all and any departure therefrom, *ipso facto*, in the direction of the normal.

A well-known psychiatrist recently went so far as to state that if a young girl attended a school where a majority of the other girls smoked and drank, while she herself failed to adopt these habits, she would be sufficiently abnormal to warrant psychiatric observation and treatment. The more completely conformable to environment, no matter how injurious the environment may be, the more normal, apparently. In this connection we might point out that the population of the insane asylums in the United States at present is rapidly increasing, although we do not know whether this movement will continue or not. Supposing it to continue, the time might come when the majority would be lunatics, at least technically ; if this time should come, the psychiatrist just mentioned would be obliged by his own definition to pronounce the lunatics normal and the rest of us abnormal. Our argument may be in the form of a *reductio ad absurdum*, but it would seem also to prophesy a serious crisis for the psychiatric profession.

Of course the current misconception of the " normal " cannot be destroyed so flippantly. Not only those who deal directly with what is now called mental abnormality, such as the psychoanalysts and other psychiatrists, but also the great majority of general psychologists seem to be oblivious to the connotation of " normal " as distinct from " average." The rapid spread of mental testing procedures in recent years has acquainted psychologists with the fact that, whenever a given population is scored for the possession of certain general kinds of abilities and the results graphed, there invariably appears what is called a " normal distribution curve." This curve simply represents the fact that the majority of a given population have certain general characteristics, such as height or mathematical ability, to a medium degree, whereas there are also small minorities that either possess very little of these characteristics or else possess them to an unusual extent. Aside from the fact that this type of curve always appears in some form or other, no one seems to know why it should be called a *normal* curve ; if one enters a certain building in Coney Island, the floor will always immediately commence to wobble under his feet, yet this is by no means a normal, or even a usual, characteristic of floors elsewhere. In the same way, the fact that certain specific abilities or traits are possessed by a majority of the persons living under the conditions of Western civilization at this particular time of the world's history, has nothing whatever to do with the other question as to whether such possession is humanly normal or not. There is good reason to believe in fact, that some of these traits, for instance the over-suggestibility which the majority of the " unthinking public " possess in high degree, are distinct symptoms of an abnormal condition. The abnormality of the hypnotic trance does not at all depend upon the number of persons who happen to be hypnotized at a given moment.

If it is incorrect to designate as normal the central portion of the usual or average distribution curve obtained, still more is it wrong to suppose that a position at the tapering ends of such a curve rather than at its bulging middle is evidence of abnormality. With the best of intentions we can see no more in this assumption than an application in science (of all places !) of the democratic belief that it is somehow creditable to run with the biggest mob, or of that other pathetic persuasion of democracy that a thousand ignoramuses are more likely to be right than is one expert. In short, we feel that this matter is important ; and we also feel that the current assumption of the identity between the normal and the average is scientifically pernicious.

An entirely different approach to the question of the normal would seem to be necessary. We believe that there is a definite standard of normality inherent in the structure and the effective functioning of each species of organism. Human beings normally have two legs ; even if by some extreme chance one were fated to pass his whole life on a remote island in company with four other humans, of whom three were freaks possessing but one leg, we still believe that a sufficiently searching biologic investigation would eventually be able to establish which were the normal and which the abnormal men. In other words, the matter is entirely one of organic structure and functioning ; it has nothing to do with the chance examples that happen to come under scrutiny. Though individuals may vary tremendously one from another, all may still be normal as long as all possess the structures native to their species, with these structures functioning in a natural and harmonious relationship to one another.

In the case of the emotions, human beings are considered by the writers to be normal if they possess the full number of emotional capacities natural to the human race, and if these emotions are so balanced and inter-related that they function together harmoniously and effectively. If any human being lacks one of the emotional capacities natural to the race, he is to be considered abnormal. And if, while possessing all, he nevertheless develops maladjustments or unnatural elationships between any two or more emotions with the result that they do not function naturally or in harmony, he is to be considered emotionally abnormal in this respect.

Normality, as we think, has nothing whatever to do with the emotional average of a group or race of human beings, nor is abnormality related to the variations of different individuals from this average. The normal person is considered to possess all the natural emotional capacities which human beings should naturally have, functioning in a 'smooth and harmonious relationship.

There is another confusion which persons accustomed to the erroneous use of the word, abnormal, may fall into. All human beings in the world probably possess some emotional abnormalities ; most of them possess a large number. We experience from time to time the abnormal emotions of Rage, Fear, Jealousy, Anger, and Hatred. But the mere fact that a man experiences Fear does not make him *on the whole* an abnormal person. Even the emotions of Dominance and Compliance which are disarranged for the moment in such a way as to result in Fear, are still usually under the control of the natural environmental influences. Therefore we say that he is on the whole normal. But we add that he is experiencing for the moment the abnormal emotion—Fear.

This psychological distinction between the individual as a whole and the separate unit response tendencies going to make up the personality of that same person, corresponds precisely to the medical distinction between normal and abnormal, or healthy and diseased, people. A physician may pronounce a man to be on the whole a healthy person. That same individual may, however, possess a slightly infected finger or an abnormally (which is not the same as an unusually) shaped eye-ball, giving rise to a slight myopia. The man as a whole is said to be normal and healthy ; but in some minor particulars he is abnormal and diseased.

It may be startling to some that no one in the world is ever completely healthy in body or normal in mind and emotions. This, however, is undoubtedly the case. Our bodies are continuous hosts to myriads of bacteria which feed upon our blood and tissues. As long as our regenerative processes rebuild these tissues fast enough, we continue on the whole to have the appearance of health. But if any human being were free from all unhealthy or abnormal physical conditions, it is probable that he would never grow old and even that he might never die. Likewise, all human beings suffer continuously from some minor emotional abnormalities, of which Fear, Rage, Hatred, Jealousy, and Grief are some of the evidences which vary in their potency and their detectability. We may even suppose that if any person could be thoroughly normal in his emotional feeling and behaviour, there would be no such thing as suffering and unhappiness in his entire experience.

Between the four Primary Emotions there may be both normal and abnormal relationships with regard to the purpose with which these emotions are connected. When these emotions do not occur simultaneously but successively, *in the normal relationship Compliance is followed by Dominance and Inducement is followed by Submission.* When we deal with Compound or Complex Emotions, we have to do with integrations that contain simultaneous combinations of the type-integrations of Compliance, Dominance, Inducement, and Submission. In such cases, *when the emotion is normal, Dominance plays the preponderant role in the Compliance-Dominance combinations and Submission plays the preponderant role in the Inducement-Submission* combinations.

There are, of course, innumerable actions which express all four Primary Emotions in their correct and normal order of succession. The following illustration describes the normal relation between the Primary Emotions. A clinical psychologist quietly questions his patient and passively observes his behaviour during many preliminary consultations. He then collects his notes and observations, concentrates his thought upon the entire case, and makes an analysis of the patient's mental difficulties and maladjustments of personality. The psychologist next begins to persuade the patient to change his course of action in accordance with professional advice. In the end the psychologist removes the patient's emotional difficulties and effects a more normal and efficient organization of his personality, thereby improving his life and increasing his happiness.

In the behaviour of the psychologist during this treatment we see expressions of the four Primary Emotions in their proper order :

1. Compliance
2. Dominance
3. Inducement
4. Submission.

The psychologist begins by complying completely with the patient's existing state of personality and emotion, a method strongly advocated by Alfred Adler among others. He accepts the patient just as he is and merely observes and records his condition. Next he analyses and reconstructs the entire personality picture. He attempts to understand the patient's personality and to master its hidden maladjustments. Here he dominates by overcoming the difficulties and resistances with which the patient is blocking his comprehension of the latter's personality. He then persuades his patient to behave in a new way prescribed by the psychologist, a process which is clearly Inducement. Finally, the psychologist, by means of Inducement, removes the patient's personality difficulties and thus serves the patient as he most wants to be served. This ultimate action expresses the Submission which is the psychologist's final purpose in undertaking the case. In this whole case Compliance made Dominance possible ; Dominance in turn furnished the basis for Inducement, while Inducement finally accomplished the ultimate purpose, which was Submission to the patient's needs and his requests for the psychologist's help.

Fear and Rage

Our subject in the present section is abnormal emotions and we have only given the above illustration in order to throw light upon what happens when such normal relationships suffer reversals. By far the commonest of the unnatural states that give evidence of such reversals are the Compound Emotions of Fear and Rage.

Fear accompanies flight or involuntary withdrawal from some threatened danger or suffering. Fear and Rage are both composed of the elements of Dominance and Compliance in the wrong relationship to each other. In the normal Compound Emotions of Desire and Satisfaction, Dominance over the environment or stimulus object is the final end of the response and constitutes the ultimate object toward which the behaviour in question is directed. In Desire, for example, the Compliance with hunger pangs or with the food that will quell them, is only temporary, and is the means to a dominant end. Similarly, in Satisfaction, though there is far more Compliance here than in Desire, Compliance is still held in check and ultimately replaced by Dominance. Dominance over our environment means that we control it ; we successfully assert ourselves over inanimate objects which either threaten or serve us.

But ultimate Compliance with our environment means just the reverse ; here the environment has the upper hand, In so far as we ultimately comply with an inanimate object stronger than ourselves, we suffer defeat which is accompanied by some degree of self-destruction or injury. Deliberately to seek compliance with our environment as the ultimate end of action is deliberately to act in such a way as to diminish our own power and defeat ourselves. Therefore, while Compliance is a necessary part of the Compound Emotions of Desire and Satisfaction, it is the subsidiary part of both these normal Compound Emotions. In any Compound Emotion combining Dominance and Compliance the latter serves the former with relation to the purpose of the action which is accompanied by the emotion in question. But when Compliance gets the upper hand, we get an emotional reversal, an unnatural or abnormal relationship between the Primary Emotions concerned. In such a case we dominate for the ultimate purpose of complying. The bare statement of this reversal shows how unnatural and even ridiculous it is, yet this is precisely the situation in both Fear and Rage.

In Fear, we feel compelled to comply with an overwhelmingly strong opponent ; we feel unable to resist it. And our ultimate purpose is to give in to this threatening object for the purpose of escaping injury or pain. In order to escape from or comply with the dangerous object we must, of course, dominate it sufficiently to comply with it.

Take, for example, the woman who sees a mouse. She shrieks, lifts her skirts and jumps on a chair. All these acts express Dominance. Yet at the same time such dominant acts have the purpose of enabling the woman to escape from the mouse with which she feels compelled to comply. She does not feel able to give battle to the mouse or to try to dominate it finally. She merely wishes to dominate it just enough to make good her escape and her compliance with its threat.

Here we see the reversal of emotional elements which gives rise to Fear. Ultimate defeat is accepted at the beginning of the action, and Dominance is used only to make good the ultimate concession to a stronger antagonist. The subject thus permits himself to feel ultimately inferior to the danger or threat in question, while at the same time he feels a mad, dominant urge to act desperately in order to carry out his Compliance with the given danger. He experiences Dominance and Compliance in a relation of conflict, the Compliance gradually defeating the Dominance that has assumed a subsidiary position in the Compound Emotion. This gradual defeat is extremely unpleasant ; and Fear is the most unpleasant of all emotional sufferings. It is far worse than the sensory pain that is threatened. And since it represents an emotional reversal or conflict, it renders the experiencing person less efficient and less vigorous. Fear in itself is definite proof that the experiencing individual is already partly defeated in his own motor-centres.

Here is a case that illustrates rather completely the bodily weakness resulting from intense Fear. A robust Alpine climber was sitting on what he supposed was the edge of a cliff, when suddenly he saw the ice swept away by an avalanche a few feet from where he sat. He thus perceived that he was dangling his legs from a thin shelf of sheer ice that might give way at any moment. He experienced a devastating Fear. He could not move for several minutes. He seemed paralyzed. Finally he managed to roll over on his stomach and to creep back inch by inch, still half paralyzed according to his own description. The moment he reached solid earth he fainted and was unconscious for about ten minutes. When he recovered he could neither stand nor walk, and it was several hours before he could proceed.

Rage is a reversal emotion in which, as in Fear, a wrong relationship is established between Compliance and Dominance with respect to the purpose of action. It has frequently been pointed out that there is a great similarity between Fear and Rage. William James emphasized the fact that Fear often turns into Rage when all hope of escape is finally cut off. The cornered rat will fight and manifest all the behaviouristic symptoms of extreme Rage. The sneakthief caught in robbery may fly into a futile spasm of Rage during which he may shoot the person interfering, merely as an expression of his fury.

There is much more Dominance present here in proportion to Compliance than is the case in Fear. But Dominance is still controlled by the forced Compliance with an object which has threatened the wrathful person. When an individual discovers that escape from a threatening object is impossible, the total situation compels him to dominate the enemy by aggressive attack in order to carry out the already accepted purpose of escape or compliance. Under these conditions, the Dominance aroused in carrying out the hoped-for compliant purpose is vastly greater than before other and easier means of escape were cut off. In fact, the entire primitive Dominance emotion of the animal or person thus trapped is called into play, still controlled by the realization that defeat has already been inflicted by the opponent. This awareness of irretrievable defeat gives a bitterly thwarted and hopeless self-abandonment to the prevailing Dominance, and this constitutes the peculiar emotional quality of Rage. Rage is Dominance expressing itself with conscious futility, turned partially back upon itself in a fury of impotent over-aggressiveness. It is a conflict between tremendous Dominance and a controlling compulsory Compliance which, though bitterly resented by the person cited, is accepted as the inevitable end of the whole behaviour pattern.

Rage reduces the efficiency of action chiefly by injecting an element of wildness and self-abandonment into the dominant behaviour of the wrathful individual. Many a prize-fighter has been defeated in the ring by a nimble-witted opponent who has deliberately excited him to self-abandoning Rage. The insult is passed while the fighters are in a clinch. The insulted boxer " loses his temper," " flies into a rage," and the spectators observe that he no longer keeps his guard up or makes any attempt to sidestep his opponent's blows. He rushes in blindly " with blood in his eye." His clever opponent welcomes this abandonment of boxing skill, increases his own defensive caution, and at the same time takes instant advantage of every weakness uncovered by the angry boxer ; he plants a well-conceived uppercut with all his reserve force, and the fight is over.

Habitually cautious or timid persons frequently come to believe that Rage is a useful emotion. This is because they cannot arouse themselves to sufficient Dominance except when they are cornered ; the only Dominance they ever experience takes the inefficient form of Rage. Occasionally the usually sweet and mild-mannered person surprises his friends by his sudden wrath, making them give way before they can recover from their astonishment. Or perhaps it happens that the Dominance-component in such attacks of Rage is sufficient to overcome an obstacle that would have been insuperable otherwise. In either case, the Dominance aroused is sufficient to accomplish its purpose *in spite of* the handicap of wildness or self-abandonment in the Compound Emotion. The habitually mild-mannered person fails to realize, however, that he overcomes these obstacles not because he flies into a Rage, but rather because he thus arouses an adequate amount of Dominance for battle. He wins in spite of the element of thwartedness or Compliance which controls his Dominance, not because of it.

Jealousy and Hatred

These are Complex Emotions, involving conflict or reversal between Appetitive-type and Love-type Emotions. Jealousy is a conflict-relationship between the Compound Emotion of Desire and the Primary Emotion of Submission ; Hatred is a conflict between the Primary Emotion of Dominance and the Compound Emotion of Captivation.

Jealousy arises in any situation wherein we experience a conflict between Desire for an object or person and Submission to the person who stands between ourselves and our possession of the desired thing. It may occur either in appetitive rivalry, such as business, or in connection with alleged love-affairs. We use the word alleged advisedly, because there can be no such occurrence as jealousy in actual love. Love is the giving and not the taking ; it is solidly based upon Submission. It is only when Desire creeps into such an emotional relationship that Jealousy becomes possible. If we wish to possess the loved one for our own pleasure more than we wish to submit to the beloved's happiness, then we have a situation in which Jealousy arises.

If we wish to possess a person, a thousand dollars, a house, or anything whatsoever, and another person proves himself superior to us in obtaining the desired object, we are confronted by two emotional possibilities. We must either submit to the person who has proven himself superior or we must continue to feel Desire for the object that we have lost. Jealousy arises when Desire is the ultimate purpose of action, for here there is a conflict between Desire for the object and Submission to the superior person who has obtained possession of the desired object. If Submission is the ultimate purpose of action, we experience the emotion customarily termed " good sportsmanship." We feel a generous admiration for the successful rival. Our desire, which has been realized by another person only enhances our admiration for that rival's demonstrated superiority, but if admiration for the rival is superficial and trifling in comparison with the continued desire for the unattained object, a conflict between Desire and Submission is inevitable under the controlling whip of the appetitive emotional elements.

Certain schools of fiction, especially Victorian ones, portray Jealousy as a proof of true love. This mistaken notion maintains that a lover can always tell when a woman begins to fall in love with him by observing when she begins to be jealous of other women. There is just enough truth in the theory to keep it alive long after psychology should have disposed of it. It is unfortunately true that, in proportion as a person becomes erotically attractive and pleasing to us, we often begin to feel a desire to possess that person for the sake of enjoying his or her body or society. Thus Desire is frequently evoked as a secondary result of " falling in love." Under these unnatural emotional conditions, Jealousy manifests itself soon after Desire takes control of the situation. But the normal conditions of love emotion are correctly shown in those quite different stories where a woman's love remains totally free from Desire and Jealousy, expressing itself in loyalty and self-surrender to the loved person even though he prove unfaithful, undependable and generally worthless. We may feel that such a woman is foolish to waste her affection upon a sot, but that it is *love* that she is wasting, no one can possibly doubt.

Hatred, like Jealousy, arises from a situation wherein the Appetitive-type emotions control the Love-type emotions toward other people. We may recall the literary axiom that " hatred is akin to love." Many writers have correctly described the turning of love to hatred when the loved person has proved treacherous or unworthy of affection. In a situation of this sort, the once-loved person arouses two separate emotions simultaneously in the injured individual.

Here is an actual case. Helen and Alice were intimate friends. They confided in each other, and each believed the other was submitting to her with the utmost loyalty and affection. Enter Gladys. She first showered her attentions upon Alice. Alice adored Gladys, and confided all her feelings to her friend, Helen. Soon, however, Helen began to win the affection of Gladys. This went on for some time until at last Alice came to believe that Helen had betrayed her confidence. She accused Helen of treachery and bad faith. (This, of course, is already evidence of Alice's abnormal emotional condition, since, except for a Desire toward Gladys, she would not have wished to possess her alone.) Alice convinced herself that during the time Helen had appeared to be her best friend, she had, in fact, been dominating her (Alice) for selfish purposes. The final act of Dominance on Helen's part was, of course, her " stealing " of Gladys affections from Alice. Whereupon Alice conceived a violent hatred for Helen, the girl whom she had formerly regarded as her most intimate and submissive friend. Alice had a conflict between the emotion of Captivation by which she believed she was holding Helen's friendship and the emotion of Dominance suddenly evoked by what seemed to Alice a deliberate injury inflicted upon her by Helen. Dominance controlled Captivation, and the result was Hatred. Had Alice continued to feel Captivation toward Helen, she would not have felt Hatred but rather a continuance of friendly interest and a sincere wish to help her give up her supposed treachery or disloyal conduct for her own sake.

When Dominance and Captivation are experienced simultaneously, this active type of emotion results. When Dominance controls, Hatred, the most destructive of all emotions, results, due to the fact that in this conflict Dominance defeats and destroys Captivation, just as the person who entertains Hatred for another, strives desperately to hurt the person hated. Indeed the person who feels continued Hatred, destroys his own peace of mind and emotional balance far more effectively than he destroys the well-being of the person whom he hates. Hatred is a two-edged emotional sword, cutting both the hater and the hated. It is responsible for the most cruel and destructive of wars. It disrupts families, communities, and nations. Civil war is notoriously more bitter than war between foreign nations because of the greater friendship or mutual Submission which existed between the two parts of the same country before the beginning of the war. The greater the love, affection, or friendship preceding the

Hatred, the more violent and destructive will be the subsequent Hatred, because of the more violent conflict between Captivation and the destructive Dominance in control.

The Objective Nature of Abnormal Emotions

We have explained and illustrated the foregoing Abnormal Emotions at considerable length because we feel that their ubiquity and prevalence in everyone's life renders them a topic of the utmost importance for the student of the psychology of the emotions. For the purpose of making as clear as possible the reversals of emotional relationship underlying them, we have put our discussion in purely subjective terms, because these will be better understood by the average reader. It now remains to show the entirely objective facts of motor functioning that give rise to the subjective experience of the reversals already described.

The principal, natural function of the self-impulses of the motor system is to maintain the organism in a state of healthful functioning by activating the muscles of the body so as to make possible the processes of food digestion, elimination of waste products, rebuilding of worn-out tissues, tonicity against gravity and air pressure, and many other similar internal processes of the self-type. The secondary function of the motor system (in general, the role of its phasic impulses) is so to activate the skeletal muscles that they respond to environmental stimuli in ways calculated to prevent the undue interference of environment with the principal motor function. All this is accomplished by the maintenance in the motor centres of a certain motor-impulse balance, in which balance the constant tonic motor discharge plays a large part. Within limits this balance may vary, permitting many motor integrations of normal type ; but when it is definitely upset, so that the normal function above described is seriously interfered with, those integrations have occurred that objectively are the Abnormal Emotions. In fact, it is not because these emotions are subjectively unpleasant, but because objectively they impair the efficient functioning of the organism, that they are to be called abnormal.

As long as the organism continues to function at all, there must always be integrations in the motor centres between the tonic discharge self-impulses and the entering motor phasic impulses, because the organism must always be in some environment or other and all environments continually stimulate the motor centres through the receptors, the sensory centres, and the correlation centres. As we have already explained, such integrations may lead to a decrease of tonic discharge when the phasic impulses are superior to the existing self-impulses, and when they are inferior to them an increase of the tonic discharge may result. But when either decrease or increase is carried beyond a definite limit, the *organically efficient* balance of the motor system is upset.

In the motor appetitive-type integration of Dominance and the motor love-type integration of Submission, the relations of the impulses within the motor centres are such that the organism is most efficiently activated. In Dominance the self-impulses are strong enough to force the phasic impulses into the patterns already existing for the benefit of the organism ; in Submission, the phasic patterns are already in harmony with, yet control, the self-patterns, and so increase the combined self-impulses and phasic impulses to maximal efficiency. But our environment is not constructed in a way that permits continually of these types of integration with their compounds and derivatives ; accordingly the motor system has developed so as to be capable of Compliance-type and Inducement-type integrations, with the result that it is thus able to meet various environmental emergencies. Whenever the latter integrations are employed, a temporary decrease in organic efficiency results, but if the effect of their employment turns out to be an eventual reinstatement of the organically efficient motor balance, they can properly be looked upon, in such temporary and subordinate guise, as contributing to the normal functioning of the organism.

It is when Compliance or Inducement either determine the ultimate result of the integrative phenomena or play the preponderant role in a given integrative process, that they upset the necessary motor balance and more or less disastrously affect the whole organism. We find the first case when Dominance is followed by Compliance ; this would occur if, for example, the clinical psychologist in our earlier illustration had begun by telling his patient that he (the patient) was sick and abnormal, and had ended by himself adopting maladjustments of personality similar to those of the patient. Again we find a wrong end-result in a succession of responses when Submission is followed by Inducement, as in the instance of the prostitute who goes through love behaviour and subsequently induces payment. The second case (wherein the wrong element plays the preponderant role in a single response) occurs in the instance of Fear, where the Compliance aspect of the integration-process predominates and the self-impulses are overwhelmed to so great an extent that efficient movements of the organism can no longer take place, heart action and digestive processes also being gravely interfered with. Many other instances will be seen by the reader when he understands the simple principle involved. In all these cases the motor balance is overturned in one direction or the other, with the result that it can no longer play its normal role in the functioning of the whole organism and that, even within its own confines, conflict and violent reversals occur.

When the wrong appetitive-type element predominates, the balance is upset in the direction of self-impulse decrease, with all the disastrous effects seen in the example of the Alpine climber overcome by extreme Fear. Here we may also see the basis underlying the usual association between severe pain and fear. It will be recalled that the impulses from the sensory pain centres cross over, probably directly, into the motor centres of the thalamic region and there have the effect of conflicting with and decreasing the tonic discharge self-impulses. When these phasic pain impulses are of intense degree, the resulting motor integration is of an extreme Compliance type, the motor balance is seriously upset so that many of the motor physiological symptoms of Fear, such as interference with metabolism, trembling of limbs, and inefficient redistribution of blood circulation, result. Due to the mechanisms of retention and so on, sensory impulses, themselves not of the pain variety, can arouse pain impulses of the imagery kind ; thus the foregoing phenomena may occur, but to a lesser extent, when the organism is confronted with an object or situation of a kind that " threatens " severe pain sensations.

On the other hand, when the incorrect love-type element controls the integration, the motor balance is upset by an over-exaggerated increase of the self-impulse patterns, with the result that the functioning of the organism and of the motor centres themselves is now just as badly thrown out of gear by this increase as it was in the other case by the decrease.

As we have seen, such reversals of normal integration relation can take place, not only between the Primary and Compound Emotions, but also when the total motor condition is of a reversed kind involving both these and also Complex Emotions.

To illustrate what we mean by the objective abnormality of the motor system, or of any organic system, let us take the crude and over-simplified example of an ordinary piece of machinery. This machine, we shall suppose, is constructed on the following principles : it consists of a complicated set of many dynamos, including of course revolving armatures ; when revolving at 1200 revolutions per minute that amount of current is furnished for which the machine is designed ; and its lubrication and other appurtenances are made to function efficiently when it is operating at or near this speed. The chief motive power for the machine is furnished by a set of cog-wheels continually engaged with its main shafts ; the force transmitted through these wheels will correspond to the self-impulses of the human motor system. There are, however, large numbers of auxiliary cog-wheels, so arranged as to be capable of engaging the individual shafts of the separate dynamos within the whole machine ; when these wheels are shifted forward and subsidiary connections are thus made, the force transmitted corresponds to the phasic motor impulses.

Let us suppose that this whole dynamo-machine is functioning at its designed, or normal, rate activated by the main cog-wheels. Suddenly a set of auxiliary cog-wheels engage with some of its separate dynamos in such a way as to reverse their direction of revolution ; within the whole machine the resulting reversed currents will oppose the properly directed currents constituting its main output, opposing armatures will jerk and jolt, and the whole machine will jangle, definitely out of gear. Also, it now delivers less current than is necessary. In this case it is functioning abnormally.

On the other hand, if the auxiliary cog-wheels engage in such a way as not to reverse the direction of revolution of the associated armatures but so as to increase the rate of their revolution in the direction previously maintained, then these dynamos commence to whirr around at a more rapid rate than necessary or desirable ; a rising hum is given out by the machine, the lubrication system is unable to supply oil and grease rapidly enough to meet the new conditions, destructive friction results, and too much current is delivered by the machine. In this case too, it is functioning abnormally.

There is also a further and more usual way in which, when the auxiliary and main shafts are applying their force to turn their respective dynamos in the same direction, the efficiency of the machine as a whole may be reduced. In this condition of alliance between the " phasic " and " self-" forces within the machine, there will be a particular state of maximal efficiency ; this state will occur when all the energy of the main shafts, i.e. all the " self " force of the machine, is being utilized for the production of the machine's proper, final output. But when part of the energy derived from the machine's main shafts has to be utilized in order to maintain the continuance of the subsidiary energy derived from the assistance of the auxiliary shafts, the efficiency of the whole machine will be reduced ; and if this condition proceeds beyond a certain limit, its efficiency may be very seriously reduced.

Let us now see how our analogy will illustrate the statement that it is normal for Dominance to follow Compliance, Submission to follow Inducement, and not vice versa. Compliance is based upon a conflict reaction ; thus in our machine the Compliance-Dominance series begins with the engagement of the auxiliary cog-wheels with the separate dynamos within the large machine. The first result is the reversal of these dynamos, since this is a conflict reaction, the immediate effect being conflicting currents within the machine. Now the machine as a whole has devices for meeting such situations, and the one now brought into play has the effect of so changing the course of the machine's own, original currents that they are brought into agreement with the disturbing currents just established. This particular reaction constitutes Compliance, but since it is effected only by changing the course of the original currents which were formerly being directed in the manner for which the machine was designed, the end-result is to lessen the effective operation of the machine.

When such an interior change in the functioning of the machine has been brought about in the manner just described, an entirely new mechanism becomes activated. This new mechanism is designed to push away from contact with the machine those auxiliary cog-wheels whose engagement with some of its dynamos has caused the change in its unit functioning. It must be made clear that this pushing-away mechanism becomes activated *as a result of* the particular manner in which the efficiency of the machine has been reduced ; the reduction is what brings it into play, for otherwise it would itself result in inefficiency by using up some of the energy of the machine for a useless purpose. The process of pushing away the auxiliary cog-wheels constitutes Dominance, and when they have been pushed away, the contrary currents no longer exist within the machine and its own currents can now return to their former, most efficient courses. This is the normal sequence of Compliance-Dominance.

It is obvious that if the process be reversed and the pushing away is followed by the setting up within the machine of adverse currents which must be complied with by a diversion of the machine's own currents, the end-result will be a reduction of efficiency, rather than a return to efficiency.

In the Inducement-Submission series the auxiliary cog-wheels turn the separate dynamos in directions such as to increase the amount of current already being furnished within the machine itself ; that is, this is an alliance reaction. In the case of Inducement the engagement of these auxiliary cog-wheels is made, not by the cog-wheels coming forward to engage the dynamo shafts, but by the shafts being pushed out from the machine to contact the cog-wheels. Such pushing out of the shafts takes up some of the energy of the machine, which is thus lessened with reference to its primary function, the production of current for a different use. It is therefore necessary for the auxiliary shafts to resume their former position but in doing so, to draw with them the cog-wheels they have engaged by means of their extrusion. This is the process of Inducement. Having successfully accomplished it, the machine will then function most efficiently when it receives the auxiliary allied forces through these shafts but without further energy expenditure of its own in order to receive them. This is the case in Submission.

On the other hand, if such a state be the first and be then followed by the inducing process of extruding the shafts and endeavouring to pull in the cog-wheels, the end-result will be the diversion of part of the machine's energies away from their designed use, with a consequent inefficient functioning of the machine.

It will easily be appreciated that the question as to whether or not the machine is, in a given instance, functioning normally or abnormally, is not by any means to be decided by the opinion of a chance onlooker. Such a passerby may have a hum in his own ears and attribute the hum to the machine, thus concluding that it is running too fast. Furthermore it will be impossible to establish the desired fact by comparing this machine with others of a similar kind or with their contemporary average operation, unless we *already* know that these other machines are now operating normally. Such a knowledge can only result from an examination by qualified engineers ; as a *a priori* assumption, it is entirely unfounded and naive. In the same way our sole means of determining whether our special machine is performing normally or not, i.e. whether or not it is a normal machine, is to have it examined by experts who will decide the matter on a basis, not of private opinion or interest, but strictly in accordance with the structural design of the machine itself.

The human organism is a very complicated kind of machine, and its efficient functioning can be impaired in delicate and complex ways. Within the motor centres certain types of integrative processes occur, as a result of which the normal, organic functioning is seriously interfered with. Objectively, the psychonic energy arising during such integrations constitutes the Abnormal Emotions.

The Physiological Expression of Emotion

We trust that by this time the reader thoroughly understands that an emotion and its physiological expression are two entirely different things. The physiological expression, whether overt or implicit, gross or subtle, is no more the emotion than a broken window is the hurling of a stone. Still less is the emotion to be confused with the sensations that occur later as a result of such physiological expression. The emotion corresponds to an integration of nervous impulses at the psychons within the motor centres, and such integrations are usually, but not always, followed by the dispatch of the *resulting* nerve-impulse patterns over the final common motor pathway of the efferent nerves to the musculature of the body. But to imagine that the original integrative processes take place *for the purpose* of the subsequent reactions is to inject a subjective and primitive philosophical factor into a scientific description, a factor moreover which is peculiarly out of place in the explanation of an automatically functioning organism. The human organism, as we know it, does not respond to environmental stimuli because of some God-like intelligence inhabiting, but because it is already of such a design that it cannot avoid responding in the ways it does.

Nevertheless, there is a very simple and direct connection between emotion and behaviour ; they stand in the relation of cause and effect, even if not in that of purpose and accomplishment. Since motor integrations usually cause the subsequent contraction of the striped or unstriped muscles in the body and thus give rise to various kinds of external and internal behaviour, we shall list here the several physiological results of the four Primary Emotions, together with illustrative examples. Such lists and illustrations could be expanded, had we the space, to include the Compound and Complex Emotions also, but this is impossible in the present book.

In this connection it should be borne in mind that any given motor integration, or emotion, can vary greatly in its physiological expression, because of the quite different external situations in connection with which such an integration can arise. The phasic motor impulses involved in the motor integration may be visual in ultimate origin, or they may be tactual, or perceptual, or conceptual, or of any complicated combination of these or other kinds. By reason of the function of the correlation centres in the final response, the resulting behaviour will bear a relation to the exciting cause, unless the organism be so far deranged in its functioning as to be considered extremely abnormal, or insane. Thus Fear, or any other emotion, may be quite differently expressed on different occasions, although, so far as the motor centres are concerned, the integrations there occurring will in all cases of Fear, etc., be of the same type. With this warning against too simple an interpretation of a very complex set of phenomena, we will now continue with the above mentioned lists.[1]

Dominance :
A. Gross Behaviour.
   1. Physiological Expressions.
     a. Contraction of tonic skeletal muscles.
     b. Aggressive, antagonistic action of any sort.

[1] Reprinted from *The Art of Sound Pictures* by W. B. Pitkin and W. M. Marston, by permission of the authors and Messrs D. Appleton & Co.

2. Illustrations of behaviour chiefly expressive of dominance.

    a. A pioneer takes up a homestead on uncultivated land, far from friends and miles removed from urban civilization. He cultivates the land, builds a house, chops down trees, and finally manages to achieve a comfort-fortable living through his masterful dominance over natural obstacles.

    b. Jack Dempsey attacks his opponent for a knock-out at the climax of a prize-fight. Every muscle in his body is tense, his arms swinging with swift force. He delivers blow after blow in rapid succession. When his opponent goes to the mat, he stands over him, bent close to the floor, his clenched fist still moving back and forth like a piston-rod.

    c. A baby howling at the top of its voice and beating the sides òf its crib with hands and feet.

    d. A husband smashing his wife's pet china because she has told him she will not do as he asks.

    e. A lawyer tearing to bits the only documentary evidence of his opponent, stolen by the lawyer's detective.

B. Subtle Behaviour.

    1. Physiological Expression.

      a. Tightening of the jaw muscles.

      b. Clinching of the hands.

      c. Dilation of the pupils of the eyes.

      d. Increased strength and rapidity of heart beat.

      e. Increased action of sweat glands.

      f. Irregular breathing with a changed ratio of inspiration to expiration, showing more exertion in every breath.

      g. Rise in arterial blood pressure.

      h. Inhibition of digestive action in stomach and intestines.

      i Dilation of the blood vessels on the outside of the body and in the brain.

    2. Illustrations.

      a. A champion boxer making his opponent wait for him in the ring.

      b. Tunney staring superciliously at an intrusive newspaper reporter who has asked him some question about his private life.

      c A man about to be shot by Mexican bandits nonchalantly lighting a cigarette and smiling at the firing squad.

d. A man lighting a cigar with a thousand-dollar bill.

f. A woman whose husband has told her that she is nothing but a woman of the streets and that he is about to divorce her, replying with a rising inflection, " Really ? "

Compliance :

A. Gross Behaviour.

    1. Physiological Expression.

        a. General adjustment of the muscular tensions and gross movement of the body in such a way as not to conflict with the harmful influences of the environment.

        b. Relaxation of any of the tonic muscles of the body which are opposed to some threatening object.

        c. Contraction of the anti-tonic muscles, as necessary to withdraw any part of the body from the opposing object.

        d. Relaxation of the grip, especially of the hand most frequently used.

    2. Illustrations of behaviour chiefly expressive of compliance.

        a. Lindbergh ignoring newspaper attacks and the jeers of his friends and calmly waiting until weather reports are favourable for his solo trans-Atlantic flight. He ignores the various inferior and harmless forces acting against him but complies with the unbeatable weather force, though still holding himself fully prepared to act at a moment's notice as soon as these irresistible forces of nature are moving in a favourable direction.

        b. Gene Tunney, after being knocked down by Dempsey for fourteen seconds in the Chicago fight, boxes the round out with consummate defensive skill. Tunney " gets on his bicycle ", runs backward and away from Dempsey, side-stepping him cleverly and never allowing Dempsey to get within a knock-out distance of his body. This action on Tunney's part is not to be interpreted as expressing fear or cowardice, but rather compliant skill in the prize-fighting game under conditions where his opponent is temporarily stronger than he.

        c. Stepping off a railroad track when a train approaches.

        d. Withdrawing the hand from a hot dish.

        e. A swimmer who has been caught by an outgoing current ceasing to swim against the current and swimming with it or across it until he is free of its power.

B. Subtle Behaviour.
   1. Physiological Expression.
      a. Decrease in the force of the heart-beat, and either decreased or increased rate of heart-beat, depending upon other bodily conditions.
      b. Decrease in systolic blood pressure in arteries, and either decreased or increased dyastolic blood pressure, depending upon other bodily conditions.
      c. Drooling at the mouth with relaxation of jaw muscles.
      d. Increased secretion of saliva and other gastric secretions.
      e. Increased blood to the stomach and digestive organs and increased parastaltic movements of the stomach and intestines.
      f. Inhibition of genital activation.
      g. Occasionally, nausea, faintness, and relaxation of the bladder or involuntary movement of the bowels.
      h. Contraction of the pupils of the eyes.
      i. Contraction of the blood vessels that supply the tonic muscles on the outside of the body. Sometimes flushing of the face, neck, chest, and even of the abdomen.
   2. Illustrations.
      a. Shrugging the shoulders.
      b. A half-circular motion from the wrist upwards and outwards of either hand or of both hands, which may be accompanied by such a remark as " Alright, you win."
      c. The facial expression known as a moué.
Submission :
A. Gross Behaviour.
   1. Physiological Expression.
      a. Voluntarily permitting another person to dictate or control the tensions and relaxations of the tonic muscles all over the body.
      b. Voluntary acceptance of another person's control by permitting him to restrain or confine the body.
      c General decrease in tension of tonic muscles all over the body, with selective increase of some tonic and some anti-tonic muscles, as dictated by the person to whom the submission is being made.
   2. Illustrations of behaviour chiefly expressive of submission.
      a. Lady Godiva riding nude through the streets of Coventry in obedience to the command of her tyranni-cal husband for the sake of relieving the townspeople

from his tyranny. In this case the woman makes a double submission of her entire body and actions. First she submits to the commands of her husband, and second to the needs of her people. She voluntarily and willingly permits herself to be controlled throughout a complicated and unusual set of actions.

b. A girl slave kneeling voluntarily at the feet of her master or mistress.

c. A small boy wiping the dishes for his mother, doing so voluntarily and gladly in order to help or to please her. If he assists her either because of threatened punishment or promised reward, his action does not express submission, but rather compliance or desire.

d. A girl giving up a party because her mother is sick and needs attention.

e. A woman working all day over the washtub or sewing machine in order to clothe and feed her children. Of course, she dominates the machine or the sewing material in order to submit to the needs of her family.

f. A man doing Christmas shopping at his wife's request, or working around the house in order to please her and make her comfortable.

g. Sending flowers to a sick friend.

B. Subtle Behaviour.

1. Physiological Expressions.

a. Decrease in rapidity of heart beat and increase in its strength.

b. General decrease in stomach and digestive organic activity.

c. Increase in activity of genital organs with corresponding constriction of blood vessels in digestive viscera and dilation of blood vessels in genital organs.

d. Moderate increase in sweat gland activity.

e. General steadying of grip tension, blood pressure, and breathing at a moderate medium level.

f. General stabilizing and harmonizing of all the internal functions of the body in such a way that the maximum alliance or co-operation between these different functions is attained.

2. Illustrations.

a. Cleopatra on first making the acquaintance of Mark Antony is reported to have jested with him in the manner of a common soldier, exchanging somewhat coarse remarks and practical jokes. Prior to this, she had been accustomed to exceedingly cultured forms of wit in her relationships with Julius Cæsar.

Without any appearance of making an effort to please, she subtly altered the entire expression of her personality in submission to the preferences and tastes of Antony.

b. Throwing away a cigarette when an elderly lady who dislikes smoke, comes into the room.

c. A woman quietly and with apparent carelessness drops an expensive dish on the floor in order to make a guest who has just broken another valuable dish, feel comfortable.

d. Smiling at the dull joke of another person.

e. A girl permitting a man to make love to her (as in *The Trial of Mary Dugan*) not because she is attracted to him, but because she wishes to make him happy.

f. Many slight gestures, such as opening the hand, palm upward, waving a person forward ahead of one, smiling deprecatingly in order to make another person feel superior and at ease, nodding consent, etc.

Inducement :
  A. Gross Behaviour.
    1. Physiological Expression.
      a. Some increase in the tension of the tonic muscles with marked increase in the blood supply.
      b. Increased tension of the tonic muscles of the body selectively to convey the suggestion or persuasion intended, and especially increased excitement in the brain and vocal cords.
    2. Illustrations of behaviour chiefly expressive of inducement.
      a. A persuasive trial lawyer, like Clarence Darrow, having little evidence to offer on behalf of his client, nevertheless persuades the jury to render a verdict of not guilty. In a case of this sort, the lawyer allies himself completely with the emotions and minds of the jury, and then proceeds to convince them that his own emotional conviction and intellectual opinions as to the innocence of his client are superior to those which the jurymen already hold as a result of the actual evidence in the case.
      b. " Lord " Timothy Dexter, the eccentric merchant of Newburyport, Massachusetts, sent warming pans to the West Indies and persuaded native molasses dealers, very much against their inclination, to buy the pans and use them for molasses ladles. Dexter sold the entire shipload at a handsome profit.
      c. Missionaries persuading native Chinese to give up their own religion and to accept Christianity.

    d. A small boy inducing his mother to permit him to go swimming by arguing that he is old enough to be a " regular fellow " and should learn how to look out for himself.

    e. A wife inducing her husband to buy her a dress by patting his cheek, cooking his favourite dish, and flattering him.

B. Subtle Behaviour.

    1. Physiological Expressions.

       a. Increase in the strength and rate of heart beat.

       b. Marked increase in the systolic blood pressure, usually accompanied by increased dyastolic blood pressure.

       c. Dilation of the pupils of the eye.

       d. Increase in the secretion of the sweat glands.

       e. Marked decrease in the activity of the digestive organs and gastric secretions.

       f. Greater than average activity of the thyroid glands ; this is probably associated with the type of person feeling inducement, especially a woman who is an habitual inducer and who takes an almost constant interest in persuading other people to do as she advises.

       g. Increased excitement and blood supply to the internal genital organs.

    2. Illustrations.

       a. A man, wishing to persuade his plump sweetheart to diet, walks along the street with her, expressing his admiration of the thin girls whom he meets.

       b. " Fishing " for a compliment.

       c. A gesture of invitation toward bottles or other refreshments on the sideboard.

       d. A girl drops her handkerchief to induce a young man to pick it up and speak to her.

       e. Many of the methods of the mother in " Mother Knows Best " were subtle inducements intended to control the conduct of the daughter.

       f. A baby holds out its arms to induce its mother to pick it up.

       g. A number of minor movements and gestures, such as the " coquettish " glances of girls, arching of the eye brows, smiling sympathetically or provocatively, tossing the head, quick movements of the body such as flicking the skirt or suddenly turning the back toward the object of inducement, shrugging the shoulders, extending the arms, etc.

The General Psychonic Theory of Emotion

So much has already been said that a succinct statement of the psychonic theory of emotion will suffice here. As we have noted, the motor centres in the head form a distinct system comparable to the sensory and correlation centre systems. Here, as in the other two main divisions of the cerebral system, phasic and self-impulses are combined, or integrated, according to the usual principles of synaptic conduction. Such phenomena give rise to a characteristic form of psychonic energy at the motor psychons, with a resulting subjective experience of emotional quality.

This general affective kind of experience we have proposed to call Motation ; Motation includes both Feelings of pleasantness and unpleasantness and the Emotions. The various emotions, together with their respective subjective qualities, result from the various ways in which the integrations in the motor centres may take place. They fall into the several classes of Primary, Compound, and Complex Emotions, depending upon the degree of complexity of the respective integrations, just as varying degrees of complexity in correlation-centre integrations correspond to Percepts, Concepts, and higher degrees of Abstract Thought. For convenience in particular instances the various emotions can also be classed as of the Appetitive-type or of the Love-type ; they may further be classified as Normal or Abnormal, and this depends strictly upon whether they are integrally connected with the normal or the abnormal, the efficient or the inefficient, functioning of the motor centres themselves and of the organism as a whole.

That all motor psychonic energy is of the same rhythm or the same physical vibration-rate, is not necessarily to be supposed. Just as may be the case with sensory and correlation psychonic energy, the motor variety may also have a range of several octaves of vibration, which nevertheless will all be included within the general motor range. Thus a vast number of subjective emotional qualities, corresponding to the various sensory modalities, are to be accounted for. The complicated integration of complex impulses will, of course, give rise to motor psychonic energies of different and various vibration-rates.

In general terms the Integrative Theory of Emotions states that, from the objective point of view, whatever psychonic or integrative energy arises at the psychons of the motor system, *per se* constitutes Emotion.

Place of Emotion in the Unit Response.

In order to see clearly just where Emotion stands with regard to the whole unit response, let us work out briefly and in general terms the course of such a response, involving all three part-reactions of Sensation, Thought, and Emotion. In the first place the response is always made to environment ; and this means that all responses are initiated by stimuli from without the organism itself. Thus the first step is the arousal of impulses in the afferent nerves leading inward from the receptors. In the sensory centres these impulses become subject to selective integration-processes which determine which impulses shall get through the sensory centres and thus take a further part in the unit response. In the correlation centres a further selectivity takes place ; not all the impulses entering from the sensory centres will escape inhibition by the existing correlation impulses already present here. Those that are not inhibited, are combined in integrations with pre-existing correlation patterns, and only some of these escape a circling movement within the correlation centres, and by so doing become phasic stimuli for the motor system. Here once again in the motor centres, the entering impulses must escape inhibition and if they do so, must combine with the motor self-impulses already in possession of the motor centres. From these combinations the impulse-patterns finally result, which gain an entrance to the final common motor paths and activate the effectors of the organism.

Thus the sensory centres first determine what sensations shall be included in the unit response. Next, the correlation-centre psychonic phenomena determine what relationships between the entering sensations and the Mental Self shall be recognized in the responses. And finally, the motor centres determine what form the muscular activity, and thus the behaviour, will take. *The final effector and bodily movement is an expression only of that energy which the part-reaction called " Emotion," lets through the motor centres.* The whole process is automatic and especially is this so in the motor centres, where Emotion occurs ; the " central stimuli " from the correlation centres entering here must follow the set rules of synaptic integration and give rise to the determined patterns of impulses that at last win through to the effector mechanisms.

We may therefore see that Emotion holds a key position in the unit response. It is the final determiner of the exact form that the response shall take. This does not mean that it is more important than the other two divisions of Sensation and Thought, however, for even before the impulse-patterns involved in the unit response have reached the motor centres, the general form of the response may have been worked out by the sensory and correlation selection of those impulses that shall be the phasic ones for the motor system. But the final determination of the exact form of the resulting behaviour, together with the furnishing of the energy for such behaviour, is the function of Emotion in the entire unit response.

We may add that emotion, if the integrative theory be true, is more directly and immediately connected with the final bodily changes brought about by a given unit response than is any other preceding part reaction of that response. This means that the detection and measurement of bodily changes furnishes a far more accurate and reliable measure of the preceding emotion than it does of the preceding part reactions of sensation and thought. If we bear clearly in mind the qualification that bodily changes are symptomatic only of the algebraic sum of the integrative motor activities which compose the emotion itself, we may state with some assurance our belief in the scientific efficacy of measuring emotions by the comparatively easy method of measuring the resulting symptomatic bodily changes. Whereas it seems to us the idea of measuring thoughts or sensations by reference to ultimately ensuing bodily reactions is little short of impossible. Too many influential part reactions, and motational integrations with other unit responses have still to occur after the sensory and intellectual portions of any unit response have been completed. Human beings who behave wrongly " see the situation as it is " more often than not, and just as frequently they know what the " right thing to do " really is. But a sudden storm of emotion intervenes, and sweeps away accurate perceptions and straight-leading thoughts. The final bodily action—perhaps treachery, seduction, or even murder—may be a direct expression of the emotional part-reaction, very little modified by the sensations and thoughts that preceded.

CHAPTER XVIII

Emotion

Part III : Bodily Symptoms of Emotion [1]

Introductory

The very earliest observers of emotion noticed certain facial expressions and bodily attitudes which, as they put it, " express the emotion felt by the subject ". Darwin and other naturalists carried these observations of emotional " expression " much further and attempted to describe systematically the bodily changes which occurred during emotional excitement. Then the James-Lange theory, which maintained that bodily changes were all important, since they gave rise to sensations of which emotion was actually composed, stimulated anew the experimental interest in bodily accompaniment of emotion. Since psychology abandoned the theory of an immaterial soul, the term " expression " of emotions has gone somewhat out of vogue, because it is thought to imply a physical expression of some intangible state of the soul. The terms, " manifestation " of emotion, or " bodily symptoms " of emotion, seem better suited to current usage, though " expression " of emotion carries a perfectly tangible and concrete meaning under the integrative theory of emotion, as explained at length in the last chapter.

Practical motives, too, have led to observations and measurements of bodily symptoms of emotion. In medieval times the idea of trial by ordeal was accepted as a valid method of determining guilt or innocence. Various tests were employed, such as grasping red hot pokers or walking over live coals. The idea seemed to be that guilty consciousness would interfere with the healing of the body after such injuries, whereas

[1] Owing to the large number of references in this chapter the reader is referred for specific information to the Bibliography at its end, where they will be found included.

the wounds would heal readily if the defendant were innocent. The well-known method of testing supposed criminals in India by making them chew rice, represents another practical attempt of the same sort to discover the bodily symptoms of the emotions of guilt. If a man were guilty it was supposed that saliva would not flow into his mouth when he chewed the rice, because of the emotions of guilt which he experienced. With the development of modern instruments for making delicate measurement of bodily changes, such as blood pressure, breathing, sweat gland activity, and the like, psychological investigators of emotion have sought, with some success, to establish practical tests for emotions of guilt, erotic repression, and other emotional states, the presence of which may have various practical implications.

From both theoretical and practical points of view, therefore, the detection and measurement of bodily symptoms of emotion is important. We shall attempt in the present chapter to summarize briefly a few of the most significant experiments along this line.

Theoretical Significance of Bodily Changes

Emotions themselves cannot as yet be measured if we accept either the physiologist's definition of emotion or the definition of emotion according to the psychonic theory of consciousness. The physiologists hold that emotion consists of the activation of a central reflex pattern or group of neurons, probably in the old thalamic motor centres. The psychonic theory maintains that emotion is the excitation of motor psychons, wherever this may occur throughout the entire nervous system. If we follow either one of these theories we can see at once that it would be necessary to measure either the central nervous energy or the psychonic motor energy in order to obtain a first-hand measurement of emotion. Unfortunately, at the present time we possess no instruments which can be applied directly to the nerve centres of the brain and spinal cord in order to measure the excitations that are going on there. Therefore, we cannot as yet measure emotion directly.

The best we can do at present is to select those bodily changes which we know to be most consistently expressive of the emotional excitement itself and to record these bodily symptoms of emotion as carefully as possible.

It seems necessary at this point to emphasize once more the fact that the final efferent nerve impulses and the bodily changes which follow do not, by any means, reflect the total excitation of the motor centres, or emotion centres, in the central nervous system. The efferent nerve impulses only represent the resultant *product* of the emotion centre integrations. Suppose, for example, two nervous impulses reach the same motor centre. One impulse, if it gained egress into the final efferent pathway, would accelerate the heart-rate and strengthen its beat. The other impulse, if allowed to escape, would inhibit both rate and strength of heart-beat. How will these two antagonistic impulses affect one another when they come together in the motor centres ? There are three possible results of their struggle to control the final common motor path :

1. The two impulses may mutually inhibit one another so that no excitation of efferent nerves occurs.

2. The two impulses, if reciprocally antagonistic, will struggle to a definite conclusion, as it were. That is to say, the victorious impulse will win through to motor expression unmodified, and the defeated impulse will become completely inhibited by the victory of its antagonist.

3. The reciprocity between the two impulses may be only partial, in which case each will modify the other in the motor centre to a certain extent and the final efferent motor excitation will represent, in the main, the stronger of the two antagonistic impulses, but modified by the motor centre contest with its antagonist.

In light of this analysis it is clear that the final efferent nerve impulses, and consequently the bodily changes which these impulses bring about, cannot be regarded as corresponding with the emotion itself or as reflecting the intrinsic energy pattern of the emotion in the same way that the aura surrounding an electric light reflects the energy pattern of the illumination from which it radiates. Rather we must consider the bodily changes resulting from emotional excitement as representing the algebraic sum of all the psychonic or nervous excitations which actually compose the emotion itself.

The above considerations, while highly technical, make important practical differences in our interpretation of bodily symptoms of emotion. Suppose, for example, a man flees rapidly away from a pursuing gangster with a gun in his hand.

2H

At first thought an observer might unwittingly assume that the fugitive's speed and energy represented the bodily counterparts of his emotional condition of intense Fear. But such is far from the case. Fear represents a conflict between unit responses of Compliance and unit responses of Dominance. The Compliance responses inhibit and modify the Dominance responses sufficiently to cause a severe conflict in the motor centre which gives the unpleasant emotional consciousness of Fear. But the Dominance responses are still strong enough to control the final efferent paths to the legs and running muscles of the fugitive. His Dominance responses cause him to run rapidly. If no conflicting Compliance responses were present in the motor centres the man would run faster yet and he would run with more skill and self control. Yet the very fact that his Dominance responses must overcome their integrative antagonists again causes mechanisms of dominant reinforcement to be called into play and so results in a secondary increase of Dominance response which once more modifies the final running behaviour. All this complex integrative struggle in the motor centres is reflected accurately and completely in the fugitive's emotional consciousness of Fear. But only the algebraic sum of his conflicting elementary emotions is revealed by the resultant bodily symptoms of speed and skill in running away.

In general, the so-called involuntary bodily changes reveal the existing state of excitation in the emotion centres much more completely and accurately than do voluntary bodily changes. If the emotion centres are intensely excited in one part of the motor system, intellectual or other excitations of other parts of the brain and spinal cord may nevertheless effectively inhibit any bodily expressions of emotion brought about by efferent impulses over voluntary motor paths. In short, voluntary movements of the body are those which are subject to inhibitions or reinforcements from other parts of the central nervous system. Involuntary movements of the body are those which are less subject to such inhibition. There are many types of involuntary bodily change which are not subject to inhibitory control from other centres at all under ordinary conditions. It is these involuntary bodily changes, therefore, which furnish us with the most reliable index of the existing state of central emotional excitation at any given moment.

The involuntary bodily changes most frequently selected as emotional indicators or symptoms are : rate and strength of the heart-beat as indicated by pulse rate and blood pressure ; rate and depth of breathing and relation between the amplitude of inspiration and expiration at each breath ; activity of the sweat glands as indicated by the psycho-galvanic reflex ; tonic contraction of the skeletal muscles such as extension of the leg or gripping of the right hand ; also, in animals, and in human experimentation under special laboratory conditions, the secretion of saliva and other gastric secretions ; the contraction of the smooth muscles of stomach, intestines, and colon ; the secretion of adrenin by the adrenal glands ; the presence of certain nitrogen excretions and other significant chemicals in the urine.

In recent years considerable experimental work has been done on these bodily symptoms of emotion. While of course it will be impossible for us to give full accounts of all this work, we will briefly discuss some of the leading experiments that have been made in this field and point out what has been learned, so far, regarding the connection between specific bodily changes and special emotional states. For convenience we will list these experiments in accordance with the bodily measures employed.

Blood Pressure

One of the most frequently employed indices of emotionality is that obtained by the various measures of heart-beat and blood pressure. Early experimenters in the field of emotion measured the diastolic blood pressure, which is the pressure of blood in the arteries at its lowest phase. Later researchers have found that the systolic blood pressure, or the maximum pressure of blood in the arteries, is indicative of specific emotion, whereas the diastolic pressure could not be depended upon to be indicative of any one emotion.

Among the early investigators of emotion to use the blood pressure method were Binet and Courtier, who used stimuli to induce surprise, fear, and pleasure in their subjects. They concluded that each individual has a definite vaso-motor reaction for each specific emotion but that all subjects do not react in the same way. They further concluded that diastolic blood pressure expresses merely the quality of emotion.

A later investigator, Marston, found that systolic blood

pressure could be used to detect deception and his results differed from those of the early investigators in that he found a typical rising blood pressure curve during *deception* for all subjects, but that during *truth* there was no typical form or marked characteristics of the curve. Marston concluded from these deception tests that the blood pressure curve is no indication of the objective truth or falsity of the subject's story, but that it is an almost infallible test of the " consciousness of an attitude of deception." These blood pressure tests of deception were used in court cases and were found to have the practical value of inducing confessions from criminals and of furnishing clues to aid police investigations.

Marston also investigated the sex characteristics of systolic blood pressure and concluded that men experience major emotional changes less frequently than do women, and that men's " fear-anger " complexes of emotion are more massive, though less numerous, than women's. Women were found to respond with greater volume and frequency to sex stimuli than were men.

Larson modified the Marston deception test by adding respiration and pulse beat instruments, and applied the test to criminal cases. This investigator reported that the deception technique " furnishes an objective method whereby permanent records may be secured and that the test can be operated successfully by police officials with 90% accuracy."

After investigating deception by means of blood pressure, Landis concluded that " blood pressure methods of detecting deception are what Marston originally claimed for them, ' highly diagnostic ' if all conditions are favourable."

Pulse Rate

The rate and strength of pulse beat was at one time almost exclusively used to test emotion. Angell and McLennan measured the pulse rate during olfactory and gustatory experiences. They found that disagreeable smell and taste caused an irregularity and depression of the pulse and that agreeable taste and smell caused an increase in pulse rate. They concluded, however, that too many factors enter in to make the peripheral blood supply an accurate test of delicate affective states, and that it is utterly futile to investigate one aspect of consciousness without due regard to *all* the aspects involved.

Binet and Courtier had more success with their pulse rate measurements, which may be due in part to the fact that they used fear, anxiety, and music stimuli. They found that fear causes almost complete cessation of the pulse, and that anxiety and music cause an acceleration of the pulse rate ; and that the quality of the emotion may change the form of the capillary pulse.

In investigating the emotion of joy, Dearborn used all sorts of pleasant stimuli and found that they gave an increase of arterial pressure with an acceleration of the pulse.

Lehmann's tests of the pulse beat showed that during concentration of attention and strain of attention the pulse would beat rapidly the first few beats and then slow down for four to eight beats, repeating this succession the whole time the experiment was in progress. Displeasure showed decrease in pulse rate, and pleasure showed a quickened pulse rate. Lehmann concluded that every mental state has a characteristic physical accompaniment consisting in a given association of organic changes, and also a sequence of such changes. He further concluded that pleasant emotions are difficult to arouse and that therefore their symptoms are weak.

Eng has probably made a more complete and comprehensive study of the effects of emotion upon pulse beat than any other investigator. Some of her results follow. During psychical work there is an acceleration of the pulse. Fright produces first an acceleration and then a retardation. Excitement causes increased and often irregular pulse beat. Depression and pleasant smells retard the pulse rate.

A most interesting study of the emotion of fear was made by Blatz in which he measured the effect of fear upon the pulse beat. He constructed a collapsible chair into which the subject was tied. For three sittings nothing happened, then at the fourth sitting the chair collapsed. The subject was alone in the room and the situation was intended to induce fear. During the fall the pulse rate increased greatly for about five seconds, then it fell. About ten seconds later another longer period of acceleration occurred but not so high as the first. There was a gradual retardation of the pulse rate with another rise to a slightly higher level which remained constant. Blatz concluded that the two components necessary for the genuine emotion of fear are an organic response of great complexity, and a gross skeletal response of adaptive nature (such as trying to save oneself from falling by flinging out the arms or legs).

Blood Volume

The fluctuations of the volume of blood in the hand, as measured by the plethysmograph (a sort of rubber glove surrounded by water, the latter being displaced by an increased volume of blood to the member due to emotion) offered another test which Angell and McLennan found useful in their study. Disagreeable taste and smell stimuli decreased the blood supply, and unexpected stimuli increased the blood supply.

Shepard found that there was little uniformity of blood volume action, since disagreeable stimuli would cause a rise in volume in some cases and a fall in others. The only uniform rise in blood volume occurred when the subject looked at his finger in the plethysmograph and was told to count his pulse. Shepard reported that feelings cannot be classified on the basis of vaso-motor and heart rate changes, and that there is no reverse relationship between agreeableness and disagreeableness.

Lehmann's experiment showed that fright causes the blood volume in the arm to rise, fall, and then rise again. Tension causes a decrease in the arm volume of blood ; during sustained mental work the volume is normal, and for simple pleasantness there is a fall in volume during the application of the stimulus, with a later rise above the original level.

Eng's results showed that fright, excitement, and pleasant smell cause a rise in blood volume ; while depression and unpleasant taste and smell cause a drop in volume.

Respiration

Changes in the rate and depth of breathing are valuable in determining the presence of emotion. The instrument which is used is called the pneumograph, a hard rubber tube which goes across the subject's chest and fastens behind at the back. A small tube connects with an opening in the pneumograph, and to this smaller tube is connected a tambour which registers the breathing on a revolving smoked drum.

Angell and McLellan found that disagreeable taste and smell produced unco-ordinated and spasmodic breathing, while the reverse is true of pleasant taste and smell. Binet, Courtier, and Vaschide used the inspiration-expiration method of comparison and reported that anxiety prolongs the expiratory pause, gaiety causes the expiratory pause to be irregular and sadness causes very deep breathing with big expiratory pauses.

Startling noises and disagreeable odours caused irregular breathing according to Angell and Thompson, while all violent emotions caused respiration to be spasmodic in rate and amplitude. Dearborn's results show that pleasant states cause the breathing to be deeper than during unpleasant states and sometimes there is an increase in the rate. Shepard arrived at the same conclusions as Dearborn but also found that fear causes shallow breathing with greater inspirations.

The experiment which started a succession of breathing tests was the one originated by Benussi and used with fair success by him in cases of deception. This experiment is important enough to be reported in full.

Method. The subject was seated comfortably in an armchair with the Marey sphygmograph adjusted upon him. The breathing changes were recorded by means of markers on a small kymograph drum. All of the apparatus was hidden from the subject by a screen. The subject was presented with cards containing letters, pictures, and numbers in a certain order. Half of these slips were marked with a red star signifying that the subject was to lie in reporting upon that slip. The subject was told to tell the contents of each card in the presence of a jury. The observers watched the subject's facial expressions, and his manner of report, and made a judgment as to whether he lied or not on each slip in turn.

Results. (It must be remembered that Benussi was concerned only with the three to five breaths before and after each question and not with the general breathing excitement.)

1. A characteristic ratio of inspiration to expiration was found which was symptomatic of internal excitement.

2. The average of the three to five I/E ratios preceding a false answer was less than the average ratios following the answer. The reverse was found in the case of a true statement.

3. The difference between the average ratios before and after the lie varied with the ability of the subject to dissimulate.

4. The observers could not tell if the subject was lying, except in cases of very poor liars where the face flushed and the speech was uncertain.

Conclusions.

1. Breathing symptoms are 100 per cent. accurate in detecting lies.

2. Poor and good liars are differentiated by breathing ratios.

3. Benussi explains his breathing ratios by reporting that the innervation of the breathing muscles was stronger before lying than after lying, but was stronger after telling the truth than before.

Using a more elaborate technique, Burtt also studied the breathing symptoms of lying and reported that the results which were diagnostic were due ·to a few crucial questions, and those which were not conclusive were due to habituation and absence of deceptive consciousness.

Experiments by Burtt, Marston, Larson and Landis show that breathing is far less effective in detection of deception than Benussi originally claimed. Marston, Burtt, and Larson agree that breathing is less diagnostic than systolic blood pressure.

Eng's work with breathing curves shows that fright causes an inhibition of respiration; depression causes retarded respiration, excitement causes irregular respiration, and pleasant odours rapid and shallow respiration (this latter might, however, be due to the sniffing of the odour rather than an emotional accompaniment of the odour). In Blatz's fear experiment the respiration was found to be retarded just after the fall with an early recovery, but some traces of retardation remained. The respiratory index

$$\frac{\text{time of inspiration}}{\text{time of expiration—time of pause}}$$

was increased and so remained.

Electrical Changes

The galvonometer is a complex instrument used to measure electrical changes within the body during emotional stimulation. The change occurring is called the " psycho-galvanic reflex " or p.g.r. The most usual explanation of the psycho-galvanic reflex is that it is a change in the electrical conductivity of the skin due to sweat gland activation and that it depends upon the number of sweat glands in the skin. It is true that a person with dry skin has a much higher resistance to the electrical current than one with moist skin.

Some writers claim that the p.g.r. is not a specific measure of anything. That it may measure general emotionality, other writers agree. However, we may be sure that the activity of the sweat glands is greatly concerned in this phenomenon and that it does register bodily changes under stress of emotional stimuli.

Wells and Forbes stimulated their subjects with various drugs to ascertain the effect of these influences upon the psycho-galvanic reflex. One of the drugs produced unpredictible results and the other, atropine, reduced the average deflection of the galvanometer. They concluded, however, that the psycho-galvanic reflex is due to sweat gland activity.

Smith's book on " The Measurement of Emotion " is a most complete study of the psycho-galvanic reflex. One of his experiments concerns the effect of affective tone on memory. He found that the best remembered words have a higher p.g.r. than those soonest forgotten, and the latter have a higher p.g.r. than the words remembered only moderately well. He also states that affective tone, as shown by the psycho-galvanic reflex, exerts its influence toward better memory or quicker forgetting.

Another of Smith's experiments concerns the effect of alcohol upon the p.g.r., and it was found that alcohol markedly reduces the p.g.r. on word association lists and that alcoholic reactions tend toward an all-or-none character. Smith concludes that the above results explain that while the subject is under the influence of alcohol, many kinds of stimuli produce little effect ; yet when once the stimulus passes a certain value, the resulting behaviour change is extreme.

Wechsler's thesis is that the galvanometric deflection is based upon four variables :

1. The sensitivity of the instrument.
2. The size of the electromotive force in circuit.
3. Body resistance.
4. The physical reaction being measured.

He concludes (1) that the p.g.r. is a sweat gland phenomenon ; (2) that there are five types of effective psychological stimuli to the p.g.r. These are outright emotion-provoking stimuli, strong sensory stimulation, mental effort, changes in concentration of attention, and affectively toned ideational processes. (3) There is no such thing as general emotivity ; (4) that the p.g.r. can be used as a practical measure in clinical work and in psychopathology to facilitate the diagnosis of different psychoses.

Nitrogen Excretion

Although the measurement of nitrogen excreted during emotional excitement is not as practical as the tests which we have just considered, it is well to look into the experiment of Benedict, who found that there is sometimes a loss of nitrogen during emotional stress even when an increased amount of nitrogen was taken into the body in various foods. But, on the whole, nitrogen metabolism undergoes no noticeable change during nervous excitement, since the deficit is almost immediately made up.

Evaluation of Psycho-Physiological Measures of Emotion

From all the foregoing mass of work it would appear to us that two definite points emerge, one negative and the other positive.

The first point is that the psycho-galvanometric measure of emotion suffers from two very serious defects. One of these is the paucity of knowledge as to just how much of this reflex is due to sweat gland influence and how much to other causes, such as action currents and so on. It is true that general opinion attributes the major influence to the changes in sweat gland activation, and this can probably be accepted. But the fact remains that we are still in some doubt as to what actual physiological factors, and what proportion of each, are really being measured by this technique. An even more serious objection is due to the extreme sensitivity of the instrument ; the fact that it responds to the most delicate changes renders its report a very complex combination of many different elements and makes definite interpretation difficult. It has therefore little practical value, since it is almost impossible, for example, to determine those factors in the p.g.r. changes that are caused by the emotions due to deception or other specific causes.

The inspiration-expiration breathing ratio suffers from a similar defect since this also is " not sufficiently susceptible of definite analysis to prove legally acceptable."

On the other hand, the systolic blood pressure changes while still being psychologically complicated in origin, appear to give reliable measurements of the characteristic changes in the subject's consciousness during attempts at deception. Larson also believes that blood pressure is most diagnostic of deception and that association and reaction times are least satisfactory.

" Psychological " Measures

So far we have discussed the measurement of changes occurring in the effectors, presumably as a result of emotion. By various psychological tests it is possible, however, to study the more subtle, interior changes brought about as a result of emotional stimuli.

Association Reaction Times

One of the best known methods of this kind is the association reaction time test. It is well established that an emotional (verbal) stimulus will evoke a delayed response. There would seem little doubt that this delay is caused by a conflict of impulses at the central synapses : there is no doubt that slowing-up of conduction is primarily a synaptic phenomenon. If we can suppose that this slowing-up takes place in the motor centres, we would have, in the reaction time tests, the most pertinent measure of emotional consciousness now available from the psychonic point of view.

This method of emotional analysis often accompanies tests of deception, but it is used frequently as an accompaniment to any or all of the psycho-physiological tests as a check on the significant bodily changes. The usual method of procedure is to give the subject a list of words one at a time, and as the stimulus word is given, the subject is asked to respond with the first word that comes into his mind. This is verbal association. For example, the list word is " cat," and the subject will ordinarily respond with " dog." Included in the list are key words which are intended to be emotion-provoking. These key words are very important in deception tests since they bear directly upon the crime. The reaction time, or the time elapsing between the giving of the stimulus word and the subject's reply, is noted and each reaction time can be compared with the general average or with any of the other reaction times. It is assumed in deception testing that the subject will take a longer time to respond to words bearing upon his guilt than he will to non-significant words, and that he will also be likely to respond with an unusual association.

Lists of the most usual responses to ordinary words have been made, against which a given subject's replies may be checked. Care must of course be taken against misinterpretation of individual (unusual), non-significant associations.

Jung has used the association reaction time test to a great extent in his analyses and finds that those reaction times which exceed the average to be expected, are caused largely by the occurrence of intense emotion. This intense emotional response depends upon "complexes" significant to the individual.

In their experiment, Henke and Eddy tested two subjects one of whom was guilty while the other was innocent. The jury and the experimenter were in ignorance of the guilty subject. All the judges picked the guilty man on the basis of his outward manifestation of emotion and his delayed reaction times to crucial words. Nothing could be told by analyzing the reaction times of the man who did not attempt to conceal his actions, but correct judgments were made on his associations.

Washburn and Leach found that the average reaction times for crucial words were longer than for the non-crucial.

In two out of four reaction time experiments according to Yerkes and Berry, the reaction times failed as criteria of judgment, since the time for crucial words was actually less than for non-crucial words.

Marston sought to analyze experimentally the frequent cases where "crucial" or emotional association times were shorter than the non-crucial or unemotional. By eliminating extraneous factors, this investigator discovered what he called "negative-type" subjects who nearly always showed shorter association reaction times on crucial words under the stress of their efforts to deceive the experimenter. This is the type of person, according to Marston, who lies faster than he can tell the truth.

It would seem to the writers that this reverse result is to be explained by the assumption that there are two types of reaction during deception ; (1) the positive type with delayed reaction times, and (2) the negative type, where the reaction time is considerably shortened. The latter is the type of person who lies faster than he tells the truth. It would further appear that the true deceptive attitude can be measured in undefeated form in the negative type liar, since it consists of increased energy applied to the task of deception. He is trying to " put one over " on the examiner. What is probably present is not a combination of guilty and apprehensive emotions (psychonic conflict), but the psychonic facilitation underlying the congenial and successful attempt at deception. As Goldstein has commented, the negative type subjects fail to get the true deceptive consciousness. The positive type liar is defeated by the skill of the examiner and the difficulty of the test, with resulting emotional confusions and inhibitions.

Responses of Children to Emotional Stimuli

Dr. John Watson has provided us with the most penetrating study of children's emotions to date. From these experiments it is easily shown how the different unit responses are built up to expression. There is more and more work being done on children's emotional reactions since psychologists now recognize that the seeds of emotional disorders and fears are sown in the infant in a great many cases.

To test the bodily symptoms of fear Watson dropped the infant on a pillow, or pulled away the blanket upon which the infant was lying. The reaction to such stimuli was a sudden catching of the breath, closing of the eyes, puckering of lips, and often crying. To induce rage Watson held the child's head between the hands or the arms closely to the sides, prohibiting movement. The child's body stiffens, the feet are drawn up and down, the breath is held sometimes until the face is blue. Love responses in babies were elicited by tickling the skin, patting, and stimulation of the erogenous zones. The infant might smile, or if crying before, would stop.

Jones, following Watson's general method, used various methods to eliminate children's fears. She tried the method of verbal appeal, that is, talking about the fear object (rabbit) until the child would talk freely about it also. However, when the rabbit was brought in the child was still afraid. Her talking about rabbits in no way accomplished any change in response to the rabbit itself.

Using the method of adaptation, Jones introduced the fear object several times. There was less fear each time the object was presented to the child. The child never became enthusiastic about the object but accepted it indifferently. In the direct conditioning method, Jones placed the fear object nearer each day to the child's plate while he ate. The hunger drive was greater than the Fear response so that the child grew less and less afraid of the fear object on successive days. Social imitation was found to be one of the successful ways of eliminating fear. The child who fears an object will investigate that object if other children show an interest in it.

Watson says " In these transferred emotional reactions (where the child has learned to be afraid) we find a reason for the widespread change in the personality of children, once even a single strongly conditioned emotional reaction has been set up toward any object or situation." He further states that conditioning " accounts for many unreasoning fears, and for a good deal of the sensitiveness of people to objects when there is no adequate ground for such behaviour."

Glandular, Visceral and Muscular Changes

Bodily changes can be induced by the addition of various glandular secretions to the blood. The effect is to give the bodily symptoms of emotion without, in many cases, the emotion being felt. This result in itself is sufficient to prove that emotional consciousness is a central phenomenon which normally causes bodily changes but is not caused by them.

Marañon injected adrenalin into the blood stream of his subjects and induced a slow, profound and irregular respiration ; a trembling of the hands and limbs ; abundant perspiration ; and all other bodily changes normally effected by motor discharge through the sympathetic nervous system. But on the emotional side the feeling of fear was rarely induced by artificial production of its usual symptoms. In cases where the emotion was felt at all it was evoked by ideas or associations of dangerous disease or other previous experiences.

Marañon gives four stages of the physiological processes of the emotions : (a) the initial psychic-emotional element, frequently following appropriate memories or ideas ; (b) the production of the vegetative emotion, trembling, sweating, etc. ; (c) the consciousness of the peripheral emotion by the brain ; (d) the authentic emotion, when consciousness of the vegetative emotion is added to the initial psychic element.

Brunswick's work on the effects of emotion on the gastro-intestinal tone shows that stimuli such as pistol shots, electric shocks, snakes, and other unpleasant experiences cause an increase in the stomach contractions and large rythmic contractions of the rectum. Pleasant stimuli cause a rise in gastric tone. Disappointment causes a tonic fall, then a rise, and finally a fall in stomach tone. Brunswick believes that this gastric change is not a specific part of the emotion, differing for different emotions, but is rather a general contribution to affective tone.

Experiments on the Bodily Symptoms of the Four Primary Emotions

All the work so far reviewed has been of a general character. The best results obtained have been in the direction of practical tests for deception and for the presence of more or less undefined emotional disturbances. Much of this vagueness seems to us to be due to the lack of any definite theory as to the real nature of emotion, and lack of any definite hypothesis as to constant psycho-neural elements of emotion.

In fact, it was not until the spring of 1928 that any results were obtained with regard to specific primary emotions. At that time, Marston performed at Columbia a series of experiments to investigate the bodily symptoms associated with the four primary emotions—Dominance, Compliance, Inducement and Submission—as defined by the Integrative Theory of Emotion. The following excerpts are taken from the preliminary report of Marston and his fellow investigators, O. B. Richard, A. E. Nissen, W. V. Clark, and Harold Brown.[1]

Compound Emotions have varying Bodily Symptoms.

According to the psychonic definition of emotion, the logical expectation would be that compound emotions would not produce constant invariable bodily changes, because the elementary emotions making up the compound would seldom be found mixed in exactly similar proportions. This coincides with experimental results. The emotion named "fear" in subject's verbal reports sometimes results in dropping of systolic blood pressure, inhibition of muscular action, trembling, general bodily weakness, and even nausea and vomiting. But under other conditions, "fear" is accompanied by rapid rise in blood pressure, violent and energetic actions of skeletal muscles, marked access of bodily vigour and tonic tension and inhibition of digestive activities.[2] Our

---

[1] W. M. Marston, "The Bodily Symptoms of Elementary Emotions," *Psyche*, No. 38, p. 70. (Excerpts reprinted by courtesy of the Editor, C. K. Ogden).

[2] W. B. Cannon, *Bodily Changes in Pain, Hunger, Fear and Rage.*

own laboratory results and clinical cases indicate that the more intense the fear experience becomes, the more of weakness and the less of strength appear in its resultant bodily symptoms.

Elementary Emotions Experimentally Determined by Ideas

But here arises a difficulty. Not only do emotions like fear, which are reported as qualitatively identical by the subjects who experience them, manifest different and changeable bodily symptoms upon different occasions, but also the same stimulus may evoke one emotional response from one subject, and another, quite different emotional response from another subject. The psychological text books explain this glibly by saying that one subject's bodily condition differs from that of another subject, that his psycho-neural set is different, or that he is differently conditioned with respect to his emotional reactions. That may be so, but it does not help us much in solving the laboratory problem of how to evoke the same elementary emotion from many subjects, in order to measure and compare bodily symptoms resulting. It has been found that different stimuli can be used effectively for different subjects to evoke the same emotion. Beefsteak, for example, may evoke appetite reactions from subject A, mince pie from subject B, and a plate of vegetables from subject C. A kiss may evoke erotic passion from X, photographs of nudes from subject Y, and a girl's tantalizing coquetry may produce the same effect in subject Z. But this method of experimentation requires considerable preliminary analysis and study of each subject. Moreover, quantitative comparisons of emotional response symptoms cannot fairly be made, since there is no proper means of equating the intensity of the different stimuli used for different subjects.

It is true that we cannot control the inner conditions of our subjects' bodies and brains before they come into the laboratory. We may now add the observation that we cannot control these conditions, as far as their effect upon emotional response is concerned, *after* the subjects come into the laboratory, merely by controlling the sensory stimuli presented to our subjects. We may be able to enforce virtually identical sensory reactions upon all subjects. That is, we may make all our subjects see blue, or taste sweet, or feel skin pressures. But these identical sensation responses are not followed by identical emotional responses.

Marañon went even further in his proof of this disparity between sensation and emotion. He enforced identical sensations, not only through the external receptors of sight, hearing, pressure, taste, etc., but also throughout the internal visceral and somatic receptors supposed by Lange to initiate emotion. Marañon administered adrenalin to different subjects, thus producing identical patterns of visceral sensations in all. But the emotional reactions experienced were not identical. Some experienced emotion and some did not. Those who did respond emotionally reported *ideas* concerning the stimulus which were appropriate to the emotion following. " A psychic motive of sad character ", Marañon says, " adds itself to the vegetative emotion ", that is, to the sensation-complex. Memories of dead friends, etc., come to mind, evidently recalled by associative connection with adrenalin sensations. In some cases it was possible to suggest affective meanings for the adrenalin sensations. The characteristic emotional quality, or " psychic " part of the emotion, as Marañon calls it, simultaneously appeared in each case. The emotion did not follow directly from the sensations, but rather from the *ideas* which served to interpret the stimulus in such a way that it became an adequate stimulus to a given emotion.

Marañon's findings are quite in accord with the psychonic theory of consciousness, and the psychonic definition of emotion. If emotion is really an integrative pattern of excitations in the psychons of the motor centres, then this emotion pattern is determined immediately by the synaptic arrangements of the correlation centres (ideas according to the psychonic theory). The integrative pattern in the sensory centres (sensations) must affect the final emotion pattern indirectly, via the correlation centres. In short, the sensations are interpreted and followed by ideas ; and the *ideas determine what emotion, if any, shall occur.*

In cases where the emotion follows immediately upon sensations, or nearly so, the variety of emotions must depend largely upon the associative connections built up by the past experience of each individual subject between certain sensations and certain emotions. In such cases, the emotional responses cannot be controlled by the psychological experimenter without a previous study of the individual subject. But if ideas can be made to intervene between sensations and emotions, and if these ideational interpretations of sensory stimuli can be controlled, then resulting emotional responses can be controlled, and the same elementary emotions can be evoked from different subjects.

Ideas Experimentally Determined by Motion Pictures

Our working hypothesis, then, was as follows. Compound emotions can produce only compound and variable bodily changes. Elementary emotions, or basic types of motor integrations, should produce relatively constant and uniform types of bodily changes, if these elementary emotions can be experimentally evoked. Identical sensations can be enforced upon different subjects, but the emotions following will not be identical, since they depend upon each individual subject's emotional associations with the stimulus sensations. But if identical ideas, or interpretations of the stimulus sensations can be enforced upon different subjects, the elementary emotions evoked should be closely similar. Our preliminary problem, then, in the experiments undertaken recently at Columbia, was to determine whether or not motion pictures could be used to evoke similar ideas, or interpretations, from different types of experimental subjects.

To investigate this problem, four motion picture episodes were presented to about 60 subjects.[1] Each person who saw these episodes was asked to characterize the theme of plot and action giving his own interpretation. The experimenters then compared these individual interpretations with respect to the predominant interpretative idea of each episode. By a simple scoring method of crediting one point for each idea or interpretation which agreed substantially with the predetermined idea which the experimenters had designed each episode to express, there was found a total average score slightly better that 80 per cent. This preliminary determination of the uniformity of ideas evoked by selected motion picture dramas is not to be regarded as possessing any final value in evaluating the efficiency of movies as an adequate emotion stimulus. It is the opinion of the experimenters that the value of motion pictures in evoking a predetermined emotion from different subjects is considerably higher than 80 per cent. when certain

[1] In still more recent experiments at Hollywood, Cal., W. M. Marston has examined the ideational effects of motion picture dramas upon more than 2,500 subjects, with results similar to those herein reported.

difficulties have been eliminated. An 80 per cent. uniformity in the interpretative ideas evoked, however, seemed sufficiently high to warrant use of the four picture episodes chosen as experimental stimuli in trying to determine the bodily symptoms of the elementary emotions corresponding to the four episodes.

Are Bodily Symptoms of Elementary Emotions Predictable ?

The next problem was to find out how far the bodily changes which occurred while each subject watched the selected screen episodes followed the physiological predictions which might be made on the supposition that each screen episode evoked its designated type of elementary emotional response.

With the generous co-operation of the motion picture producers, four screen episodes were designed. Each episode contained action and plot depicting relationships between the screen characters and the stimuli to which they reacted which corresponded as nearly as possible to the four basic types of elementary emotional response which we have designated as the Primary Emotions.

These four elementary emotional responses are : Compliance, Dominance, Inducement, and Submission.

In Compliance response the subject reacts to a stimulus which he interprets to be antagonistic and stronger than himself. He responds by reflex weakening of tonic energy, directing his behaviour toward avoiding further conflict with the stimulus. For Compliance stimulus there was used the Metro-Goldwyn-Mayer feature film, "Student Prince." The film was cut and the titles and sequences were changed in such a way that only those portions of the picture showing Compliance activities were shown. Both the individual actions and the plot of the episode showed the Student Prince complying with circumstances and environmental forces stronger than himself. He was compelled to give up his student friends, his life of artistic freedom, and his girl. He was compelled to undertake, unwillingly, the dull and dreary duties of a figure-head sovereign. He *complied* throughout with antagonists stronger than himself.

In Dominance response the subject reacts to a stimulus which he interprets to be antagonistic to and weaker than himself. He responds by a spontaneous surging of tonic energy directed toward overwhelming the stimulus. For

Dominance stimulus several fight pictures, combined in unified sequence, were used. The fighting was done in the prize ring, in the days of bare knuckles and fights to a final knock-out. The hero was shown overcoming obstacles, beating opponents, and eventually winning the "world's championship." Throughout this episode the principle character *dominated* opponents whom he showed to be weaker than himself.

In Inducement response the subject reacts to an allied stimulus, a person, whom he regards as weaker than himself. He responds by spontaneous increasing of tonic energy, directed toward influencing the stimulus person to follow his commands. For Inducement stimulus there were combined scenes and action from two popular feature pictures, " Love," and " Flesh and the Devil." John Gilbert and Greta Garbo, both specializing in love scenes of seductive character, were the principles. Each took the initiative in inducing the other in different parts of this episode. Each *induced* an attractive person, weaker than himself, or herself, to yield to the inducer's commands.

In Submission response the subject reacts to an allied stimulus, a person, whom he regards as stronger than himself. He responds by spontaneous decrease of tonic energy, permitting his behaviour to be controlled by the stimulus person's dictates. For Submission stimulus there was used a dance by Gilda Gray, filmed by United Artists. In this dance the girl is represented as a captive of Tibetan priests, by whom she has been taught to express the submission of the people to their Gods. The dancer's costume, as well as her dance movements, express admirably a willing devotion to her masters.

These four episodes were presented in the order named to 56 subjects, 28 of each sex, a man and a woman being tested simultaneously in each case. The subjects ranged in age from 15 to 60, and also varied widely in education and occupation. We tested a prize-fighter, a professor, an unskilled labourer, editors of *Encyclopaedia Britannica* of both sexes, stenographers, clerks, a dentist, writers, chorus girls, etc. Due to considerations of space we shall not attempt to include here the experimental technique in detail. We measured simultaneously systolic blood pressure, tension of the right hand grip, psycho-galvanic reflex (when satisfactory apparatus adjustments could be made), and respiration (including amplitude, frequency, and inspiration-expiration ratios). For an illustration of our *modus operandi* see Fig. 45 (Frontispiece) : " Experimental Set-up for Measuring Bodily Symptoms of Emotion."

Since most definite and significant predictions could be made in connection with systolic blood pressure behaviour, the present account will be confined to blood pressure measurements alone. The general principles of rise and fall of systolic blood pressure are fairly simple, although the bodily mechanisms involve certain complications which have been pointed out elsewhere. In general, we may assume that rise of systolic blood pressure is a result of *increased* tonic motor discharge over various systems of efferent nerves, notably the sympathetic branch of the autonomic system. The heart beat is strengthened, and very possibly also accelerated, while appropriate vaso-motor changes tend to enhance the rise of systolic pressure and blood volume in the arteries and arterioles serving the skeletal muscles, brain, and other organs of strenuous action. Conversely, we may assume that drop in systolic blood pressure is symptomatic of *decreased* tonic motor discharge, which, in emotional situations, is oftenest the result of increased nervous excitation of antagonistic efferent systems, such as the vagus nerves, the entire cranial branch of the autonomic system, and also the sacral ganglia connected with the functioning of the autonomic system. Combining these general principles of systolic blood pressure change with the types of integration of motor impulses postulated as the bases of primary emotions, it becomes possible to make theoretical predictions of the directions of blood pressure change to be expected during Compliance, Dominance, Inducement, and Submission, if these elementary emotions be successfully evoked during the corresponding screen stimulus episodes. Of course, even under maximally efficient conditions, one could not expect 100 per cent. of the ideas evoked by a given screen episode, throughout the entire episode, to conform in type to the predetermined primary emotion. That is to say, even if the theme of *compliance* in " The Student Prince Episode," were maximally effective, we should anticipate a certain amount of wandering of attention throughout the 16 minute episode, with ideas not adequate to Compliance emotion thereby creeping in. We should also expect a considerable number of irrelevant associative ideas to be evoked by the actions on the screen. Since the nature of these ideas would be determined by the subject's individual experiences, and not by the nature of the screen episode at all, we should expect the blood pressure changes to vary accordingly from the pattern predicted. We could logically predict, therefore, that perhaps 15 or 20 per cent. of the blood pressure changes would not follow theoretical predictions of direction of change ; or, if they did so, would do so by chance, and not as a result of the primary emotions intended to be called forth. The chance of coincident effects would, of course, tend to be neutralized in the large group of subjects by an equal likelihood of opposite effects. Altogether, the preliminary prediction was made that from 80 to 85 per cent. of the blood pressure changes might be expected to follow theoretical predictions, if our experimental conditions were maximally controlled.

Compliance episode should produce preponderance of drop in systolic blood pressure. The episode used contained other action relationships besides sheer Compliance, however, notably Dominance in Appetite compound.

Dominance episode, though similarly compounded with Compliance, should cause a preponderance of *rise* in systolic blood pressure.

Inducement episode should produce *rise* in blood pressure. An unavoidable complication here, however, consisted in the fact that while the man, John Gilbert, was inducing (or really captivating) the girl, Greta Garbo, Greta was correspondingly submissive and vice versa. Alternating types of ideas of Inducement and Submission might be evoked, depending upon which screen character was followed at the moment.

Submission episode should cause a preponderance of drop in systolic blood pressure. But even greater likelihood existed here that subjects watching the dance of a girl captive would ignore the picture audience before whom she was dancing, and regard *themselves* as the audience to whom she was submitting, thus themselves experiencing *Inducement* (erotically compounded into Captivation emotion) instead of the *Submission* intended to be evoked.

Results

Table I

	Compliance	Dominance	Inducement	Submission
Total systolic b.p. change per minute for all subjects	858 mm.	830 mm.	742 mm.	566 mm.
Change in accordance with prediction	699 mm. (drop)	583 mm. (rise)	545 mm. (rise)	227 mm. (drop)
Change contra to prediction	159 mm. (rise)	247 mm. (drop)	197 mm. (drop)	339 mm. (rise)
Percentage of total change following prediction	81.4%	70.2%	73.4%	40.3%

These results seem fairly definite and clear cut. The blood pressure changes during three episodes preponderantly follow predictions. During the fourth episode the blood pressure changes appear preponderantly contra to prediction. The percentage of preponderance, in both cases, is probably sufficient to be regarded as significant. The total average percentage of changes following predictions in the Compliance, Dominance, and Inducement episodes was 75 per cent. This percentage obtained with stimulus episodes imperfect as indicated, compares favourably with the possible 80 per cent. or 85 per cent. predictibility judged possible under maximally favourable conditions.

With regard to the Submission episode, we find about 60 per cent. blood pressure changes opposite to prediction. Apparently this reversal is due to the fact—which we partially anticipated—that the ideas evoked by watching a captive girl dance submissively are predominantly ideas of *Inducement, based on the relationship felt between the subject and the girl*, rather than ideas of Submission based upon the relationship between the girl and her captors or the gods she was supposedly worshipping. This reversal was due, chiefly, to an interesting sex difference in attitude toward the girl. The *women*, and not the men, were the subjects who regarded themselves as the mistresses or captors of the girl dancer, according to their verbal reports. About 80 per cent. of the women subjects reported this attitude, with corresponding ideas of *Inducement* rather than ideas of Submission. (They liked the girl as much as the men did ; several " loved her ", they said). The women's total blood pressure changes per minute, correspondingly showed 70 per cent. *rise*, predictable for Inducement. A majority of the men, on the other hand, reported ideas of Passion (in which predominant Submission controls, and is erotically compounded with passive Inducement) as predominating over ideas of Captivation (in which active Inducement controls).   53 per cent. of the men's blóod pressure changes, correspondingly, followed prediction. The total result for the episode contra to prediction, therefore, seems plainly attributable to controlling ideas of Inducement (in Captivation compound) evoked by the dancer in women subjects. An adequate Submission stimulus episode is extremely difficult to obtain, we discovered, in commercial films passed by American censors.

Another phase of predictability of emotional responses may be mentioned briefly at this point. This concerns predictions as to the relative pleasantness of the four stimulus episodes. There have recently been examined at some length the comparative pleasantness of the four primary emotions. The conclusion placed Submission as most pleasant, Inducement as next, Compliance as slightly pleasant, or indifferent, and Dominance as predominantly unpleasant prior to its final successful termination. Thus our prediction would be that subjects would give highest pleasantness rating to the Submission episode, ranking Inducement second, Compliance third, and Dominance fourth. All subjects were accordingly asked to rank the four stimulus episodes in order of their pleasantness. The results, as shown in the following table, are very closely in accord with prediction.

Table II

	Submission.	Inducement.	Compliance.	Dominance.
Number of First Choices	27	16	13	8
Number of Second Choices	22	19	14	9
Number of Third Choices	9	22	19	14
Number of Fourth Choices	6	7	18	33
Total score (4 for 1st choice 3 ,, 2nd ,, 2 ,, 3rd ,, 1 ,, 4th ,,)	198	172	150	120

The chief point which this exact conformity between results and predictions in pleasantness value of the four primary emotions leaves open for discussion, is the confusion between Submission and Inducement emotions during the stimulus originally designed for Submission. In our previous discussion we concluded that this dance episode evoked Inducement emotion preponderantly, rather than Submission. Yet we find, in the above table, that this episode nevertheless gives greatest pleasure to subjects of both sexes, if their own pleasantness ratings are to be relied upon. Closer consideration of the relative proportions of Submission and Inducement emotions evidently compounded in the episodes originally designed for Inducement and Submission, however, shows that the largest proportion of Submission emotion was evidently evoked by the dancing captive girl episode, even though Inducement predominated in this episode. Assuming that the percentages of blood pressure change in accordance with prediction may be taken as approximate measures of the relative proportions of corresponding primary emotions evoked, we find that the Inducement episode evoked 73 per cent. Inducement, and 27 per cent. something else, perhaps partly Submission ; whereas the Submission episode evoked only 60 per cent. Inducement, with the remaining 40 per cent. probably largely given over to Submission (love passion). At least we seem justified by the subject's reports in concluding that this dancing episode evoked more Submission emotion in Passion compound with Inducement, than any other episode. The prediction for it, in that case, would be first place in pleasantness value ; which, in fact, turned out to be the actual result obtained.

Control records of systolic blood pressure changes were, of course, taken on 30 subjects, 15 of each sex, while reading Woodworth's text-book in psychology, a stimulus which, supposedly, contained little provocation to emotional response. The total blood pressure changes per minute, for all subjects were less than 5 per cent. as great as those occurring during the experimental stimulus episodes averaged together. The blood pressure changes during the control records were almost evenly divided between rise and drop, with slight preponderance of drop in blood pressure.

Sex Differences

For the purpose of bringing out possible sex differences in bodily symptoms of primary emotions, we tested one man and one woman subject simultaneously in each experiment, thus ensuring identical test conditions for each sex. Since previous work had shown that subjects of both sexes react emotionally with least restraint when their blood pressure is taken by an experimenter of opposite sex, we assigned our researchers accordingly. Miss Alice Nissen, a graduate student at Columbia, recorded the male subject's blood pressure using the discontinuous auscultatory method. Mr. Walter V. Clark, also a Columbia graduate student, recorded women subjects' blood pressure by the same method. With experimental conditions thus equalized between the sexes, several significant sex differences appeared.

Table III

Women's total systolic b.p. change (all episodes) per minute	1729 mm.
Men's Total systolic b.p. change (all episodes) per minute	1268 mm.
Excess of women's total changes per minute over men's.	461

It would appear from the above table that women show significantly greater bodily symptoms of primary emotions under the conditions of this experiment, than do men. Women's total blood pressure changes were, in fact, 136 per cent. of those shown by men. Our supplementary reports concerning the frequency with which subjects of both sexes attended motion pictures, their enjoyment of the cinema, etc., did not reveal any corresponding sex differences in the subjects' habits and tastes with regard to screen dramas, which might be regarded as accounting for the sex differences in quantity of bodily symptoms shown.

Interesting sex differences in pleasantness ratings of the four stimulus episodes also appeared, as shown in the following table :

Table IV
Sex Differences in Pleasantness Ratings

	Submission Men Wmn		Inducement Men Wmn		Compliance Men Wmn		Dominance Men Wmn	
1st Choices	17	10	3	13	4	9	8	0
2nd Choices	9	13	12	7	6	8	5	4
3rd Choices	3	6	12	10	10	9	7	7
4th Choices	3	3	5	2	12	6	12	21
Total Score (computed on same scoring method as above)	104	94	77	95	66	84	73	47

From this comparison between men's and women's preferences in stimulus episodes, it appears that women derive greatest pleasantness from Inducement emotion, and least

from Dominance. Men on the other hand, find Submission
(in love passion compound) decidedly most pleasant, while
at the same time they prefer Dominance to Compliance by a
margin of 73 to 66. It seems most clearly significant of all
that out of a total of 32 women subjects who gave pleasantness
ratings, not one woman gave the Dominance episode first
choice. Apparently we may conclude, in everyday life, that
women find fighting, competitive struggles, and dominant
battling for appetitive rewards least pleasant of all activities.
Apparently also, these results indicate that men do not find
the love pursuit and capture of women, which primarily
involves Inducement emotion and which males are popularly
supposed to enjoy above all else, nearly so pleasant as Submission emotion in situations where a beautiful woman holds
the whip hand by exciting the male to uncontrollable passion.
Our results plainly suggest that *women prefer captivating men,
and that men prefer to be captivated.*

In connection with this comparative study of sex differences
in pleasantness-rating of the four stimulus episodes, it may
be interesting, also, to glance briefly at the comparative
amounts of blood pressure change shown by subjects of both
sexes during each episode. The next table shows this
comparison.

Table V

	Men	Women
Total b.p. change per min for *all* episodes	1268 mm.	1729 mm.
B.p. change during *Submission* episode :	254 mm.	312 mm.
Percentage of total change, all episodes :	20%	18%
B.p. change during *Inducement* episode :	265 mm.	477 mm.
Percentage of total change, all episodes :	21%	28%
B.p. change during *Compliance* episode :	373 mm.	486 mm.
Percentage of total change, all episodes :	29%	28%
B.p. change during *Dominance* episode :	376 mm.	434 mm.
Percentage of total change, all episodes :	30%	26%
Order of pleasantness of episodes :	S, I, D, C	I, S, C, D
Order of magnitude of bodily symptoms	D, C, I, S	C, I, D, S

Little or no correspondence appears between the order of
pleasantness of the four stimulus episodes and the order of
magnitude of bodily symptoms of primary emotion with either
sex. Submission emotion, found most pleasant by male
subjects, and ranked second in pleasantness by women subjects,
appears to produce the smallest quantity of blood pressure
changes in subjects of both sexes of any episode in the series.
A greater percentage of male blood pressure changes occurred

during the Dominance episode than during any other episode, while women showed greatest and equal percentages of change for Inducement and Compliance. A certain marked difference in male responsiveness seems to exist between the appetitive primary emotion elements of Dominance and Compliance, and the love elements of Inducement and Submission, with the appetitive emotions clearly in the ascendency. No such noticeable difference appears in the women's bodily symptoms of emotion between Appetite and Love emotion elements, although there is much more difference between women's Inducement and Submission symptoms than in the case of male subjects.

Two practical implications may be found, perhaps. First, our evidence indicates that men respond more strongly with appetitive emotion elements than with love emotion elements. That is to say, men have developed more capacity for responding with emotions designed to take selfish advantage of persons and things than have women. And this despite the fact that men, as well as women, find these self-seeking emotions least pleasant.

Second, there appears some indication that women have developed Inducement emotion at the expense of Submission. Practically speaking, this fact suggests that what appears to be Submission, and Submissive love passion, in women's love affairs with men actually consists for the most part of Inducement. Woman's submissive appearing behaviour may be regarded in the light of an Inducement technique designed to propitiate male Dominance. Which reminds us, of course, of Bernard Shaw's " Man and Superman ".

Conclusions

From the entire data of this series of experiments, a small part of which is briefly summarized above, we drew the following conclusions :

1. That elementary emotions may be predictably evoked if an experimental stimulus can be devised capable of evoking similar ideas, in different subjects, appropriately interpreting the relationship between stimulus and subject.

2. That motion picture episodes, properly devised, constitute such an experimental stimulus to a very promising extent.

3. That the direction of bodily changes during Compliance,

Dominance, and Inducement responses, thus evoked, followed theoretical predictions in a significant proportion of their total volume.

4. That women subjects show a significantly greater total response to elementary emotion stimuli than do men.

5. That men rate both Dominance and Submission emotions relatively higher in the pleasantness scale than do women ; while women rate Inducement relatively higher than do men.

6. That men respond more strongly with appetite emotion elements than with the elements of love emotion.

7. That women's erotic emotions, which appear predominantly submissive, actually consist, for the most part, of active Inducement emotion.

Future Experimental Work on Emotion

To us it would seem that the results obtained from the foregoing experiment offer some suggestions for future experimental work in the field of emotions. In the first place we believe that such experiments will profit by being conducted upon the basis of a definite theory as to the nature of emotion. Much previous work, it would appear to us, has been of a general exploratory character, and the conclusions reached have been correspondingly vague, more related to general emotionality (a term which may mean almost anything), than to definite data respecting specific emotions. The employment, as an experimental starting-point, of any theory, whether the psychonic theory or another, may be expected to yield more definite results than in the past, provided such a theory meets the objections already discussed which are attendant upon the previous confusion between Sensation and Emotion.

We do not ourselves know of any present theory except the integrative theory which meets these objections and offers a clear-cut basis upon which further experimentation may be built. With regard to the integrative or psychonic theory of emotion, the above experiment has suggested several lines for future refinement and improvement. One of the main difficulties encountered and already discussed was the difficulty of obtaining maximally adequate stimuli for the primary emotions. Motion picture episodes appear to be an advantageous form of administering such stimuli to the subjects, but it is evident that the best results will be obtained if such pictures can be privately produced for the psychological laboratory to meet the exact requirements of the experiment. The Eastman Kodak Company's amateur moving picture equipment would seem to render this possibility within the easy achievement of any well equipped laboratory.

A careful study of the experiment described above will suggest many other refinements of technique and procedure, and it should prove possible to investigate Compound, and perhaps even Complex, Emotions to some extent by means of the general procedure already outlined. In the final outcome, however, there is little doubt that a direct measure of the activity within the centres where emotion actually originates, will prove the eventual necessity either for complete confirmation or final refutation of the psychonic theory or of any other theory of emotion. We do not feel that it is at all hopeless to expect the future development of precision instruments that will make this type of measurement possible.

BIBLIOGRAPHY.

ANGELL (J. R.) & McLENNAN (S. F.) "Organic effects of agreeable and disagreeable stimuli." *Psychol. Review*, 1896
ANGELL (J. R.) & THOMPSON. "Organic processes and consciousness." *Psychol. Review*, 1899, VI, 32-73
BENEDICT (F. G.) "Excretion of nitrogen during nervous excitement." *Jour. Physiol.*, 1902, VI
BENUSSI (Vittorio) "Die Atmungsymptome der Luge," *Archiv. fur die gesamte Psychol.*, 1914, 244-73
BINET (A.) & COURTIER (J.) "La circulation capillair." *L'Année Psych.* 3, 1896
BLATZ (W. E.) "The cardiac, respiratory, and electrical phenomena involved in the emotion of tear." *Jour. Exp. Psych.*, 1925, VIII, 109-23
BRUNSWICK (D.) "The effects of emotional stimuli upon the gastro-intestinal tone." *Journ. Comp. Psy.*, 1924, IV, 19-80
BURTT (H. E.) "The inspiration-expiration ratio during truth and falsehood." *Journ. Exp. Psy.*, 1921, IV, 1-23
BYRNE (O.) *A History of Theory and Research on Emotion* (Columbia University Master's Thesis), 1927
CANNON (W. B.) *Bodily Changes in Pain, Hunger, Fear, and Rage*
DEARBORN (G. Van N.) *The Emotion of Joy,* 1899
ENG (H.) *Experimental Investigations into the Emotional Life of the Child compared to that of the Adult*, 1921 (tr. 1925)
JONES (M. C.) "Elimination of children's fears." *Journ. Exp. Psych.* 7, 1924, 382-90
JUNG (C.) "The association method." *Am. Journ. Psych.;* 1910, 219 ff.
LANDIS (C.) & WILEY (L. E.) "Changes in blood pressure during deception." *Journ. Comp. Psych.*, 1926, VI, 1

LARSON (J. A.) " Modification of the Marston deception test." *Journ. Crim. Law and Criminol.*, XII, 3, 1921, 390 ff.
"The cardio-pneumo-psychogram in deception." *Journ. Exp. Psych.*, VI, 1923
" Present police and legal methods for the determination of the innocence or guilt of the suspect." *Journ. Crim. Law and Criminol.*, XV, No. 2, 1925, 219 ff.

LEHMANN (A.) *Die Hauptgesetze des menschlichen Gefühlslebens.* Aufl. Reisland, Leipzig, 1914

MARAÑON (G.) " Contribution a l'etude de l'action emotive de l'adrenoline." *Revue Francais d'Endocrinologie*, 1924, 2, pp. 301-25
" La Reaccion emotiva a la adrenalina." *La Medicina ibera*, XII, Agosto, 1920
" Breve ecsayo sobre la edad y la emocion." *Archivos de Medicina cirngia : y especialidades de Madrid*, Avril, 1921

MARSTON (W. M.) " Systolic blood pressure symptoms of deception." *Journ. Exp. Psych.*, 1917, vol. II, pp. 117-63
" Reaction time symptoms of deception." *Journ. Exp. Psych.*, 1920, III, pp. 72-87
" Sex characteristics of systolic blood pressure behaviour." *Journ. Exp. Psych.*, 1923, VI, pp. 387-419
" Negative type reaction time symptoms of deception." *Psych. Rev.*, 1925, 241-47
Emotions of Normal People, Kegan Paul & Co., London, Harcouit, Brace & Co., New York, 1928, Chapters VII, VIII, XI, XII.
" The Art of Sound Pictures " (with W. B. Pitkin), D. Appleton and Co., New York, 1930

SHEPARD (J.) " Organic changes and feeling." *Am. Journ. Psych.* 1906, XVII

SMITH (W. W.) *The Measurement of Emotion*, Kegan Paul, London ; Harcourt, Brace & Co., New York, 1922

WASHBURN (M.) & LEACH. " Tests of association methods of mental, diagnosis." *Am. Journ. Psych.*, 1910, 163-7

WATSON (J. B.) & WATSON (R. R.) " Studies in infant psychology." *Scientific Monthly*, 1921, 494-515

WECHSLER (D.) *The Measurement of Emotional Reaction : Researches on the Psycho galvanic Reflex.* New York, 1925

WELLS (F. S.) & FORBES (A.) " On certain electrical processes in the human body and their relation to emotional reactions. *Archives of Psych.*, 1911, 16

YERKES (R. M.) & BERRY. *Am. Journ. Psych.*, 1909, 20, 22·37.

CHAPTER XIX

PERSONALITY

PART I: PERSONALITY PATTERNS AND THE LOVE TYPE

Introductory

HAS a mechanical man any personality? Suppose it were possible to construct a robot capable of performing mechanically all the acts which a human being performs. Would you say that such a robot possessed personality? Probably the average person would deny that a mechanical device possessed personality no matter how similar the robot's actions were to those of the human being. A machine, somehow, is popularly regarded as the exact antithesis of human personality. We may say of a man, in everyday life, " he is only a machine, he lacks personality."

On the other hand, suppose a pet dog comes into the room and licks his master's hand. We speak of the dog as " affectionate." We think of him as having an attractive canine personality, perhaps more limited and primitive than our own, yet somehow resembling it very closely. What attribute does the dog possess that entitles him to a " personality? " What was lacking in the machine that is present in animals as well as in human beings, and which gives the popular suggestion of " personality? "

It seems to be a current concept that persons who are bubbling over with energy and activity, which has its source within such individual's organism, possess a great deal of personality. At the other extreme, persons who are seclusive and who go away from their fellows to ponder and day-dream by themselves are said to have " shut-in " personalities. The implication in this term would seem to be that these persons possess a great deal of personality within themselves which is nevertheless shut off from outward expression. Personality, then, is a term which seems to refer to certain energies or activities *within the organism* which are present to a large degree in human beings, to a lesser degree in animals, and which are absent altogether from mechanical devices.

What then is the internal activity, the sum total of which is termed " personality ? " Evidentally it is the activity called " consciousness." More especially, according to popular ideas, the term " personality " is associated with emotional consciousness. The temperamental prima donna, the captivating entertainer or social hostess, and the intensely emotional poet are regarded as individuals with " lots of personality." But it would not do to limit the definition of personality to emotional consciousness alone. Human beings with giant intellects like Einstein, Newton, and Edison would also be regarded as possessing a great deal of intellectual personality in the opinion of most thoughtful writers. Also, confessed sensualists like Petronius, Mark Antony, and Lord Byron have certainly been regarded as possessing striking personalities whose chief characteristic was the marked amount of sensory consciousness which they constantly sought to enhance. The real meaning of the word " personality " therefore, as this word is currently used, would seem to be the sum total of sensory, intellectual, and emotional consciousness possessed by a given individual.

To identify personality with consciousness would be a dangerously unscientific proposal if consciousness itself were not objectively defined. According to our preceding definitions of consciousness as psychonic energy, it is not a mysterious attribute of the soul but rather consists of a special type of energy generated in the brain and central nervous system. When we say personality is consciousness, therefore, we really define personality as the sum total of that energy within the individual organism ; consciousness, in fact, is the energy which is most influential in determining and directing all the organism's unit responses and part-reactions. Personality, according to this suggestion, is identical with the determining factor in each individual's life behaviour.

Perhaps a hundred years from now psychology may have devised instruments to study psychonic energy or consciousness directly. Perhaps some sort of ray may be discovered capable of illuminating the various centres of the human brain so that photographs of what is going on there may be recorded. In that event human personality can be studied directly by measuring and analyzing the psychonic energy which occurs in various parts of the central nervous system under all the possible experimental conditions representing situations to which the individual is exposed in everyday life. Were such measurements and analysis of personality possible, we might say that X's personality was of such and such a type regardless of what X's personality seemed to be in the opinion of various casual observers of X's behaviour. X's behaviour, in fact, would be predictable from the results of our study of X's personality. We could then say naturally that X's personality was one thing and his bodily behaviour another.

At any given moment X's outward or external behaviour might be expressive of his personality or it might not. It might be that certain parts of X's body were quiet or inactive. We could not say from casual observation whether this inactivity was brought about by central inhibition or merely by a local condition of subliminal nervous excitation. Even if X's body were extremely active we could not tell from external observation how many different types of nervous excitement were being integrated together to produce the visible activity. In short, mere observation of X's bodily activities at any given moment might reveal very little information about X's true personality.

Nevertheless, in the present condition of our psychological laboratories, we are forced to depend upon such objective observations of behaviour as are now possible in order to form judgments about our subject's personalities. In other words, the only way psychology can objectively determine personality at the present time is to study the individual's unit responses according to the best available methods, and then try to discover further how the unit responses are put together in the general life behaviour of the individual.

Personality Patterns

So far we have talked about unit responses ; now we have to talk about the unit person. Unit responses bear certain definite relations to one another within the total behaviour of an individual. They are put together in certain *patterns*. No matter whether unit responses occur simultaneously or whether they occur successively, there is almost always some degree of pattern discernable in their inter-relationship.

For example, let us return to the illustrations cited in

Chapter I. There we noted that a " born republican " manifested various unit responses of Submission to his parents and Compliance with the opinions of his individual family group in early life, by endorsing the Republican party. These unit responses may have begun to occur at the age of five or six and probably continued up to voting age. Thus habits of reaction were formed by repeated unit responses of a given type. Later, when this man voted, for the first time, his unit response to the ballot was to mark the Republican nominees for election. This unit response was clearly related to the responses which preceeded it throughout childhood and youth. The unit response of voting the Republican ticket was, in fact, caused by the preceding responses. Here we find a casual relationship between successive unit responses. This relationship is part of the total pattern which goes to make this man's personality.

Again let us analyze the case of the man who kicked his dog because he had to get his own supper. Here we have two unit responses simultaneously occurring, namely, the response to the absent-wife-supper-getting situation, and the unit response to the dog jumping up on his master. Evidently in this case the Rage response controlled and directed the response to his dog which ordinarily would have been an affectionate one. An inter-acting relationship between these two responses was evidenced by the man's behaviour. And this relationship helps to indicate a part of his total personality pattern.

Types of Personality Patterns

Granted that unit responses become organized into a unit person or unit personality pattern, it becomes very convenient to postulate certain general types of personality which may serve to simplify what would otherwise be an impossibly complicated study of all possible personality patterns. This postulation of personality types has been attempted in a number of different ways. Different criteria for differentiating types of personality have been used in different systems of classification. We may safely assert that none of these systems of personality classification have proved very useful, because none of the criteria adopted have been sufficiently definite or objective.

Some of the early Greek philosopher-psychologists suggested personality types called " sanguine," " phlegmatic,"

" choleric," and " melancholic." These suggested classifications were probably based in reality upon everyday observations of expressions of emotion or emotional attitude. Persons who appeared habitually optimistic would be classified as sanguine, those given to sudden violent temper fits, as choleric, etc. In an attempt to rationalize this system of classification and give it some physical basis, early writers attempted to find various conditions of the internal bodily secretions, such as bile, which would account for the class of personality observed.

The system of personality types which has received most popular attention in recent years is that proposed by Jung. This system is extremely simple, consisting of only two types, the introvert and the extrovert. The introvert is an individual whose attention is habitually directed inward toward his own subjective states, his thoughts and feelings. The introvert builds his conscious life about these subjective states as a centre. The extrovert is a person with precisely opposite tendencies. His attention is directed toward the outer world, and his conscious life centres about his perceptions of external reality. Extroverts may be mechanically inclined with their chief focus of attention upon material *things* ; or they may be gregariously inclined with their chief attention focussed upon *people*. This idea of Jung's is especially valuable in making psychopathic studies. The degree of extroversion or introversion serves as an excellent practical criterion, in certain border line states, between the mentally normal and the mentally abnormal. But it tells us very little indeed about the ordinary unit person whose attention is fairly well distributed between internal and external phenomena. Nor does Jung's classification furnish any objective criterion whatsoever for analysis of personality pattern.

A large number of other classifications of personality have been proposed which we shall make no attempt in the present volume to describe, beyond referring the student to the bibliography at the end of this chapter.

In our own approach to this subject in the preceding section we noted that personality pattern might be indicated in a rough way by psychological study and analysis of behaviour. We also noted in the two cases taken from Chapter I that behaviour thus studied reveals certain chronic or habitual relationships existing between different types of unit responses.

If, then, we can discover in this way the most general and most stable types of unit response relationships characteristic of different types of personalities, we shall have before us an objective classification of personality peculiarly revealatory of the innermost nature of the unit person.

Let us repeat our reasoning as follows. Personality is really the unit organization of consciousness. Flashes of consciousness accompany nearly every unit response. Practically all unit responses are related in some way to other unit responses occurring simultaneously or successively. These relations between unit responses are determined by more or less permanent types of connection between different types of unit responses. If these types of connections can be determined, then the corresponding types of more or less permanent organization of consciousness can be determined for any given individual. Therefore personality, which we have defined as unity of consciousness, can be objectively classified according to the types of connection, or integration between unit responses. These types of connection, then, which are to serve us as our types of personality, must be discovered from a comprehensive study of any individual's total behaviour.

For the sake of convenience let us group all unit responses into two classes—responses of love and responses of appetite. Love responses are normally evoked by *people* and appetitive responses are naturally evoked by *things*. Love responses include Inducement, Submission, Passion, Captivation and the combination of Passion and Captivation into unit Love response. Appetitive responses include Compliance, Dominance, Desire, Satisfaction and the combination of Desire and Satisfaction into the unit response of Appetite.

Now there are three different types of relationships which the writers have actually found existing in different human personalities between love responses and appetitive responses. These three relationships are as follows :

1. Love responses may control appetitive responses. This is the type of personality organization which results in creative activity, as described in preceding chapters. No matter what type of creative work is accomplished, the ability to do such work is derived from a type of personality organization wherein the unit love responses are in control of the appetite responses.

2. Love responses and appetitive responses may have

no fixed or permanent relationship one to the other. Certain types of people and all material objects may be responded to appetitively. A few people may call forth love responses on nearly all occasions. Or it may be that, in the case of selected individuals, love responses control responses of appetite while, in the case of all other persons, appetitive responses control love reactions. In any case there is no definite unification of personality pattern with either love responses or appetitive responses in control.

3. Appetitive responses may control love responses. This is the type of personality organization which habitually uses other people for the subject's own selfish benefit. This type of person controls other people by manifesting love behaviour toward them and subsequently utilizes other people's love responses, thus evoked, by changing his behaviour into an appetitive pattern. All the emotional reversals mentioned in the fore-going chapters, as well as various disintegrations of the personality pattern itself, inevitably result from this type of personality organization.

We now have before us three proposed personality types based upon the writer's observations and case studies. For brevity's sake we may name our three personality types: 1. the love type, 2. the duplex type, and 3. the appetitive type. Let us now discuss each of these types in further detail with illustrative examples and cases.

The Love Type

We must first emphasize the fact that our three personality types are only intended to classify individual personalities according to the type of relationship between love and appetitive responses, which most frequently prevails. If we classify a person as belonging to the love type, for example, we do not in the least imply that such an individual's love responses will control his appetitive responses upon all occasions and under all possible circumstances. We only mean that, in the main, love responses are predominant. Under favourable conditions of the environment and on occasions when the personality is fairly well integrated to make a unit person, love responses will prevail. But under peculiar emotional stresses and strains, under markedly unfavourable environmental conditions, and during activities when the personality is not functioning as a unit, appetitive responses may frequently gain the ascendency. This precaution against placing too comprehensive an interpretation upon our proposed personality types is especially necessary in considering the love type of personality, since this type represents the most complicated and highly evolved behaviour pattern attained by human beings, and consequently, like other highly evolved states of biological balance, it is extremely difficult to maintain. Love personalities require, for the most part, a protective environment, or at least a highly selective one.

What sorts of individuals possess love type personality? For the most part love personalities are limited to women, creative artists, intellectual originators, inventors, a few creative teachers and religionists, and, in general, very many young people of both sexes who have not yet been compelled to earn their own living, and still possess " youthful idealism ".

The love type personality of creative artists, and originators such as inventors and commercial pioneers, is impersonal in its focus. That is to say, such individuals, though possessing love responses strong enough to control their appetitive responses and so fuse them into a creative pattern, nevertheless direct their resulting creative activities, not toward their fellow human beings, but rather toward inanimate materials and material creations.

The above list of people likely to possess love type personalities is by no means exhaustive. There are, for example, humble fathers, country doctors, faithful supporters of large families, and truly altruistic philanthropists who possess real love type personalities. In general, we may say that all these love type individuals either live in an environment removed from business and social conflict or else possess sufficient resistance to withdraw emotionally from appetitive stimuli for a great part of the time.

Women

Women, as a sex, naturally possess love type personalities. Let us see what this means. It means, primarily, that nature has devised woman's body in such a way that its organs and stimulus mechanisms tend to build up love responses at the expense of appetitive responses. In a previous chapter we have studied the procreative drive together with the compound love responses which this drive automatically builds up. We discovered that the stimulus mechanism concerned with menstruation and childbearing naturally evoked the unit responses of Passion, Captivation, and creative responses of both types. We also had occasion to note that the love responses, when thus evoked by woman's natural stimulus mechanisms, actually assume control over her appetitive responses in connection with the bearing and bringing up of children. A woman desires and dominates food material for the purpose of submitting to her child and caring for him. She satisfies the child's needs rather than her own. And she satisfies her own needs during the nursing period in order to make proper nutriment for the baby. Throughout all these natural activities of motherhood it is plain to be seen that the mother's love responses control her appetitive reactions in such a way that whatever she acquires is passed on to the child and is acquired for his sake rather than for her own. This relationship between love and appetite constitutes the love type of personality as we have defined it.

The love life of most women with their husbands similarly indicates control of the appetitive responses by the love responses within the protective environment of the home. A wife is able to devote practically all her time and attention to serving the needs and comforts of her family. Wives of wealthy men, of course, are able to procure a sufficient number of servants to relieve themselves of all physical work, even including care of the children. But the life of a poor woman with a husband and several children to care for, represents a long career of drudgery the results of which are almost exclusively devoted to the husband and the children and not to the wife herself. Under modern conditions the average wife is not compelled to drudge in this fashion since the manual labour of housework has been greatly lightened by modern inventions and various commercial services such as laundries, bakeries, etc. Nevertheless a modern wife most frequently devotes a large share of her energies to pleasing her husband and serving his interests and those of her children. She does these things, apparently, for the most part as true love responses and not as acts of compliance with necessity.

It will probably be conceded without lengthy argument that a large majority of women devote themselves spontaneously to the service of their loved ones along the lines just discussed. But it is also obvious that these same women frequently act selfishly and appetitively. When the appetitive responses, for example, are uppermost in a woman's behaviour she may dominantly scold her children, berate her husband, make herself as disagreeable as possible for the purpose of accomplishing some selfish end of her own. Again, she may battle appetitively with other men's wives for social prestige and recognition. She may frequently attempt to dominate women more fortunate than herself in some particular by making " catty " remarks about them and spreading malicious gossip about their alleged shortcomings. All these reactions clearly evidence a control and complete subordination of the love responses by the appetitive behaviour elements. But with the average woman these appetitive lapses represent but a comparatively small part of her total behaviour. Moreover her appetitively controlled acts are more or less sporadic and unorganized as contrasted to the continuous and highly organized love behaviour which centres about her husband and home. Therefore, on the whole, we may still classify a majority of women as the love type of personality despite their variations from this pattern at frequent intervals.

A more serious question arises, however, in the case of the well-fed, socially prominent wife of a wealthy man after she reaches the age of 45 or 50. Such a woman's bodily love drives no longer compel her to seek love rather than appetite. She has continuously trained herself to seek physical possessions, social prestige, and æsthetic surroundings. In short, she has deliberately trained and developed her appetitive responses while the natural power of her love responses has been steadily diminishing. It seems probable that a great many women as they reach middle age definitely shift from the love type of personality to the appetitive type pattern for the reasons mentioned.

Youths

The scope of the present volume does not permit comprehensive discussion of other types of love personalities like youthful idealists, creative artists, creative teachers, and religionists whose general and better organized life behaviour is controlled by the love responses in much the same way as the behaviour of women just discussed. It may be said, however, that only youths during adolescence and immediately following are activated by a tangible bodily erotic drive comparable to that of the female organism. At puberty, of course, the gonads undergo certain changes which result in a total alteration of the entire endocrine balance of the body. An excess of erotic hormones apparently appear within the organism which result directly and indirectly in building up love responses in much the same way that a woman's love responses are activated. This condition frequently lasts up to the age of twenty or even later. In a majority of cases this temporary erotic drive is not strong enough to control the entire personality. Youths, during adolescence and immediately following, are frequently selfish, thoughtless, and rebellious against all authority. Nevertheless their intellectual interpretations of human beings frequently indicate a belief that love responses control human behaviour, or should control it. Youthful idealists believe that it does, and youthful radicals and pessimists become violently rebellious because they subconsciously feel that love should control the human personality but does not. This particular period of youth, therefore, is a peculiarly interesting one for the psychologist in studying the evident conflict between love and appetitive responses for the eventual control of the personality pattern.

Intellectual Originators

Let us consider for a moment, by way of contrast, the manner in which love responses control the behaviour of intellectual originators.

Here we pass into a somewhat different category of love type personalities. In the instances so far considered, the personality type is not only based upon love responses but these responses are directed *emotionally* toward other people. The unit love-type responses of these personalities obviously include their own emotional part-reactions as their most predominant elements. This need not always be so ; there are other love-type personalities in which the unit responses are chiefly composed of, or determined by, their own correlation or sensory part-reactions. The objective criterion as to which subdivision of the love-type we are dealing with in any particular case, will be the *class of end result* toward which the unit responses are directed, whether emotional relationships with other persons, the solving of intellectual problems of science or philosophy, or the procuring of new sensory experiences. Under the present heading we have to deal with those in whose unit love-type responses the mental part-reaction plays the predominant role, as evidenced by the character of end result (intellectual construct) toward which these responses are directed.

We have already noted in the second chapter on Thought-Processes, that intellect possesses two characteristic types of activity which we termed Knowing and Realization. We may now go a step further and consider the creative activities of intellect when the appetitive intellectual responses of Grasping and Comprehension (Knowing) are combined with the intellectual love-type responses of Imagination and Explanation (Realization).

We have already seen how the Passion response of a creative artist controls his Desire response so that he literally gives *himself* to the material that he desires to mould and re-shape into his own pattern. The true creative artist, in short, passionately surrenders himself to his art, to his work.

In exactly the same way the intellectual creator surrenders himself completely to the task of re-shaping the data he has grasped, into his own pattern. The task of intellectual creation becomes for him an end in itself. He forgets everything else for the time being in the sheer joy and intense effort of creating new intellectual masterpieces, new ideas, and new systems of thought. It matters not to the truly creative intellectual whether or not his creation will ever serve a practical purpose. It matters not to such a man that the same amount of mental work applied to money-making activities would make him rich. This type of person, for the very reason that his intellectual love responses control those of Appetite, devotes his whole intellect without stint to the creation of new intellectual material.

The entire creative process, however, begins and ends in his own brain. The intellectual creator is not concerned with objectifying his creation in tangible, concrete form, such as a mechanical device or invention. He is satisfied with his *idea* for a mechanical device, as soon as he feels assured that the *idea* is perfected. Of course, some experimentation may be necessary to perfect the intellectual creation, as in the case of Newton. But Einstein, for example, once he became satisfied that his intellectual creation of the Relativity Theory was perfect, secured the services of a collaborator to work out the mathematical formulation of his theory. He has been content, moreover, for the most part, to leave the actual experimental proof of relativity to astronomers and other experimentalists. Thomas Edison long ago conceived the idea of talking pictures, introducing the pictures as an accompaniment to his phonograph. But Münsterberg and many practical picture producers maintained that sound and sight could never be combined to give a popular form of entertainment. Edison appears to have accepted this verdict without contest. He was perfectly satisfied with the perfection of his idea, which he felt assured was sound. Whether the idea was applied in the field of practical showmanship was a matter of trivial importance to the great intellectual creator. It is rarely indeed that an intellectual creator manifests any considerable interest in anything outside the realm of ideas.

Further insight into the intellectually creative type of personality may be gained by contrasting this sort of individual with other intellectual workers in scientific and practical fields. Several modern text books of psychology, for example, state frankly that the study of science in general and of psychology in particular, is motivated chiefly by the practical desire to control human behaviour for appetitive purposes. This assertion is doubtless true with regard to the writers of these text books. Perhaps a majority of psychologists, for example, shrewdly judging that psychology, as the newest of the physical sciences, offers the greatest opportunity for individual achievement, proceed to elect psychology as their life-work in accordance with this practical judgment. This type of individual most frequently selects a subject for research that is closely connected with some lucrative commercial field. One may guess that most intelligence tests, vocational tests, and similar practical devices have had their origin in motives of this kind. Again, the scientist's appetitive motivation may be of a more subtle sort. He may undertake researches calculated to bring him academic preferment. He may publish his research results without any serious attempt to interpret them or to use his material for the creation of a new scientific theory. Such an individual's intellectual love responses are not in control of his intellectual responses of appetitive type. He is not an intellectual creator or originator.

The Inventor

Finally, we may consider still another type of creative personality, the inventor. The typical inventor " thinks with his hands." He does not retire to his study with blue prints and mathematical data piled high on his desk and proceed to think out his proposed invention mentally. He goes to his shop and begins handling and manipulating the various tools and existing mechanical devices that he hopes to use in working out something new.

Many inventors, when called upon to explain the principles and commercial advantages of their inventions, are unable to do so. Their attempted explanations are apt to be incoherent, inadequate, and even ignorant. Yet the same inventor who fails to explain his device in coherent terms, can always *see* how the machine works in minute detail. His sensory perceptions apparently arrange themselves in original and creative patterns while he is working over his apparatus. His emotional part-reactions may be dull, his intellectual part-reactions may be missing almost altogether, yet his sensory part-reactions will always be found keen, sensitive, and prolific. The suggestion follows that our typical inventor is a creative person of *sensory* type. That is to say, an inventor is an individual whose sensory part-reactions play the most prominent part in his unit responses and whose love-type responses predominate over and control his responses of appetitive variety.

One objection to this classification of the typical inventor's personality pattern will arise immediately in the minds of many students. The inventor, who works largely with his hands as we have seen, appears to be predominantly a man of action. He might be described, in fact, as a " motor type " person in many psychological classifications of personalities, especially in behaviouristic ones.

Why, then, should we classify him as a sensory type personality ? Our answer to this objection must refer once again to our initial definition of personality. Personality was defined as the pattern of consciousness. Gross bodily behaviour is not in itself conscious, except in so far as it is brought about by unit responses that include part-reactions of consciousness. The inventor's physical activity over his machine, therefore, is not really a part of his personality, but only a symptom or a result of his personality. To describe the inventor as a motor type personality would be to classify him according to his bodily behaviour and not according to his prevailing type of consciousness.

There is a further objection to be met. The inventor, in common with the athlete, the physical labourer, and other physically active types, must possess an organism whose " hidden machinery " on the motor side is peculiarly active. The motor excitations of a physically active individual must be relatively more intense than is the case with other types of persons. If the inventor's nervous system is intensely activated on the motor side, and if motor psychonic energy is actually motation or emotional consciousness, why should the inventor prove a relatively unemotional type of individual ? Why, in fact, should the athlete, the mechanic, the peasant working in the fields, and nearly all other classes of physically active persons, reveal themselves as comparatively unemotional in their consciousness ?

Many students in classroom discussion of the psychonic theory of emotion as motor consciousness, have advanced arguments similar to those contained in the last paragraph. The answer is simple, although not obvious. Intense physical activity depends, not upon the complexity of impulse integration in the motor centres of the brain, but rather upon the simplicity of such integrations. Schematically speaking, the motor type of person is one whose motor centres afford the clearest and most uninterrupted paths between the correlation centres and the efferent nerve trunks. The more rapidly and easily the nervous excitations, or impulses, are permitted to pass through the motor centres and out into the motor nerves leading to the muscles and other effector organs, the greater will be the muscular and effector activity. In short, the simpler the integrative pattern in the motor centres, the greater and more constant the bodily activity will be. Now motor consciousness, or motation, does not depend upon efferent nerve excitation, but rather upon the *amount* of integrative activity in the motor centres, according to the psychonic theory of consciousness. The more complex the integrative pattern, therefore, the more varied and complex will be the emotional experience of the individual. And the simpler the integrations, the simpler and less varied will be the emotional consciousness.

According to the predictions of the psychonic theory, then,

we should expect to find " motor type " individuals possessing intense but very simple emotions. The nervous excitement in their motor centres might at times become intense, but must at all times remain integratively simple and direct. The moment motor integrations become complicated with numerous conflicts and alliances of psychonic impulses having their origin in various and different parts of the central nervous system, the moment, that is, that emotional experience becomes varied and complex, at that moment bodily activity must become irregular, variable, and less smoothly co-ordinated. Expressing this in psychonic terms, we would say that the more emotional a given unit response became, the less efficient and the less extensive the final bodily action would tend to be.

The actual facts, therefore, appear to bear out the psychonic theory. Inventors and other action-type people show smooth, quick, and effective bodily actions and movements. Their emotions are apt to be strong but very simple. When their emotions become more complicated and more varied in pattern, their physical activities become correspondingly interrupted and less efficient. In fact, so many observers have noted the correspondence between emotionality and diminution of final bodily activity that many theories have described emotion as due to the blocking of motor impulses in the central nervous system. The early psychologists frequently attributed feeling and emotion to the blocking of instinctive action. These observations are quite in accord with the psychonic theory of motor consciousness as emotion.

Having discussed our justification for classifying " action type " people as possessing preponderantly sensory personalities, let us complete our analysis of the typical inventor. It is especially obvious that in his case the sensory part-reaction is highly determinative of the entire response ; what he does, in fact, is to combine the sensory impressions he receives from the inanimate objects he deals with, into new and original patterns, and thus he originates novel, mechanical devices. The devising of these contrivances essentially represents new combinations *of sensory impressions.*

In this activity there are two elements, the sensory awareness *per se* and the perception or synthesizing of many sensations into a unit group or pattern. Sensory acuity itself may be compared to the Grasping activities of the intellect ; while perceptive synthesis seems comparable to the intellective process of Imagination. The inventor, according to our analysis, represents a type of individual whose sensory responses and perceptive responses are combined in a creative pattern. Perception responses would represent the love type reactions while sensation itself would represent the acquisitive or appetitive type responses. We would not, however, insist too strongly upon this analogy, since perception, after all, is a correlation function and the inventor is a sensory type. However, he is not only a sensory type, but a creative or love type as well ; what makes him a love type is the creative synthesis of his sensations, and what makes him a sensory type is the fact that this synthesis uses as its materials, not concepts or emotional relationships, but *sensory impressions.*

The inventor devotes himself to his own variety of creative task as unreservedly as the intellectual creator surrenders himself to ideational creation or the creative artist to creations of an emotional kind. The inventor is thoroughly content to work out his invention for its own sake. He is oblivious to practical matters as a rule and prone to neglect domestic duties and interests. His personality outside his inventive activities is likely to be childish and simple. Inventors are proverbially impecunious and usually make little money out of their own inventions. All these behaviour characteristics indicate an exclusive absorption in their inventive creations. This surrender of the entire personality to creative work regardless of all other considerations seems to be the outstanding behaviour characteristic of all personalities whose love responses predominate over responses of appetite and control them for the most part throughout the personality pattern.

The Subdivision of Personality Types

In the foregoing sections we have analyzed a few examples of the so-called love type of personality. Our analysis revealed that there is a large class of persons whose love type responses in ordinary circumstances do control their appetitive responses ; and that this is particularly true in those type situations that furnish the key to the consistent pattern of their life behaviour and activities. We have also found that this love response control can occur in the three different cases when any one of the three basic divisions of consciousness predominates and determines the *direction in which* the love-controlled behaviour is to be focussed.

In all three divisions of conscious predominance we found that control of appetite by love responses resulted in some sort of creative behaviour, the sort being determined by which kind of consciousness was most influential in the entire unit response. The inventor was cited as an example of love type personality with sensory part-reactions predominating in a majority, or in the most typical instances, of his unit responses. The scientific or intellectual originator was used as an example of a love type personality with intellectual part-reactions predominating throughout the characteristic pattern of unit responses. Women, creative artists, youthful idealists, and altruistic teachers and religionists, were mentioned as examples of love-type personality whose emotional part-reactions predominated throughout their most important groups of unit responses. In reviewing all the subdivisions of love type personality we may note that the behaviour fields of their typical activities seemed accurately to reflect the division of consciousness predominating within the personality.

Our behaviouristic criterion, therefore, of the love type in general would be genuine creative activity indulged in for its own sake. Our behaviouristic criterion for the sensory, intellectual, and emotional types within the general love type personality, would be the class of material or stimuli dealt with during the creative procedure. We shall meet with these same three subdivisions again in considering the other main personality types, and thus we may outline a simple scheme for classification of personality, in the following table (p. 514):

FIGURE 46
Classification of Personality Patterns

CLASSIFICATION OF PERSONALITY PATTERNS			
Sub-Classes	GENERAL TYPE OF PERSONALITY		
	Love Type	Appetitive Type	Duplex Type
Sensory	Inventors Creative artisans Sport-loving amateur athletes Many architects, interior decorators, etc.	See Figure 47	See Figure 48
Intellectual	Creative scientists Constructive philosophers Intellectual creators and originators in fields of sociology, economics, political economy, literature, etc.		
Emotional	Majority of normal women Youthful idealists Creative artists Constructive religionists		

CHAPTER XX

PERSONALITY

PART II: APPETITIVE AND DUPLEX TYPES

Appetitive Type Personality

BEFORE discussing the duplex, or intermediate type, it seems advisable to analyze the appetitive type of personality which stands in most extreme contrast to the love type just considered. In our discussion of the love type we noted throughout that both Appetite and Love responses were present and united in an habitual behaviour pattern with the Love responses in control. In just the same way, during our discussion of the appetitive type personality we must remember that responses of Love are present but are controlled by responses of Appetite. The appetitive type personality is not to be confused with less unified personalities where simple Appetite responses most frequently occur by themselves without any subservient love response.

In considering love type personalities we noted that a majority of this type were women, since nature's stimulus mechanisms for bringing about love control of the appetitive responses appear most prominently in the female organism. We may now note that a great majority of appetitive type personalities are men. The only reason which we can give for this observed fact seems to be a negative one, that is to say, the absence of special procreative drive mechanisms in the male organism. It may be also that male hunger hormones are more potent than female and that male hunger pangs are more intense and of somewhat longer duration. The writers have accumulated some evidence indicating such conclusions but not enough to support a definite assertion to that effect. Not all men, by any means, have appetitive personalities, and many women, on the other hand, possess personalities distinctly belonging to this type. Nevertheless there would seem to be an inherent tendency in the male organism to develop appetitive type personality.

Besides a great many men of all classes and occupations we might suggest the following classes of individuals as examples of appetitive type personality. Pleasure-seekers of both sexes who obtain their pleasure by using other people, as in prostitution and pleasure-seeking sex affairs without love ; " society " people, where the social company of other people is used to promote the society person's own prestige and reputation ; " gladhanders," gigolos, " yes men," sycophants, " gold diggers," and persons who entertain, go to church, and join clubs and societies for the purpose of reaping appetitive benefits from the people thus contacted ; destructive critics of art, many politicians and a majority of business people of both sexes ; habitual gossips, scandal mongers, and persons who pry into other people's affairs and personalities and obtain confidences merely to gain superiority or appetitive ascendancy of some kind over the other individuals, this class of persons including many social workers, psycho-analysts, and psychologists ; finally, all dependent relatives, wives, and other dependents who manifest affection toward their patrons in order to be supported by them, but do not love the patron for his own sake regardless of financial advantage.

This is only a partial list of the many classes of individuals whose life behaviour is organized on the principle of using a love control of others for their own self interest. It will, of course, be impossible to analyze in detail any considerable number of these different classes of appetitive type personalities. We may, however, consider briefly one example of each of our subdivisions of appetitive type personalities, namely, emotional type, intellectual type, and sensory type.

Sensory Appetitive Types

A unit person of this type reacts ultimately to money, or things. The controlling reactions in every response pattern consist of Desires to possess material property but this is not all of the response. Appetitive type personalities do not seek to deal directly with the material objects to be acquired or manipulated. Appetitive type personalities almost invariably attempt to use other people to do the actual acquiring or manipulating of material objects and themselves profit by the results of other people's labour. Responses of genuine love type are shown toward the people to be used. But unit responses of Desire and Satisfaction toward money and possessions predominate over and control the love responses to people, so that when the behaviour pattern is complete the love type relationship with people is continued or discontinued according to the degree of material profit obtained from the relationship. Thus Love responses become an essential part of the profit-seeking pattern but always under the control of appetitive responses.

Perhaps a majority of business men possess a typical personality pattern of this class, which, whether justly or not, is typified in the popular mind by the Hebrew man of business. Jewish merchants and moneymakers have been noted throughout history for their complete self-absorption in business as well as for their success in driving sharp and profitable bargains. This type of business man, moreover, is not a pioneer like the miner, the rancher, the cattle man, or the farmer. On the contrary, the Jewish business man is found almost exclusively in densely populated areas where a maximum of contact with other people is assured. He is essentially social in his habits and methods of business. He is an habitual and very successful inducer of other people. Throughout his business career he uses this Inducement or persuasive ability to persuade other people to buy his goods and pay the price demanded for them. Business men of this type seldom if ever try to force their wares upon other people by dominant methods. There is another type of business man who constantly seeks monopolies calculated to compel other people to pay high prices, and who, if necessary, attempts actually to destroy the property of those who do not submit to his demands. But the Jewish business man does not do this. He relies habitually upon high-power sales talk and persuasion, often of a very subtle variety.

This type of business man also is quite willing to submit to other people if he can make a profit or avoid a loss by so doing. If the owner of some desirable merchandise demands an unreasonably high price for it, the Jewish business man will pay the price provided the seller convinces him that the goods are in great demand. He does not seek as a rule to determine the demand by a careful scientific survey of the market. He bases his judgment almost altogether upon the personal appeal of the seller's arguments, i.e. his unit response is a submissive one when the seller's Inducement is strong enough. He frequently uses, as a secondary criterion, the degree to which other business men are willing to submit to this same seller. That is to say, if a Jewish business man becomes convinced that some of his business rivals are sufficiently impressed with the seller's argument to submit to his demand, his own submissive response is greatly intensified. He tends to submit both to the seller and to the judgment of those of his business rivals whom he particularly admires.

One actual instance of this type of reaction which has come to our attention is as follows. A magazine story had been on the market for a number of years at a nominal price. No one wanted to buy it. At last the wholly individual needs of a large motion picture producing company caused this company to make an offer for the story. Immediately the Jewish executive of another company who had turned the story down several times and who had no especial need for it, bought the story at about ten times its former market price. The essential point to be noted in this behaviour is the fact that the story was not judged on its own property evaluation with respect to the business needs of the purchaser. Instead, the purchaser showed a unit response of personal Submission to the judgment of a business rival for whom he had great respect. The fact that this rival's judgment in wanting to acquire the story was not based upon the general value of the story but rather upon special and peculiar business needs was not known, of course, to the purchaser. In cases of this kind the Appetitive combination of unit responses could not stand alone without making use of a personal Love reaction to another individual. Instances of this type show the extreme stability and closeness of integration of the typical appetitive personality pattern.

There is another interesting response element prominent in the behaviour described, and that is over-compliance. The extensive use of Submission ultimately controlled by Appetite turns a good part of the Submission into Compliance response. The purchaser who paid a high price for a worthless story no doubt *complied*, to a great extent, with what seemed to him to be the necessity of paying dearly or losing an article which might bring him a big profit if purchased. This over-compliance development, in this particular type of personality, frequently results in Fear, and this type of personality is commonly subject to states of almost chronic Fear emotion.

It also results in frequent yielding to antagonistic threats which might easily be disregarded if considered objectively on their own merits.

This appetitive type of personality frequently expresses itself in business in still another fashion. A younger or less influential man attaches himself personally to the service of another man who bids fair to become successful and wealthy. In such cases the unit Love responses are knit into a pattern which might properly be called Passion response, though without any implication of erotic physical relationship. A shrewd young business man of this type frequently detects potentialities of success in his patron long before success is actually achieved. At the beginning it may look to the outsider like a case of spontaneous friendship and admiration, but in the cases investigated by the writers the younger men have readily explained that they had attached themselves to the other man because they believed in his success and therefore felt that their own careers lay in that direction. Several cases of this sort also have been observed wherein the patron's business hopes were frustrated, the younger man immediately deserting him and forming personal attachments to someone else. In these cases it is very plain that appetitive responses were always in control, but that Love responses always appeared to be a necessary and essential part of the unit behaviour pattern. The writers have found in several cases that the young men just described considered that an appetitive purpose for their attachment to another individual must always be present in order to justify their Submission to the patron. This indicates that the appetitive type personality pattern is a deeply inwrought one and does not consist merely in isolated actions performed for reasons of temporary expediency.

We may now generalize with respect to the outstanding characteristics of the appetitive type personality above described. Throughout the behaviour considered two distinct sets of unit responses appear. The first group of unit responses are reactions to people. The second are reactions to things. These two groups of unit responses are only successively connected together. They are not fused into a single new type of complex unit response possessing new characteristics and attributes as in the Love type personality previously considered, where Love and Appetite responses unite to form creative behaviour. In the appetitive type of combination, reactions to things control reactions to people, yet people are not treated as things, as they were, for example, by the early Roman military conquerors. People are properly reacted to with Love responses just insofar as they are able to serve the ultimate appetitive purposes which control the entire behaviour pattern. The moment a person ceases to serve this ultimate appetitive purpose he is either completely disregarded or else reacted to dominantly as an antagonistic thing or obstacle.

The appetitive type personality is an eminently successful one, within limits, with respect to its acquisitive accomplishments. Persons of this type are able to acquire much money and material property because that is the single purpose toward which the entire behaviour pattern is directed. Moreover, this type of personality is able to accomplish its single purpose with a minimum of effort and conflict, because other people are not treated dominantly but are induced and submitted to in ways calculated to make them serve the ultimate purpose of the appetitive type individual.

The limitations in the objective efficiency of this type of personality lie almost wholly in the degree to which other people are able to perceive the ultimate purposes of the appetitive type individual. Appetitive type persons understand one another's ultimate purposes quite thoroughly but still accept them as legitimate. A thorough-going appetitive type person does not resent the fact that another individual of the same type is seeking to use him for an ultimate end. That seems to him justifiable and natural. His only concern, therefore, is to attempt to control his dealings with the other fellow in such a way that the balance of advantage will be on his own side. But Love type personalities and duplex type personalities do not react in this way to appetitive type persons. They do not accept as legitimate the use of one person to serve the appetitive purposes of another. Therefore, when they detect the presence of an ulterior purpose they cease to respond with Love reactions to the persuasions and Inducements of the appetitive type person. They then cease to deal with the appetitive person altogether or else begin to react dominantly to him as though he were not a person at all but a thing. It would seem to the writers that this mutual misunderstanding of two fundamentally different types of personality is the true psychological cause underlying the age-old conflict between Jews and Gentiles. When persons who do not themselves possess appetitive type personality perceive that they have been used without their knowledge for the appetitive benefit of another person, their dominant resentment knows no bounds. Themselves lacking the requisite personality traits to master the appetitive type individual by his own methods, a non-appetitive type person resorts perforce to Dominance and physical violence.

There is a rare type of duplex personality which possesses sufficient psychological insight to discover the ultimate purposes of the appetitive type person before these purposes are accomplished. The duplex person then resorts immediately to Dominance. This dominant attitude effectively prevents the appetitive type person from using the duplex person. Also the appetitive type individual, true to his personality pattern, finds himself unable to deal with his opponent by methods of direct Dominance. Again running true to his complex type of behaviour, he attempts to propitiate the dominant duplex person by increased use of both Submission and Inducement, which methods of treatment are totally ineffective as long as the duplex person maintains his dominant attitude. The duplex individual in this case wins his point and the appetitive type person, running true to form, admires him for it. This would seem to the writers to explain the frequently successful business partnerships between Jews and Irish, the Jews representing the appetitive type personality and the Irish the duplex personality with very strongly developed Dominance responses.

There remains to discuss our justification for classifying the appetitive type business man as an essentially sensory personality. We may admit, in the first place, that many persons of this type are extremely emotional. But the more successful persons in the class described exhibit a fundamental coldness which characterises their most successful business behaviour and which is lost most frequently when their business responses are thwarted or unsuccessful. The typical appetitive person, while frequently manifesting the appearance of emotion for the purpose of making his Inducements of other people more impressive, nevertheless appears to maintain a predominant sensory consciousness responding with extreme flexibility to sensory changes in the stimulus situation. In act, his business efficiency is to a great extent dependent upon this sensory control of behaviour. Furthermore, nothing is more obvious than that the interests of this personality type are primarily concerned with money, in the sense that their subjective scale of values uses money as its fundamental criterion of value.

What, then, is money? It is, of course, a medium of exchange and thus a symbol representing other things. Before the invention of money, the appetitive sensory type personality dealt with actual objects such as cattle, sheep, clothing, shoes, corn, and other material commodities. These were dealt with directly; the man who accumulated the largest number of objects, such as herds of cattle and merchandise caravans in actual operation, as his personal property, was considered by the sensory appetitive type as the most successful. When it was found more convenient to do away with the system of direct barter, money was invented to stand for and represent any and all of the objects formerly dealt with directly. Thus money is directly translatable into cattle or clothing, or any of the vast number of commodities toward which the energy and behaviour of this type of personality is directed. Money, in fact, is only a symbol for things ; and thus we may say that he whose primary interests are monetary, is a sensory type, since his activities are characteristically focussed upon sensory objects.

With regard to this type, emotion represents an impeding factor which must be minimized at all times to make his behaviour successful. This type of individual also frequently manifests a large amount of intellectual consciousness but when the personality balance swings from the sensory to the intellectual we find the appetitive type person deserting his business pursuits and devoting himself to scientific or academic interests. In the main, we may safely say that the eminently successful appetitive type business man possesses a predominantly sensory personality with quick decisive physical action and strongly developed, intense, but simple emotions, which we previously noted as characteristic of the inventor or sensory Love type personality.

Emotional Appetitive Types

We may next consider the emotional class of appetitive type persons, because this class overlaps considerably the sensory appetitive type. The controlling reactions in the important unit response patterns of emotional appetitive type personalities consist of Desires to obtain pleasant emotional stimulation. A unit person of this type seeks ultimately to experience the emotions of Dominance and Satisfaction. A stimulus to Desire also may be the ultimate purpose of such individuals' behaviour. But the ultimately desired appetitive emotions must be obtained, as in the sensory type personality, by control of other people through their Love responses. It seems to be a curious fact repeatedly observed by the writers that appetitive type persons who seek emotional gratification above all else seldom seek such gratifications by mere eating, drinking, or possession of beautiful objects, devoid of any accompanying and subsidiary emotional contacts with other human beings. The appetitive emotional type individual may revel in food and drink but to obtain his ultimate enjoyment he must eat and drink with other people and if possible at their expense. In the same way the emotional appetitive type person of male sex habitually uses the Love responses of women to establish Dominance mastery over them and then throw them aside after they have served the pleasure of the moment. Actual enjoyment of the process of seduction of a woman means that Captivation or Passion responses are being used by the man to put the woman in a situation where he can dominate her.

In this respect, enjoyment of seduction for its own sake so to speak, is to be clearly distinguished from mere Captivation or Passion emotion which is so intense that scruples and consequences are forgotten. Cruelty and sadism are personality traits which naturally associate themselves with appetitive behaviour of the type just mentioned. Another form which this same appetitive use of Love responses frequently takes in this class of personality, is use of parental affection for the ultimate purpose of experiencing egotistical Satisfaction in the successful accomplishment of the offspring. This appetitive type personality trait is found in men who indulge and pamper an only son, exaggerating his abilities and successes not because they are genuinely devoted to the son's welfare but because the son's success may carry on the father's and reflect added glory and prestige upon the father's ego.

The same trait is also found in mothers of the appetitive emotional type, whose Love responses toward their daughters are governed by the persuasion that these daughters are their possessions. The daughter, if physically presentable, may constitute an ornamental possession and be used to increase the mother's social prestige (Dominance) over her associates and, as she calls them, friends. This use of the daughter is accomplished by means of Love responses in which flattery and actual care for the daughter's appearance and advantage may play leading parts. These responses, however, are ultimately directed toward the daughter, not as a human person, but as a thing, the possession of which continues to inhere in the mother. The controlling element in this Appetite-Love combination response toward the daughter becomes exceedingly apparent when it is no longer possible for the mother to make use of the daughter for appetitive purposes. This may occur if the daughter marries a man possessing neither social ambitions nor abilities, or if she eventually decides that she has a better use for her time and energies than the continual furtherance of her mother's appetitive interests. In such cases the mother's Love responses become reversed, and frequently a bitter Hatred pattern replaces the former Love element in her responses.

So far we have only mentioned illustrative personality traits belonging to the appetitive emotional class under discussion. Let us now seek an example of a unit personality whose principal behaviour consists of Appetite responses dominating over and controlling Love responses. A certain type of stage performer exemplifies the personality type under discussion. In an earlier chapter we have distinguished between creative artists who originate stories, plays, and other works of art, and the transforming artists who enact these original creations in such a way that they are impressed effectively upon the minds of the public. Some of these actors and actresses whom we have classified as transforming artists are genuinely creative individuals with Love type personalities. These performers are known in the profession as " good troupers." Their primary purpose on the stage is to give the public good entertainment ; no matter what their own private grief or suffering may be, they compel themselves to follow that basic ethic of the stage, " on with the show." In other words, the public is to be considered first and it is up to the stage performers to give the audience the best that is in them, regardless of their own personal feelings. The type of personality which is habitually capable of this creative attitude is a Love type personality closely resembling that of the mother who is ready at all times to take care of the welfare and happiness of her child, regardless of her own interests or appetitive enjoyment.

But there is another type of stage performer who really cares nothing for his audiences except insofar as they serve to inflate his already over-developed ego. On the stage this type of person may appear gracious, charming, and of an altogether delightful personality ; the audience responding to this stage or screen personality applauds vociferously and lauds the actor to high heaven. With the aid of the proper publicity such an actor or actress may receive an incredible amount of hero worship from multitudes of people, yet the moment the curtain is down or the camera is " cut ", the controlling appetitive side of such personalities appears. The same person who has used his Love responses on the stage to captivate an audience, now becomes rude, " up stage ", and utterly bombastic toward his fellow performers, business associates, and friends. He talks only of his own ability and success. He demands the most servile flattery from those who wish to associate with his greatness. He exhibits extreme jealousy toward other performers who seem likely to share his glory in the slightest degree. He insists, for example, upon facing the camera throughout all the big scenes of the motion picture drama regardless of the appropriateness of such grouping to the story. Even on the stage he may curse fellow actors in an undertone in order to throw them off their balance and render their performance comparatively less effective than his own. Actors and actresses of this type frequently demand revision of the play in order to give them bigger scenes and deprive other performers of any chance to shine. Off the stage such individuals are uniformly vain, inconsiderate of others, and egotistical to an extreme which is almost unbelieveable.

In the behaviour described above it is easy to see that the controlling responses are appetitive and also that the emotional element in the total unit response tends to predominate. The charming affability which this type of actor or actress expresses on the stage, is used to control the people in the audience and to make them render emotional tribute, in precisely the same way that Inducement and Submission responses are used by appetitive type business men to control their customers and make them pay money tribute to the successful inducer. The appetitive type personality pattern is essentially the same in both cases. The chief difference lies in the type of appetitive tribute ultimately sought. The business man wants money, the actor wants praise which will give him the emotional experience of dominant superiority over his fellows. Of course, the business man may incidentally desire prestige, and the actor incidentally desires a high salary. But the publicity value of a high salary frequently means more to an actor of an appetitive type than the money itself, and he nearly always spends his earnings lavishly and even generously, to purchase still more dominant prestige from those on whom the money is spent or before whom his extravagant possessions are exhibited. There seems little doubt about the fact that appetitive type emotional values constitute the ultimate purpose of this very marked class of personality.

We may note incidentally that appetitive personalities of emotional type are likely to be successful in attaining their ultimate objects in precisely the same way that appetitive type business men are successful. Also they are subject to precisely the same limitations in their success. If the theatre-going and motion picture public discover the ultimate appetitive personality traits of a favourite actor or actress, that performer's popularity immediately begins to wane. A single story in the newspaper or magazine relating some cruel, snobbish, or meanly selfish act performed off stage by a popular idol, may precipitate the idol's fall from popular favour. Of course this is less likely to be true if the appetitive type individual thus unmasked is a character actor who usually plays the part of a villain or " heavy ", but on the other hand such an actor is never likely to attain the greatest heights of popular adulation, nor is the actor or actress who is willing habitually to play the villain, likely to possess an appetitive type personality. In general we may lay down the rule that the success of the appetitive type actor in winning popular favour depends fundamentally upon concealment from the public of his ultimately controlling appetitive personality traits.

Intellectual Appetitive Types

It is difficult to discover an intellectual appetitive type person whose intellectual activities and achievements are of a deep or weighty nature. Most persons of really profound intellect appear to be of either duplex or love type personalities, their intellectual output being either frankly iconoclastic or definitely creative correspondingly. There is, however, a certain type of distinctly intellectual person who does not delve too deeply into the mental subject matter at hand, whose personality type seems to be distinctly appetitive. This sort of personality is found in many different intellectual and semi-intellectual fields. There is, for example, the newspaper reporter whose ultimate ambition is to learn more facts than his rivals, but who proceeds to gather these facts on most occasions by making himself affable and friendly to those persons whose information he wishes to acquire. There is also the essayist and special writer who seeks the friendship of distinguished people in order to acquire their ideas and knowledge to enhance his own writings. There is the psychoanalyst and social worker who wins the confidence and perhaps the love of a patient or applicant for charity, not with the creative purpose of rendering help, but rather from the motive of learning the innermost secrets of the other person's private life, for his own intellectual profit. There is also the writer of popular books on various scientific and intellectual subjects who does no work of his own in the field he is writing about but quietly acquaints himself with the ideas of the creative workers most widely known at the moment, and appropriates these ideas to his own purposes without giving any credit for them. There are many popular lecturers at women's clubs and the like who systematically obtain their information in this way from others more learned than themselves.

One step higher in the intellectual scale we find some college professors, and men who have managed to get themselves ranked very near the top in various fields of science, whose personality traits and method of procedure shows precisely the same trend. Such men become very friendly with their colleagues and systematically glean from them original ideas and suggestions. They attend scientific conventions and make a point of becoming as intimately acquainted as possible with new and distinguished leaders in their own field. By means of all these friendly contacts with creative men of science they acquire for themselves a great store of well assorted knowledge ; and this knowledge they incorporate into their own books, lectures, and articles, usually without giving any credit whatsoever to the sources of their information. All these examples, selected from various intellectual occupations, show fundamentally the same appetitive behaviour pattern of acquiring knowledge for selfish purposes by friendliness or Love behaviour toward other people who possess the knowledge desired.

The appetitive control and use of Love responses by intellectual type personalities seems, on the whole, so simple and obvious that no single example need be studied at length. Appetitive type personality would seem, according to the observations of the writers, to occur very frequently among persons who earn their livelihood by some form of intellectual activity, with the single exception of those truly profound intellectual workers mentioned. These people are not very seriously handicapped by the possibility of being found out, for the simple reason that the great majority of people with whom they come in contact are less appetitively developed than themselves. Creative intellectualists are apt to be so completely devoted to their subject that it never occurs to them to doubt the motives of fellow scientists who question them about their discoveries and methods of research. Therefore, within the scope of the intellectual field, appetitive type persons are apt to enjoy a success that is virtually unlimited by any likelihood of their supply of information being cut off.

Differences between Love Type and Appetitive Type Personalties

In the section on Love type personalities we noted that control of Appetite by Love responses invariably resulted in some sort of creative behaviour, because of the apparent fusing of Love and Appetite into a new type of behaviour possessing characteristics not contained in its component reactions. In the present section on appetitive type personalities we found that no such fusions between Love and Appetite responses existed. As a matter of fact we noted the repeated appearance of conflict between the first and second stages of the behaviour pattern. Love responses by which appetitive type individuals induce other people to give them what they want, must always be definitely cut off and replaced by antagonistic appetitive reactions at the moment the appetitive object is actually obtained.

Love type personalities habitually endow inanimate materials with human values derived from themselves. They use inanimate objects for the benefit of human beings. Appetitive type persons, on the other hand, use human beings for the purpose of obtaining inanimate objects. They endow their own personalities with values derived from things which

FIGURE 47

Appetitive Type Personalities

Sub-Classes	
Sensory	Majority of business men in centres of population
	" Gold-diggers "
	Prostitutes
	" Joiners," clubmen, church-goers, etc., with ulterior money-making purposes
Intellectual	Ruthless newspaper men
	Parasitical and plagiaristic essayists, special writers, etc.
	Insincere psychologists, psycho-analysts, and social workers
	Scientists, teachers, and professional men who base their reputations upon the ideas and knowledge of others
Emotional	Seducers
	Sadists
	Parents who exploit children socially or for personal gratification
	" Society " people and would-be " society " people
	Actors who are not " good-troupers "
	Publicity seekers
	Habitual gossips and scandal mongers
	People who habitually use others for their pleasure

they have obtained. It is not unheard-of for them to imagine that the person who merely possesses the greatest number of things, is, in derivative fashion, the greatest person. In other words, Love type personalities place human values uppermost, while appetitive type personalities are controlled primarily by material values.

Finally, as a result of the two differences already noted, we find that Love personalities attain greater harmony of functioning within themselves, while appetitive personalities, on the average, obtain larger and more valuable material possessions. Love type personalities are compelled by their existing behaviour patterns to sacrifice material objects in order to obtain internal peace and harmony. Appetitive type persons, in following the behaviour pattern which they have developed, are compelled to sacrifice the internal harmonies of other people and of themselves to the manipulation of material objects.

The objective contrast between these two types of personality consists, in a word, of happiness versus success.

Duplex Type Personality.

The duplex personality is a perfectly definite type, with marked characteristics of its own. It is not to be confused with a mixed, or borderline group, invented only for convenience, to include personalities which lie part way between the love type and the appetitive type. The duplex personality represents a type of individual whose love and appetitive responses seem to be of approximately equal strength. Which type of response controls the personality at any given moment, therefore, depends upon the nature and strength of the environmental stimuli with which the organism is confronted. The duplex person may be thought of, roughly, as an individual who loves when he loves, and fights for what he desires when Desire is preponderantly evoked.

Perhaps a majority of duplex persons would become love-type people were it not for the necessity of earning a living in an appetite-controlled world. To remain truly creative, in society as it is, requires a considerable amount of sacrifice of appetitive rewards, and a personality with powerful appetitive drive is incapable of this sort of sacrifice. Many duplex persons studied by the writers began their careers by studying some form of creative art. When these persons discovered the hardships and sacrifices which their fellow artists were obliged to endure in order to attain even a modicum of recognition and success, they abandoned the artistic career as impractical. Duplex persons possess such an even balance of love and appetite development that it is impossible for them to sacrifice either one or the other. To starve in a garret for the sake of creating an artistic masterpiece entails an abandonment of appetitive satisfaction of which they are incapable.

Faced with the world as it is, therefore, and with the necessity, imposed by their own personalities, of extracting from life both love-type and appetitive-type experiences, duplex persons work out a double system of living, harmonized by alternating love behaviour and appetitive responses. These persons go after money, power, and material success in a more or less ruthless way, treating other people, for the most part, as inanimate things to be dominated and used for appetitive gain. On the other hand, they select a small group of individuals—a wife and children perhaps, a mother, lover, or life-long friend—whom they regard in a very idealistic way as persons worthy of complete love and faith. For these chosen few a typical duplex person will give himself, his possessions, and even his life without stint. Love relationships with these people represent the inner core of life, the pleasantest part, and therefore it becomes a matter of rigid principle with the duplex person to maintain these love relationships on a pure love level without permitting any self-seeking attitude to creep in. If the selected loved ones die, or prove unworthy of love, the duplex person is likely to become a bitter cynic, yet always cherishing a sort of abstract love ideal secretly in his mind, as a substitute stimulus for love responses which are as necessary to his personality as are the appetitive responses.

A second type of stimulus met with in everyday life turns many potential love-type personalities into duplex persons. The Christian religion is based upon a very interesting psychological theory of reforming humanity by loving people no matter how they may treat the Christian in return. For example, we find this doctrine explicitly set forth in the commands of Christ, " Love them that hate you, and do good to them that despitefully use you." And the promised result follows : " For great is your reward in Heaven." Now the duplex person doesn't care about rewards in heaven. He must have his rewards here and now. Moreover, when the cheek of a duplex person gets slapped, his Dominance response is so strong, for the moment, that all possibility of love behaviour is swept aside for the time. Instead of offering the other cheek, the duplex person is compelled by his personality type to hit back.

Intellectual duplex people reason in this way about the underlying theory of Christianity set forth in the last paragraph. If you try to kiss a person who hits you, he (or she) will only hit you harder. An individual whose love responses are not developed sufficiently to respond with love to a love stimulus, interprets love treatment at the hands of an enemy, not as love but as trickery or as confession of defeat. According to either interpretation a response of increased Dominance results. If the apparently loving opponent is attempting a trick, his trickery must be destroyed before it has a chance of succeeding. If the opponent is confessing defeat, he can now be pushed safely to the wall, to insure the spoils of victory. So, reasons the duplex intellectualist, it is the height of futility to love a person who hates you. Whichever way he looks at your behaviour he will only hate you worse and injure you more. Thus the doctrine of "Christian sacrifice," or loving unlovable people, appeals to the duplex person as false and impractical. The writers have even heard a duplex person assert that this doctrine is only serviceable as propaganda on behalf of appetitive-type people. It seems designed to make love-type persons, they argue, return again to the slaughter after having once been fleeced by an appetitive-type person who deliberately utilizes their love behaviours for his own appetitive benefit. A duplex person would maintain that the only way to make an appetitive person respond with true love is to first put him forcibly into a situation where he cannot react any other way.

For the reasons discussed, therefore, the duplex type of personality persists in maintaining two distinct and opposite varieties of response, with a relationship of reciprocal alternation between the two. Of the two, the love responses are likely to be inherently stronger, but the appetitive reactions are likely to be set off more frequently by environmental stimuli, and control, therefore, a larger proportion of the duplex person's life behaviour.

In the duplex type of personality we may place the "early American" type of business man, ruthless and very practical in his commercial enterprises, yet generous and completely controlled by sentiment in his home and love relationships. We may also include a certain type of prize-fighter (and other aggressive athletes and physical labourers) ably depicted by Jack London in *Valley of the Moon*. In this personality class, too, belong "hard" women, money-makers and pleasure seekers, who nevertheless respond with the purest sort of love to their lovers, their children, or perhaps a dependent father or mother ; a few strong military conquerors like Julius Cæsar, credited with killing a million men, yet never once disloyal to a loved woman or to a personal friend ; a certain type of

" ward-boss " politician and regular army officer, utterly ruthless toward rivals and opponents, yet generous, kindly, and
paternal toward their constituents and soldiers ; and, finally,
many female prostitutes and women of the world, and male
criminals of yegg and gangster types, who professionally rob
other people yet give themselves and their ill-gotten gains
without thought of self to lovers, children, or friends of their
own profession. (These people are not " honest " or conventionally reliable towards lovers and friends, but they do
seem to be spontaneously generous and to respond sporadically
with the purest of love responses towards certain selected
individuals).

The outstanding characteristics of duplex personalities
seem, then, to be the following. Duplex people possess love
and appetitive response patterns in such relationship one to the
other that neither is capable of controlling or eliminating the
other. When confronted by an appetitive social environment,
duplex persons react appetitively. But they also tend to seek
out a few, selected individuals toward whom they can respond
with pure love-type reactions, thus maintaining alternating
activity in both love and appetitive behaviour patterns.

For purposes of further illustration of the duplex-type
personality, let us consider examples of sensory, intellectual,
and emotional duplex persons.

Duplex Sensory Types

The business of prize-fighting necessarily requires that
opponents be physically attacked and dominated. The
prize-fighter need make little or no attempt to control his
opponent's behaviour in any way, by treating him as a human
being. His job is to force the other fighter to defeat by
hitting him as hard as possible. To accomplish this purpose
he must regard his antagonist as a *thing*, to be destructively
dominated. Prize-fighters differ, of course, in the degree of
Dominance toward opponents, but the most popular and
consequently the most successful fighters are said to possess
" the instinct of the killer."

In most cases, men who adopt physical fighting as a
profession like to fight. At least boxers of the " killer " type
find their appetitive responses adequately taken care of by
the activities of fighting, and making money by beating
opponents. Here we have the most primitive and direct

expression of appetitive Dominance, free, for the most part, from any admixture of love behaviour designed to control the responses of other people or utilize them for appetitive ends. Nor do love responses control the appetitive responses to result in any form of creation. The two types of behaviour are quite separate, thus constituting a true duplex pattern.

With many fighters the personality pattern stops just at this point. Their relations with women, like their relations with other fighters, are largely appetitive, with sex responses of the type known as " lust." But in the cases of several fighters studied by the writers there appears " another side " to the personality. These men show a very pure and unsophisticated type of love response toward their wives, girl friends, children, sparring partners, and trusted managers. Toward these selected individuals they frequently manifest a childlike confidence, faith, and Submission. The wife or chosen girl friend may be utterly adored, and her commands are frequently accepted as unquestioned gospel in all matters save those pertaining to the profession of fighting. True to the duplex type, however, self-interest always governs in appetitive affairs, just as love interest is permitted to govern in all other matters. The failure of " Billy's " wife to understand this duplex alternation of control (in Jack London's *Valley of the Moon*) reveals a frequent source of friction between love-type and duplex-type personalities.

Interesting side-lights on the basic balance of the duplex personality sometimes occur in the form of a struggle between the fighter's wife and his manager for the right to exercise a controlling influence over his affairs. The wife usually wins. Why ? Because, in the first place, she constitutes a much stronger stimulus to love responses than does the manager. Thus we may note that the appetitive reactions of a duplex person may frequently yield to love control, if the love stimulus is strong enough ; suggesting that the love response pattern may sometimes be intrinsically stronger than the appetitive pattern.

In the second place, the wife is frequently able to demonstrate conclusively that the manager is not a love stimulus at all, but is really the fighter's worst enemy posing as a friend. In other words, the wife proves to the fighter's satisfaction that his manager is disloyal to his interests. Instantly the fighter's type of behaviour toward his manager shifts from one extreme to the other. Whereas he previously trusted the manager implicitly and regarded him as his best friend, the fighter now quarrels with everything his manager says or does, and begins to regard the other man as his worst enemy. As soon as possible the boxer gets rid of his manager, not because he is controlled by love for his wife, but because he is controlled by Dominance toward a person newly revealed as an antagonist. This complete shift from love response to appetitive response invariably occurs, in the typical duplex personality, whenever a person formerly loved is discovered to be an antagonist in disguise.

A word remains to be said concerning our sub-classification of the duplex prize-fighter as a predominantly sensory type of personality. Like the creative inventor and appetitive business man, the prize-fighter is essentially a man of action. He cannot waste time on emotion, though both his Dominance and his Love emotions may be very intense as far as they go. His vocabulary and education are seldom adequate to permit any considerable amount of intellectual activity, even if his native tendencies ran in that direction. As a matter of fact, prize-fighters are proverbially " dumb " and unintellectual. (This duplex sensory type of prize-fighter does not include a fighter like James Joseph Tunney, who may be duplex but appears more intellectual than sensory). Thus we find in the duplex fighter type " a man of action," with simple, strong emotions, and little intellectual activity. For reasons previously set forth at length, it is our conclusion that persons of this type possess a preponderant amount of sensory consciousness, and are largely governed by it. For this reason, they are enabled to act swiftly, and with a precise adaptation in changing sensory stimulus situations.

Duplex Emotional Types.

Many women teachers and business women, both married and single, belong to this class. Apparently because of their sex characteristics, it is not so much money or power that they seek as a result of their commercial activities, but rather emotional experience mainly of appetitive type. These women will tell you that they must have " independence," " active interests," " a life of their own." They say they " enjoy the struggle of business," or " like being on their own." Also, we usually discover that such a woman enjoys various appetitive satisfactions of an emotional rather than an intellectual sort. These emotional experiences may be sought in possession of a beautiful home, clothes, objects of art, travel, clubs, entertainments, music, or merely in little constantly added luxuries and possessions of everyday life. Appetitive responses designed to secure these appetitive emotional experiences form a necessary and unescapable part of the behaviour pattern of women of this type. To give up the job and settle down to love in a cottage, or to give up the annual summer travel, for instance, in order to write a book, seems too much of a sacrifice to persons of this class.

Duplex personalities are generally incapable of curtailing their appetitive responses to make more room for love or creative behaviour. And duplex personalities of emotional type are controlled by responses seeking emotional experiences of appetitive nature.

But these duplex emotional women also possess a " love side." In rare cases, the principal love stimulus may be a husband or lover. When such is the fact, the husband will frequently be found to be an invalid, or person of weak character unable to earn a living for two. Duplex emotional women are unlikely to respond strongly in love to a person whose economic activities are likely to conflict with or control their own. Like other duplex personalities, they seek to establish and maintain a complete reciprocal alternation between appetitive and love behaviour ; and a successful, high-powered husband is " instinctively " recognized as likely to interfere with the wife's independent appetitive activities.

A significant variation of this same behaviour pattern occurred in the case of a young and attractive woman of distinct duplex personality type, studied by the writers. This girl was a Roman Catholic by birth and conviction. No less than four times, according to her own statement, she loved Protestant young men sufficiently to entertain seriously their proposals of marriage. But each time the question of agreeing to bring up the children in the Roman faith was met by refusal on the man's part. That meant, each time, that the girl must herself give up her religion, or else give up her love affair. Religious conviction to her was a precious emotional possession, defended by all her dominant responses. She *could* not yield love control of herself to a man who would deprive her of

religion and refuse to let her train her children religiously as she
sincerely believed they ought to be trained. So she gave up
her love affair, in each case. The typical duplex personality
is incapable of yielding to a love response which entails sacrifice
of important appetitive behaviour patterns. The duplex
personality seeks objects for its love responses which can be
reconciled with its chief appetitive activities. Duplex people
insist upon having both love and appetite, free from mutual
interference and inhibition.

In a majority of cases, the love behaviour of a woman of this
type is centred about children, sisters, a widowed father, a
beloved mother, or about an appetitively weak, love-type
husband. The writers have observed cases where duplex
emotional women, holding positions as teachers, devote
themselves " heart and soul " to the children in their classes.
Toward their pupils, such teachers manifest a pure, creative
type of love response. They help their little friends in school
hours and out ; they are patient, kind, and always generous
of themselves in every way. But they are likely to work out
of hours only in response to some human need of the child
himself ; they are not likely to work overtime correcting papers
because that would be felt as work for their employers, and not
as a love response to the children. These same teachers, in
their relations with the school authorities who are their
appetitive superiors, are almost invariably "independent,"
critical, and sometimes disrespectful and openly rebellious.
For this reason, duplex emotional teachers seldom attain high
rank or special privileges in a closely organized urban school
system. They adore their children. But they act dominantly
toward the school authorities who hire them. That is the
inevitable result of duplex personality, especially when
preponderantly emotional.

In another case of this same type, the writers found a group
of sisters utterly devoted to one another, and to their mother.
The unselfish love of each for all the others was a beautiful
thing to see. Yet at the same time all these sisters possessed
hard, egotistical, " property-loving," and dominant personality
patterns, habitually evoked toward matters of money and
business. They were all excellent business women, could
" make a dollar serve them twice," and handled property with
marked cleverness, skill, and obvious enjoyment. Toward one
another they expressed love ; toward outsiders they behaved

appetitively. This type of behaviour may be regarded as evidence of an underlying duplex emotional personality pattern.

Duplex Intellectual Types.

Male college teachers and professors, who are very kindly and paternal toward their students, yet sharply critical and intellectually dominant toward the work of other men in their own intellectual field, may serve to exemplify this class of duplex personality. The class is not an especially important one, since comparatively few individuals fall into it according to the observations of the writers. It would seem that a majority of destructive intellectualists belong to the appetitive type of personality pattern rather than of the duplex type.

One case observed by the writers may be cited as illustrating the intellectual duplex type. A college professor of high standing in his field had won his reputation primarily as a critic. His criticisms were keen, penetrating, and intellectually destructive. He sometimes admitted that he had discouraged many young men to the point of driving them out of the field altogether by his destructive criticisms of other authorities. He appeared to gloat over his critical virulency.

Yet to his students he was kindness personified. He helped them on all occasions, gave generously of his time and vast store of intellectual knowledge, and encouraged even the most stupid ones to persevere and get everything they could out of his courses. He was an intellectual egotist toward his colleagues, but a kind intellectual father to his students.

Again we may note the true duplex personality pattern. To this professor other men in his own field were rivals and opponents, like other championship contenders to the prize-fighter. He responded dominantly, like the fighter, and achieved international fame by knocking out his rivals intellectually. Yet his students constituted an entirely separate and distinct type of stimulus. To them he reacted with combined creative and love responses—both constituent parts of a strongly developed love pattern of behaviour. Love and Appetite alternated in the expression of this duplex personality, neither interfering with the other, and both predominantly intellectual in the type of stimuli responded to.

FIGURE 48
*Duplex Type Personalities**

Sub-Classes	
Sensory	" Early American type " of business man
	Many prize-fighters, aggressive athletes, and physical labourers
	Some women prostitutes, some gangster-type criminals
	Many " hard " and impersonal types of money-makers of both sexes
Intellectual	Critical college professors with paternal attitude toward students
	Atheistic propagandists, like Robert Ingersoll, with alternative constructive moral teachings
	Many " radicals " and socialists like Debs
	Many playwrights, authors, cartoonists, and other artists whose work, though destructively critical, is yet creative
Emotional	Many part-time pleasure-seekers
	Paternal-type politicians, and some Army officers
	Some outstanding military conquerors, notably Julius Cæsar
	Many women teachers, and other women who earn money to be " on their own "

Summary

We have suggested a new classification of personality pattern, based upon the type of relationship existing between appetitive responses and love responses as evidenced by the general behaviour of the individual. Love type personality means that the love responses tend to control the appetitive responses under average favourable conditions. Some sort of creative behaviour furnishes objective evidence that the love responses are in control.

Appetitive type personality means that the appetitive responses tend to control and utilize the love responses, under ordinary environmental conditions. Some sort of love control of other people for the subject's own appetitive benefit invariably reveals the existence of appetitive personality pattern.

Duplex type personality means that appetitive and love responses are so balanced and interrelated, that both seek

* Since it is difficult accurately to describe duplex individuals in succinct terms, reference should be made to the text for more accurate description of examples indicated in this table.

reciprocally alternate expression, toward selected stimuli. Two distinct types of behaviour of love and appetitive varieties respectively, characterize this personality type.

We have further subdivided each personality type into sensory, intellectual, and emotional classes, according to the type of part-reaction which seems on the whole to predominate within the total unit response pattern. The objective criterion for this classification is the type of environmental stimulus predominantly sought out and reacted to. Thus sensory class personalities react prevailingly to stimuli productive of much sensation ; emotional class people to stimulus situations adequate to bring about rich emotional experience ; and intellectual class persons to stimuli of a markedly mental or intellectual nature.

The reader is especially asked to note the fact that the cases and examples cited are only intended as illustrations used to help explain the personality classification proposed. These illustrations are not intended as a complete listing or cataloguing of all the personality patterns which compose the types and classes under discussion. Such an attempt to delineate the entire scope of each type and class would require an entire volume devoted exclusively to the subject of personality classification.

Nor do we claim that we have cited the best or most striking cases under each type. We have, however, used actually observed cases in every instance, selected from our own studies according to our own judgment of their illustrative value for the personality classifications proposed.

The writers sincerely believe that the personality classifications suggested may be used in a practical way in everyday life by the student of psychology with considerable success and benefit in understanding the general trends of unit personalities.

Finally, we may urge another precaution upon the reader. Human personalities are very complex and many-sided. In our experience it is rare indeed to find a person who fits squarely into one of the personality pigeon-holes suggested, with nothing left over to go into some other class or type. Then, too, there are any number of border-line and in-between personalities, partaking of two or more types or sub-classes. No attempt to indicate these overlapping and intermediate cases can be made here. But the reader should certainly anticipate some overlapping and some intermediate variations of type in every case which he attempts to classify. Despite their incidental variations from type, a clear-cut understanding of the basic type and class of personality pattern, in each case, should give the same practical knowledge of how the personality, in general, may be expected to work, that the student of anatomy derives from his knowledge of the human skeleton, and the chief muscular pulls exerted upon it. There may still remain many important parts of the human organism to be described ; but the most important directions and scopes of movement become practically predictable.

FIGURE 49

Summary of Contrasted Personality Types

SUMMARY OF CONTRASTED PERSONALITY TYPES			
	TYPE OF PERSONALITY PATTERN		
	Love Type	Appetitive Type	Duplex Type
Unit Response Character-istics	Love Responses controlling Appetitive Responses, the two combining	Appetitive Responses controlling Love Responses, the two in conflict	Love and Appetitive Responses of equal strength, the two appearing in reciprocal alternation
Typical Behaviour Resulting	Creative Work	Using other people for purposes of self-aggrandisement	Unselfish love toward selected individuals; appetitive conduct toward rest of world
Optimum efficiency of unit response pattern	Internal psychonic harmony within the organism	Strong development of appetitive responses through internal psychonic conflict with love responses	Development of both love and appetitive responses without either psychonic harmony or conflict
Optimum efficiency of resulting behaviour	Happiness	Success	Alternating Happiness and Success

FIGURE 50—*Summary of Illustrative Examples*

Sub-Classes	TYPE OF PERSONALITY PATTERN		
	Love Type	Appetitive Type	Duplex Type
Sensory	Inventors	Majority of business men in centres of population	" Early American type " of business man
	Creative artisans	" Gold-diggers "	Many prize-fighters, aggressive athletes, and p h y s i c a l labourers
	Sport-loving amateur athletes	Prostitutes	Some women prostitutes, some gangster type criminals
	Many architects, interior decorators, etc.	' Joiners,' club-men, church-goers, etc., w i t h ulterior money - making purposes	Many " hard " and impersonal types of money-makers of both sexes
Intellectual	Creative scientists	Ruthless newspaper men	Critical college professors with paternal attitude toward students
	Constructive philosophers	Parasitical and plagiaristic essayists, special writers, etc.	Atheistic propagandists, like Robert Ingersoll, with alternative constructive moral teachings
	I n t e l l e c t u a l creators and originators in fields of sociology, economics, political economy, literature, etc.	Insincere psychologists, psychoanalysts, and social workers	Many "radicals" and socialists like Debs
		Scientists, teachers, and professional men who base their reputations upon the ideas and knowledge of others	Many playwrights, authors, cartoonists, and other artists whose work though destructively critical, is yet creative
Emotional	Majority of normal women	Seducers	Many part-time pleasure-seekers
	Youthful idealists	Sadists	Paternal-type politicians and some Army officers
	Creative artists	Parents who exploit children socially or for personal gratification	Some outstanding military conquerors, notably Julius Cæsar
	Constructive religionists	" Society " people and would-be " society " people	Many women teachers, and other women who earn money to be " on their own "
		Actors who are not " good troupers "	
		Publicity seekers	
		Habitual gossips and scandal mongers	
		People who habitually use others for their pleasure	

INDEX